EMERGENCY CARE
SURGICAL AND MEDICAL

APPLETON
CENTURY
CROFTS
EDUCATIONAL DIVISION
MEREDITH
CORPORATION

EMERGENCY CARE

SURGICAL AND MEDICAL

seventh edition

Warren H. Cole

> *Emeritus Professor, Department of Surgery, Abraham Lincoln School of Medicine, The University of Illinois at the Medical Center, Chicago, Illinois*

Charles B. Puestow

> *Emeritus Clinical Professor, Abraham Lincoln School of Medicine and The Graduate School, The University of Illinois at the Medical Center; Chief, Surgical Service, Veterans Administration Hospital, Hines; Senior Surgeon, Medical Director and Director of Medical Education, Henrotin Hospital; Consulting Surgeon, Rush-Presbyterian-St. Luke's Medical Center, Chicago, Illinois; Colonel, M.C., A.U.S.*

With 28 Contributing Authors

Copyright © 1972 by MEREDITH CORPORATION

All rights reserved. This book, or parts thereof, must not be used or reproduced in any manner without written permission. For information address the publisher, Appleton-Century-Crofts, Educational Division, Meredith Corporation, 440 Park Avenue South, New York, New York 10016.

791-1

Library of Congress Catalog Card Number: 74-150215

Under the title *First Aid: Diagnosis and Management* this book in part was copyrighted as follows:

Copyright © 1965 by Meredith Publishing Company
Copyright © 1960 by Appleton-Century-Crofts, Inc.

Under the title *First Aid, Surgical and Medical* this book in part was copyrighted as follows:

Copyright © 1951 by Appleton-Century-Crofts, Inc.
Copyright © 1942, 1943, 1945 by D. Appleton-Century Company, Inc.

PRINTED IN THE UNITED STATES OF AMERICA
390-20206-1

Contributors

William A. Altmeier
Christian R. Holmes Professor and Chairman, Department of Surgery, University of Cincinnati College of Medicine, Cincinnati, Ohio

Curtis Price Artz
Professor and Chairman, Department of Surgery, Medical University of South Carolina, Charleston, South Carolina

Walter L. Barker
Clinical Associate Professor, Department of Surgery, Abraham Lincoln School of Medicine, The University of Illinois at the Medical Center; Assistant Chief of Surgery, Chicago State Tuberculosis Sanitarium; Attending Physician, Cardiothoracic Surgery, Cook County Hospital, Chicago, Illinois

Edward J. Berkich
Instructor, Department of Surgery, University of Cincinnati College of Medicine, Cincinnati, Ohio

Warren H. Cole
Emeritus Professor, Department of Surgery, Abraham Lincoln School of Medicine, The University of Illinois at the Medical Center, Chicago, Illinois

Ormond S. Culp
Professor, Department of Urology, Mayo Graduate School of Medicine, University of Minnesota; Chairman, Department of Urology, Mayo Clinic, Rochester, Minnesota

Joseph D. Farrington
Chairman, Sub-Committee on Emergency Services, Prehospital Committee on Trauma, American College of Surgeons; Chairman, Sub-Committee on Ambulance Services, National Academy of Sciences, National Research Council, Washington, D.C.

William T. Fitts, Jr.
Professor, Department of Surgery, University of Pennsylvania; Chief, Surgical Division B, Hospital of the University of Pennsylvania, Philadelphia, Pennsylvania

Archer S. Gordon
Department of Thoracic Surgery, L.A. County/University of Southern California, Los Angeles, California

Oscar P. Hampton, Jr.
Assistant Director (Trauma Activities), American College of Surgeons; Associate Professor of Clinical Orthopedic Surgery, Washington University; Consultant in Orthopedic Surgery, Veterans Administration Hospital, St. Louis, Missouri

William H. Harridge
Late Clinical Professor, Department of Surgery, Abraham Lincoln School of Medicine, The University of Illinois at the Medical Center, Chicago; Late Attending Surgeon, St. Francis Hospital, Evanston, Illinois

Gerrit L. Hekhuis
Brigadier General, USAF, MC; Director of Professional Services, Office of the Surgeon General, USAF, Washington, D.C.

Robert J. Joplin
Consultation Board, Massachusetts General Hospital; Attending Orthopaedic Surgeon, Veterans Administration Hospital, Boston, Massachusetts

Burton C. Kilbourne
Clinical Associate Professor, Abraham Lincoln School of Medicine, The University of Illinois at the Medical Center; Attending Surgeon, Rush-Presbyterian-St. Luke's Medical Center, Chicago, Illinois; Attendng Staff, Ripon Memorial Hospital, Ripon, Wisconsin

John J. Kovaric
Colonel, M.C., USA Medical Advisor, Office of the Secretary of the Army, Office of Civil Defense, Pentagon, Washington, D.C.

Hiram T. Langston
Clinical Professor, Department of Surgery, Abraham Lincoln School of Medicine, The University of Illinois at the Medical Center, Chicago; Chief, Department of Surgery, Chicago State Tuberculosis Sanitarium; Consultant in Cardiopulmonary Surgery, Veterans Administration Hospital, Hines, Illinois

Bernard J. Leininger
Assistant Professor, Department of Surgery, Loyola Medical School, Chicago; Attending Physician, Veterans Administration Hospital, Hines, Illinois

William A. Mann
Late Emeritus Professor, Department of Ophthalmology, Northwestern University Medical School; Late Emeritus Chairman, Ophthalmology, Chicago Wesley Memorial Hospital, Chicago; Late Consultant, Veterans Administration Hospital, Hines, Illinois

Max M. Montgomery
Major, M.C., A.U.S.; Emeritus Professor, Department of Medicine, Abraham Lincoln School of Medicine, The University of Illinois at the Medical

Center; Attending Physician, University of Illinois Hospitals, Cook County Hospital, and Veterans Administration West Side Hospital; Consulting Physician, Henrotin Hospital, Chicago, Illinois

Rudolf J. Noer

Professor, Department of Surgery, University of South Florida College of Medicine, Tampa, Florida

Eric Oldberg

Professor, Department of Neurology and Neurological Surgery, Abraham Lincoln School of Medicine, The University of Illinois at the Medical Center; Senior Attending Neurological Surgeon, Neuropsychiatric Institute of the University of Illinois Hospitals; Senior Attending Neurological Surgeon, Rush-Presbyterian-St. Luke's Medical Center, Chicago, Illinois

Eudell G. Paul

Active Staff, St. Margaret's Hospital, Hammond, Indiana; Consultant, South Chicago Community Hospital, Chicago, Illinois

Robert M. Poske

Captain, A.F.R.; Professor, Department of Medicine, Abraham Lincoln School of Medicine, The University of Illinois at the Medical Center; Attending Physician, University of Illinois Hospitals, Veterans Administration West Side Hospital, and Cook County Hospital, Chicago, Illinois

Charles B. Puestow

Colonel, M.C., A.U.S.; Emeritus Clinical Professor, Abraham Lincoln School of Medicine and The Graduate School, The University of Illinois at the Medical Center, Chicago; Chief, Surgical Service, Veterans Administration Hospital, Hines; Senior Surgeon, Medical Director and Director of Medical Education, Henrotin Hospital; Consulting Surgeon, Rush-Presbyterian-St. Luke's Medical Center, Chicago, Illinois

John H. Schneewind

Professor, Department of Surgery, Abraham Lincoln School of Medicine, The University of Illinois at the Medical Center; Chief, Emergency Service, University of Illinois Hospitals, Chicago, Illinois

Sam F. Seeley

Retired Brigadier General, M.C., U.S. Army; Professional Associate, Division of Medical Sciences, National Academy of Sciences, National Research Council, Washington, D.C.

Christopher H. Southwick

Chief of Surgery, Blodgett Memorial Hospital; Attending Surgeon, St. Mary's Hospital and Butterwork Hospital, Grand Rapids, Michigan

Harry W. Southwick

Professor of Surgery, Chairman of the Department of General Surgery, Rush Medical College; Attending Surgeon, Rush-Presbyterian-St. Luke's Medical Center, Chicago, Illinois

Preface

The tremendous number of injuries sustained in industry, in the home, by automobile accidents, by military activity, and in various civilian accidents constitute a high percentage of patients treated by the first aid workers and by the medical profession. For this reason the authors have felt that emergency care should be included in a single volume that could be available to advanced first aid workers, to hospital emergency rooms, doctors' offices, as well as to military installations.

The first edition of this text entitled "First Aid: Surgical and Medical" was published in 1942. It was planned as a text for a course in first aid given at the University of Illinois College of Medicine and all contributing authors were members of its faculty. It was geared at that time to advanced first aid workers, instructors in first aid, nurses and physicians, as well as to policemen and firemen and others interested in emergency care. A Seventh Edition of this text has been changed considerably from its original intent. Many new authors have been added who were selected from outstanding authorities in the field of trauma throughout the United States. Approximately half of the present authors are not connected with the University of Illinois and a large number are members of the Trauma Committee of the American College of Surgeons. They also include outstanding military authorities. Although emergent care is described in detail, great emphasis has been placed upon definitive care of traumatic injuries and medical emergencies. Because of the expanded discussion of definitive care and the addition of many outstanding authorities it was felt that the title of the book should be changed to "Emergency Care: Surgical and Medical." The term "first aid" is more elemental than the scope of this book.

We are most grateful for the excellent cooperation of our contributing authors.

Contents

Contributors / v

Preface / ix

1. Precautions and Limitations in First Aid Work / 1
   Warren H. Cole

2. General Principles of First Aid, Common Conditions Requiring First Aid; Materials Needed / 5
   Warren H. Cole

3. Disaster Planning and Triage / 17
   John H. Schneewind

4. Anatomy and Physiology / 23
   Charles B. Puestow

5. Bandaging / 50
   Warren H. Cole

6. Wounds / 68
   Rudolf J. Noer

7. Surgical Infections / 91
   William A. Altemeier
   Edward J. Berkich

8. Shock and Hemorrhage: Electric Injury / 103
   William T. Fitts, Jr.

9. Injury to Large Blood Vessels / 115
   William H. Harridge

xii / Contents

10. Thermal Injury: Burn, Chemical Burns, Electric Injuries, Heatstroke, Heat Exhaustion, Cold Injury / 123
    Curtis P. Artz

11. Transportation of the Injured / 139
    Joseph D. Farrington

12. Special Weapons Effects / 149
    Gerrit L. Hekhuis

13. Fractures, Dislocations, and Sprains / 161
    Oscar P. Hampton, Jr.

14. Cardiorespiratory Emergencies / 196
    Archer S. Gordon

15. Injuries of the Chest / 235
    Hiram T. Langston
    Walter L. Barker
    Bernard J. Leininger

16. Abdominal Emergencies / 252
    Charles B. Puestow
    Sam F. Seeley

17. Injuries of the Scalp, Skull, Spine, and Nervous System / 266
    Eric Oldberg

18. Eye Injuries / 286
    William A. Mann

19. Head and Neck / 299
    Christopher H. Southwick
    Harry W. Southwick

20. Genitourinary Trauma / 310
    Ormond S. Culp

21. Care of the Injured Hand / 322
    John H. Schneewind

22. The Feet / 329
    Charles B. Puestow
    Robert J. Joplin

23. Medical Emergencies / 356
    Max M. Montgomery
    Robert M. Poske

24. The Prostrate Patient / 398
    Warren H. Cole

25. First Aid in Industry / 405
    Burton C. Kilbourne
    Eudell G. Paul

26. Military and Civil Defense Aspects of Mass Casualty Management / 420
    John J. Kovaric

    Index / 429

EMERGENCY CARE
SURGICAL AND MEDICAL

1 / Precautions and Limitations in First Aid Work

WARREN H. COLE

Since accidents occur without previous knowledge as to time and place, it will be purely accidental if a physician is immediately available for first aid care. Therefore lay individuals should have training in the principles of first aid. The type of first aid care rendered the victim of an accident often determines whether the patient lives or dies. For this reason alone, skillful first aid care is essential. Another reason for extending and improving first aid care is that in spite of innumerable precautions to prevent accidents, we continue to see them, and in increasing numbers. In addition to emergencies created by accidents, emergencies created by disease are, of course, quite common. The need for expert knowledge in the care of these patients is emphasized by the fact that in most emergencies we have no time for extended deliberation looking for the correct action and therapy. Even well-trained physicians will make mistakes. For the above reasons it appears there will always be a need for training in first aid.

Necessity of Knowing Limitations of Ability

The first aid attendant must always recognize his limitations; much first aid care requires medical training. In this volume we shall present many phases of first aid which are obviously *beyond the capabilities of one not possessing medical training*. However, we shall describe the complete first aid therapy for its educational value, so that the lay person may know the correct treatment even though often he cannot carry it out; at least this knowledge may prevent the lay person from carrying out erroneous therapy and inflicting damage to the patient. With few exceptions we state when this treatment is beyond the capabilities of nonmedical personnel. The question regarding limitations may be clarified to a great extent by the warning that *operations and anesthetics are not first aid procedures* and are therefore outside the realm of first aid care. We wish forcefully to remind the first aid worker of the old proverb which warns us, so truthfully, "A little knowledge is a dangerous thing." The first aid worker must *know his own limitations in knowledge and ability, and abide by them.*

Necessity of Performing Proper Treatment

The first aid attendant must always be aware of the fact that erroneous therapy may be not only detrimental but *even fatal;* he must be cautious and reasonably sure of the indications before he performs some type of treatment which may be harmful if incorrect. The needless performance of a tracheotomy (usually performed only by physicians) under difficult circumstances without aseptic precautions and adequate instruments leading to serious complications is an example of the necessity of proper indications. It will usually be far wiser not to administer the treatment which is doubtful and possibly harmful, and to expend that energy in obtaining the services of one more highly trained or of a physician. The first aid attendant must, therefore, be certain that his proposed action is not foolhardy and damaging, rather than courageous and helpful as he had hoped and planned. The indiscriminate use of a tourniquet, of which first aid workers are so frequently guilty, likewise represents an error in judgment. This precaution is particularly important because the need for a tourniquet in first aid work is in reality quite uncommon, since pressure dressings will control any hemorrhage except that from a large artery. This point must be borne in mind constantly because *much harm can result from tourniquets;* the pressure of the tourniquet may *damage the tissue locally,* but of still more importance is the possibility of *development of gangrene if the tourniquet is left in place too long.*

Importance of Proper Priority of Treatment

Minor injuries may require only a limited knowledge of first aid. Often there are several injuries, and the first aid worker may not be sure which injury deserves attention first. For example, we must not initiate our first aid care by spending time on the care of a minor wound when the patient's airway is obstructed. This would constitute a serious error in judgment. Likewise we must not allow our attention to be diverted away from the control of a serious hemorrhage by a painful fracture.

Errors in Technique

Just as serious as errors in judgment are errors in technique, such as application of bandages so tightly to badly injured tissue that the blood supply (already impaired) is obstructed completely, with consequent gangrene. The application of bandages around a fracture without adequate splinting represents one of the most common errors made by the first aid worker. The effort to stop bleeding with a tourniquet instead of a pack and pressure bandage is another common example of an error in technique.

Prevention of Accidents

Industry has become very effective in preventing accidents to their employees (see Chap. 25). However, we have not been as effective in preventing them while driving automobiles, or at home. The police force is important in minimizing careless driving. Their role is outside the scope of this text, but as individuals we should increase our efforts to drive carefully and conscientiously.

It appears appropriate that we give consideration to home accidents especially since in 1969 there were 27,000 deaths from home accidents, and 4,000,000 disabling injuries (Accident Facts, 1969; Nat. Safety Council). In 1969 falls accounted for more deaths (11,200) than any other single cause among home accidents; carelessness is the most important cause of such accidents. These figures are approximately five percent less than in 1968, due presumably to continued education in accident prevention.

Innumerable precautions in prevention of home accidents may be listed as follows:
1. Keep drugs out of reach of children, and in well-labeled containers.
2. Do not store poisons in areas near food.

3. Double check your gas burners, especially to make sure the flame has not gone out while the valve is turned on.
4. Make sure that electric wiring is not worn.
5. Be very careful when climbing ladders; make sure the lower ends of the ladder are firmly placed on the floor or ground.
6. Extreme care must be utilized while in the shower or bathtub; use mats.
7. Keep your medicine cabinet well stocked with first aid supplies.
8. All people, especially elderly ones, must use special care while climbing up and down stairs; use the handrail and watch the steps to prevent tripping.
9. If you must hurry, watch where you are stepping.
10. Children must be taught how to avoid injuries.

2 / General Principles of First Aid; Common Conditions Requiring First Aid; Materials Needed

WARREN H. COLE

Immediate and effective emergency care may be lifesaving, and may be performed by lay individuals as well as physicians. First aid may be defined as the assistance rendered before definitive treatment can be carried out; it is usually performed at the scene of the accident.

It must be remembered that not all patients requiring first aid are the victims of injury; some will be stricken suddenly with an acute illness of a nonsurgical nature. First aid in military life differs considerably from that in civilian life, just as the practice of medicine differs in the two situations. For example, a very few instances of acute disease of the heart or uremia from severe kidney disease will be encountered in military life, at least in a form requiring first aid treatment. In civilian life proportionately many more patients with these diseases will be found helpless or unconscious (on the streets or elsewhere), and first aid will be necessary before a physician is available.

Since bombing of cities and industrial areas will perhaps be an important phase of future wars, civilians and military personnel alike will be directly involved. Needless to say, many of the principles of first aid in civilian life are very similar to those employed in war. In war, first aid procedures at the front lines will be limited almost exclusively to wounds and their complications. The prominent differences between the two types of injuries are discussed in Chapter 26.

CONDUCT OF FIRST AID PERSONNEL. When an accident is encountered, one of the first things to consider and ascertain is whether or not anyone is conducting first aid. If not, it will presumably be up to you to volunteer your services and perhaps take charge of the first aid work—at least until more competent assistance arrives. Find out whether or not a physician has been called. If not, ask an observer to do so. In such emergencies you must remain calm and conduct yourself in a tactful manner. You should act quickly but not with too much haste, and speak in a natural voice. An air of commanding efficiency inspires confidence in the patient and bystanders. Silence exciting remarks of spectators, and reassure the patient if he is apprehensive. The crowd should be dispersed from the injured person, primarily to give him air. If it is warm, it may be advisable to have one or two spectators fan the patient while you are conducting your examination and first aid. This will keep some of the spectators occupied and at the same time will have a beneficial effect upon the patient.

OBSERVATION OF SURROUNDINGS. Make a quick survey of the conditions related to the injury or accident. Accurate observations may lead to discovery of the type of injury. The position of the body may determine the mechanism and type of injury. A few glances about the scene of the accident should determine whether or not any weapons are present—thereby obtaining information as to a possible suicide or homicide. If the patient has been injured and it appears that the injury was inflicted intentionally by the patient or other persons, the police should be called. Inquiry should be made of the spectators as to whether or not anyone knows the patient. When identification is obtainable, relatives should be notified. The data obtained from observers, as mentioned, will require only a few seconds in its accumulation. Naturally, precious time should not be wasted on such data when the patient may be in need of immediate attention. Much of this information may be obtained while the first aid volunteer is working on the patient.

COMMON SYMPTOMS AND SIGNS ENCOUNTERED. Naturally the lay individual will be greatly handicapped in conducting first aid, especially when an acute medical disease has caused the emergency. For this reason he should become familiar with some important symptoms and signs of acute medical diseases. To assist the first aid worker in assaying the important features of injuries and acute illness, many of the important manifestations are listed below.

One of the most alarming and serious manifestation presented by the patient is *hemorrhage*, which is discussed in detail in Chapter 8. If the hemorrhage takes place at the site of an open wound, it will readily be detected. Hemorrhage may take place under the skin with formation of a palpable mass known as a hematoma, the skin over which usually develops a purplish tint within a few hours. Hemorrhage may also take place inside body cavities—for example, peritoneal cavity, thoracic cavity, and cranium. It should be remembered that crushing injuries may not break the skin but may be sufficiently serious to produce death with a relatively small amount of associated hemorrhage.

Absence of breathing (see Chap. 14) is of course associated with cessation of life, but it should be emphasized that on numerous occasions the heart is still beating and life can be saved with proper therapy primarily artificial respiration performed immediately. Numerous conditions, including electrical shock, cardiac arrest, deep shock due to hemorrhage, foreign body in the larynx or bronchi (air passages to lungs), drowning, aspiration of vomitus, and carbon monoxide poisoning, may result in cessation of breathing. An *increase in respiratory rate* may be produced by numerous conditions, the most common emergency conditions being fright and exhaustion. Heart disease may produce an increase in the rate. Obstruction of the respiratory passages may increase the respiratory rate, but there usually will be an accompanying audible stridor indicative of obstruction. *Irregular breathing* is encountered in numerous emergency conditions, such as uremia, injury to the brain, and apoplectic stroke.

Unconsciousness is a serious manifestation and may be defined as insensibility to all stimuli. Unconsciousness may be caused by head injury, cerebral thrombosis, diabetic coma, hypoglycemia, heart disease, and numerous other conditions. These are discussed in detail in Chapter 23.

Paralysis is a serious manifestation and perhaps is most commonly observed in apoplexy, i.e., rupture or thrombosis of a blood vessel in the brain. In this condition the paralysis usually is limited to one side, including perhaps the arm, leg, and face. Such a type of paralysis likewise may be found when a hemorrhage has occurred within a brain tumor, and in brain injuries. If the paralysis includes both lower extremities, most likely the explanation is injury to the spinal cord. The height of the paralysis will vary depending upon the site of injury. Details of spinal cord and brain injuries are discussed in Chapter 17.

Any change in the *color and condition of the skin* should be noted. A cold, clammy skin is encountered in shock of all types, including true surgical shock due to injury, and psychic shock as well.

Fainting might be classified as a type of mental or psychic shock. Pain itself may produce a cold, clammy skin and other manifestations of shock. Bluish discoloration (cyanosis) is perhaps most frequently encountered in acute heart disease. Cyanosis also may be produced in poisons, obstruction to respiration, and so on. Flushing or cyanosis of the skin may be noted in certain types of gas poisoning. It should be remembered, however, that exertion, excitement, fever, and alcoholic intoxication may produce flushing.

Much information can be gained from the *appearance of the pupils*. Marked bilateral dilation accompanies death, but it may be encountered in atropine or belladonna poisoning. Contraction of the pupils is suggestive of opium or morphine poisoning. Inequality may be encountered in brain lesions.

Hemoptysis, or coughing of blood, suggests one of two major conditions: 1, injury to the lung; or 2, pulmonary hemorrhage due to tuberculosis, cancer, or some other disease process. The history of an accident would of course differentiate these two conditions. The most common cause of hemoptysis caused by injury is puncture of the lung by a fractured rib. Contusion of the lung or the air passages could also produce it. At times injury to the mouth or nasal cavity producing hemorrhage may result in aspiration of blood into the trachea and bronchi. This stimulates the cough reflex with consequent evacuation of the blood by the cough.

Vomiting may be encountered in numerous conditions. Shock of any type might induce it, particularly if the patient has eaten a hearty meal shortly before the accident. Children are particularly prone to vomit with slight provocation. Chemical poisoning and acute food poisoning (usually due to bacteria) also may produce vomiting. Vomiting of blood is usually indicative of a hemorrhage in the stomach or duodenum, but it should be remembered that blood arising from the mouth or nasal cavity may be swallowed and later vomited. True hematemesis, that is vomiting of blood, usually is encountered in acute injury affecting the upper intestinal tract or a bleeding peptic ulcer. It must be remembered that vomiting is one of the important symptoms of many acute intraabdominal diseases requiring immediate operation.

Examination for *abnormality in the radial or temporal pulse* will give a fairly accurate and quick estimation as to the immediate state of the circulatory system, reflecting in general the heart action. Naturally, the pulse will be absent if the patient is dead. It may also be absent in shock of various types. In general, therapy must be immediate and efficient to save life if shock is so pronounced as to produce an absent pulse. These features are discussed in Chapters 8 and 9. Acute heart attacks may produce various types of abnormalities in the pulse including absence, weakness, tachycardia (increased rate), and irregularity (see Chap. 23). Irregularity of the heart rate is not often produced by injury except when the injury has resulted in hemorrhage in the pericardial sac surrounding the heart (cardiac tamponade). It must be remembered that simple conditions such as fright and exertion may produce an increase in the heart rate. A decrease in the heart rate, below normal, will be encountered in relatively few conditions in first aid work. Perhaps the most common condition is injury to the brain resulting in increased pressure within the cranial cavity, and in certain types of acute coronary disease and heart block.

Convulsions may have a number of causes, most of which will not be related to injury. However, almost any type of brain injury can produce convulsions. Certain types of poisons, such as strychnine, will produce convulsions. Children particularly are prone to have convulsions, sometimes with slight provocation; often high fever in itself will cause convulsions in children. Convulsions are common in attacks of epilepsy, during which the patient usually loses consciousness, froths at the mouth, and frequently bites his tongue.

The presence of *fever* usually indicates that the patient's difficulty is not due to accident. Very few accidents, including brain injuries, can produce fever in a short time. In general, the presence of fever indicates some sort of infection.

IMMEDIATE AID TO THE PATIENT. The first aid worker must immediately *determine if the patient is bleeding* and *if the airway is open*. At times it may be necessary to extricate the victim from a wrecked automobile before these important points can be determined. If hemorrhage is present it must be stopped immediately, since the loss of blood from a large artery may be sufficient to produce death in less than a minute if uncontrolled. Hemorrhage can be stopped by one of four methods: 1, *pressure over the wound with a dressing;* 2, *digital pressure in the wound;* 3, *pressure over the artery above the wound;* and 4, *application of a tourniquet.* If bleeding is mild, simple pressure over the wound will probably be sufficient to control it. One should not do this with the bare hand (except in massive hemorrhage), since this would contaminate the wound. A freshly laundered and ironed handkerchief, towel, or sheet is reasonably sterile and in an emergency can be used for this purpose, if sterile surgical dressings are not available. Details of the care of the wound are discussed in Chapter 6, and control of hemorrhage in Chapter 8.

As stated, the first aid worker must determine immediately whether or not there is any obstruction to the airway. In reality, this is just as important as hemorrhage. With few exceptions, the function of respiration will be present as long as the heart is acting sufficiently to produce a hemorrhage. *Circumstances of the emergency will often determine what type of aid should be applied first.* For example, if the patient is unconscious and has just been retrieved from the water, attention must be directed immediately to respiration. If the patient is bleeding from a wound and respirations have also ceased, the bleeding may be controlled in 10 or 15 seconds by a pack, and artificial respiration begun. Such a combination of circumstances will be rare. More common will be *cardiac arrest* and cessation of respiration often developing spontaneously without accident. Although nonmedical personnel may carry out artificial respiration, medical assistance will be necessary to treat the cardiac arrest (see Chap. 14). Respiration may be detected in numerous ways—for example, by watching and palpating the chest and abdomen for respiratory excursions and by watching the alae of the nose for movements. The age-old method of detecting life by holding a mirror in front of the nose or mouth is neither practical nor accurate. Another effective method of detecting expired air is to hold one's face or hand close to the patient's nose or mouth. The skin of the face is more sensitive than that of the hand and will perhaps detect more readily the air current set up by exhalation. However, this method is not as effective as the two just mentioned. If there is indication that breathing has just ceased, artificial respiration usually will be indicated until one is convinced that the patient is dead. Artificial respiration, as will be discussed in detail in Chapter 14, must be conducted for a period as long as 30 minutes or so before giving the patient up as dead. Naturally, the type of wound or injury may make it apparent that the patient is dead.

Any acute distortion of the body should be corrected, but care must be utilized in doing so lest a fracture be present and damage done by the manipulation. Determine whether or not the patient is unconscious by talking to him and asking him questions. If he is unconscious and vomiting, turn his head to the side to prevent aspiration of stomach contents. *Aspiration of stomach contents* can readily occur in patients who are only partially conscious, and *is extremely serious* because of the danger of suffocation and of the development of aspiration pneumonia later. *Do not let the patient see his own injuries.* Place him in a comfortable position with his head slightly elevated if he is not unconscious. If he is unconscious, place his head level with his body. If he is in shock, the head should be kept lower than his body (see Chap. 8). *Under no circumstances have him sit up or stand* until it is ascertained that his injury or illness is trivial.

If there is any abnormality in respiration, open the mouth and examine with the finger for foreign bodies. Loosen tight clothing such as collar, vest, belt. The various phases of respiratory obstruction will be discussed in detail later, but the subject is mentioned here because it represents one of the first points to investigate.

Naturally it may be necessary to remove clothing to examine the patient or treat his injuries. If it is necessary to obtain access to a wound immediately, the clothes should be cut or ripped, particularly over an extremity when there is evidence of fractures. If there is no hurry about exposing the injured part, the clothing may be removed in a normal way, removing the clothes from the uninjured part first.

If the patient is cold (particularly if the temperature is below "room" temperature), apply warmth. If bystanders are present, they may be asked to obtain hot blankets or hot water bottles. To obtain the proper warming effects of blankets, they must be placed *under the patient as well as over him.* The blanket under the patient serves also to make him comfortable.

Do not be in a hurry to move the patient. If he has a fracture he should remain recumbent where found until a splint is obtained to immobilize the fracture. One should endeavor to make the patient comfortable until some sort of equipment for splinting is obtained.

Be very slow to give the patient stimulants by mouth. Alcoholic beverages are contraindicated. Hot coffee or tea are acceptable, but *no liquids or food of any kind should be given* until it is ascertained that an operation will not be necessary. If an operation is necessary, liquids by mouth will *complicate the anesthesia* by encouraging vomiting, and perhaps result in aspiration of vomitus into the bronchial tree of the lung—a complication which is serious because of the danger of pneumonia.

EXAMINATION OF PATIENT. After completion of the first aid procedures indicated by the initial survey of the patient's condition, the examination of the rest of the body must be completed, to determine if additional care is indicated, particularly if the physician has not arrived. Naturally the history leading up to the patient's illness or accident will be extremely important and may lead to the exact diagnosis or discovery of additional injuries. For example, if the injured person landed on the buttocks, fractures of the vertebrae or base of the skull might be sustained. The examiner should smell the patient's breath carefully, since certain odors may lead to the diagnosis. For example, an acetone breath may be indicative of a diabetic coma, and an alcoholic breath may be indicative of inebriation. However, we cannot emphasize too strongly that the presence of *alcohol on the breath is not proof* that the patient's half-conscious or unconscious state is due to alcohol. It is a very serious error to attribute a comatose or unconscious state to alcohol when the real cause of unconsciousness is intracranial (brain) injury.

In order to make the examination complete and not omit some part of the body, a systematic examination should be made. Before carrying out the examination a thorough inspection should be made. The examiner has already determined whether or not the patient is conscious and has likewise probably palpated the radial or temporal pulse.

In his *examination* the examiner should start at the head. Ordinarily this examination will not be very meaningful unless carried out by a physician or advanced medical student. Palpation is carried out, particularly over the scalp, to detect bruises, bone irregularities, or asymmetry. The ears are examined, particularly for the presence of blood; this is important, as will be discussed in detail later, because bleeding from the ears often is indicative of a fracture of the base of the skull. Bleeding from the nose is not so serious and may indicate nothing more than a buckling of the cartilage in the nose. The mouth particularly should be examined for the presence of foreign bodies, including broken teeth or loose dentures. It is very essential that foreign bodies of any type be removed from the oral cavity, since the unconscious or half-conscious patient is apt to aspirate these foreign bodies. Examination of the mouth is also indicated for the possible presence of burns which might be inflicted by poisons.

The examiner palpates the back of the neck, the clavicles (collar bones) and shoulders for tenderness, bone irregularities, or asymmetry. The chest and abdomen are examined for bruises and tenderness, as will be discussed in detail in a subsequent chapter. One of the most significant features about the abdominal examination is to determine whether or not muscle spasm is present. Muscle spasm is highly suggestive of serious intraabdominal injury.

It is particularly important that the back be examined for the possible presence of fractured vertebrae, especially since such injury is so serious and so commonly overlooked, even by competent physicians. Undue tenderness or malalignment of the spinous processes in the midline of the back may be indicative of fracture. As will be discussed later, *patients with fractured vertebrae should be moved with extreme caution*, lest serious damage be inflicted upon the spinal cord.

Each extremity is palpated gently for tenderness and bone irregularities. Carefully rotate all extremities, as movement of joints will detect significant injuries. Frequently it will be impossible to determine by history and examination alone whether or not a fracture is present. On such occasions an x-ray should be taken later by the physician—in fact *an x-ray should be taken of all bones which might possibly be the site of a fracture.*

Common Conditions Requiring First Aid

The accidents or illnesses which may require first aid are numerous. Frequently there will be difficulty in arriving at the correct diagnosis. In order to give the student a preliminary idea as to the scope of first aid work, some of the important conditions requiring first aid will be mentioned now, but details will be presented in subsequent chapters.

These conditions can be separated into two broad groups: 1, civilian; and 2, military emergencies. More details of military emergencies are discussed in Chapter 26, but a few will be presented here so that certain principles can be emphasized. Many aspects of the two groups of emergencies will be identical. Open wounds will be the primary emergency encountered in military first aid but will constitute only a portion of civilian emergencies. *Hemorrhage* and *shock* may be encountered in either group. Manifestation and treatment will differ only slightly in the two groups except that more plasma than blood will be used for therapy in military than in civilian shock. *Blast shock* of war rarely will be observed in civilian life. *Fractures* will be very common in either group. Open (compound) fractures will be more common in war because of the force producing them, that is, bullets, shrapnel, and so on. *Automobile accidents* are a frequent cause of injury in civilian life and may result in almost any type of injury. *Fracture of the skull with intracranial injury* will be common in civilian or military life, but in war fracture of the skull is more apt to be of the open type because of bullets, shell fragments, and flying debris. *Bullet wounds* involving any portion of the body will be encountered in either group. In World War I the majority of wounds were due to bullets or shrapnel; but in World War II the incidence of such wounds was smaller except on the Russogerman front. *Blast injury* may be trivial or fatal; it may be fatal without any evidence of an external wound. *Burns* are common in either group and in general are serious. They may be caused by numerous agents, usually fire, explosives, or inflammable solutions. *Respiratory emergencies* are relatively uncommon and are seen most frequently in near-drownings. Children are apt to aspirate foreign bodies, some of which lodge in the larynx requiring immediate removal or tracheotomy. In war, massive wounds involving the mouth and neck may block the respiratory passage with blood or torn tissue. War wounds of the chest may leave large defects in the thoracic wall, and the consequent pneumothorax may be fatal unless immediate aid is available to close the defect with some type of dressing or by operation. Numerous *medical emergencies* are encountered in civilian life, but few in war. Of this group, *fainting* is the most common. Acute *heart failure* is also common and unfortunately associated with a high mortality rate. *Poisoning* due to ingested chemicals or to inhaled gas is relatively common and serious.

Material Requirements for a First Aid Kit or Station

- 2 ounces of 2 percent aqueous solution of iodine (USP)
- 6 ounces alcohol (70 percent)
- 6 sterile cotton pads (covered with gauze)
- 24 sterile square gauze compresses
- 1 roll 3-inch adhesive plaster, also 1-inch
- 4 gauze bandage rolls of each size, 1, 2, and 3 inches wide
- 2 cloth slings, 1 yard square
- 2 tourniquets (rubber tubing or equivalent)
- 1 Thomas or half-ring splint for leg
- 3 pairs small hemostats (artery forceps)
- 1 bandage scissors
- 2 dozen safety pins; 2 dozen tongue blades

2 ampules antivenin
4 ampules tetanus antitoxin serum (1,500 units each)
2 morphine tablets, grain ¼ (or 2 syrettes of morphine)
1 hypodermic syringe with needle
2 vials procaine 30 ml
1 scalpel with blade
1 pair surgical scissors
4 small straight and 4 curved cutting needles
1 mouse-tooth forceps
1 small needle holder
2 tubes each 0000 silk and 00 silk, preferably with needle attached
1 tube #1 chromic catgut and 000 chromic catgut
6 ampules penicillin (300,000 units each)
1 bulb syringe, large
1 gastric lavage set—Ewald tube, bulb, basin
16 ounces 1/10,000 potassium permanganate solution
2 universal hand splints
3 aluminum splints, 18 x 4 inches
1 cotton roll, 3-inch (sheet wadding)
4 rolls plaster of Paris (3-inch and 4-inch)
1 package petrolatum gauze 1 x 36 inches and 1 package 3 x 18 inches
1 package petrolatum gauze ½ x 72 inches (for nosebleed)
3 rolls bias cut stockinet 3 inches and 3 rolls 6 inches
6 sterile towels
2 pairs, size 8 rubber gloves (sterile)
1 vial epinephrine 1/1000, 30 ml
1 adult and 1 child airway
2 Senn retractors, small

Antiseptics

Although numerous effective antiseptics are available, there is no substitute for the cleanliness afforded by soap and water. Practically all antiseptics are irritating to raw tissue; consequently they are not advised for routine use in deep wounds, even minor ones. If the wound is shallow, i.e., of the abrasion type, the entire area including 2 or 3 inches of surrounding skin may be cleansed with soap (bland) and water. A mild antiseptic may be applied over superficial wounds of this type.

Summary of Immediate Measures which May Be Necessary

Always treat first the conditions which create the greatest immediate threat to life, e.g., obstruction to breathing and hemorrhage. We have enumerated below a list of first aid measures which may be necessary:

1. Determine whether or not the injured person is breathing. If not, begin artificial respiration immediately.
2. If breathing is unimpaired, look for bleeding; if profuse take steps immediately to stop it.
3. If no impairment to respiration, or bleeding, look for signs of shock and fractures.
4. If the injured person is conscious talk to him and find out about pain and injuries.
5. If injury is serious, have someone call a doctor and ambulance; if no one is available, you will have to do this yourself *after* you have taken care of the urgent first aid measures.
6. Loosen tight clothing, especially the collar and waist band or belt.
7. Work quickly but carefully, being sure not to move fractured bones.
8. If the patient vomits, lower his head and turn it to one side to prevent aspiration.
9. Remove loose objects such as artificial dentures from the mouth of an unconscious person.
10. Do not attempt to give an unconscious person anything to drink.
11. Do not give a conscious person anything to drink until you have found out an operation will not be necessary.
12. Keep the injured person quiet and warm, but do not overheat him because this may increase shock.
13. Apply splints to fractures before moving the patient.
14. If a fracture of the spine is suspected fix the patient to a back board before moving.
15. Do not urge or allow the patient to sit up, stand, or walk, until you are sure he can safely do so.

3 / Disaster Planning and Triage

JOHN H. SCHNEEWIND

The fundamentals of a Disaster Plan are similar for most hospitals, but the details in every hospital are quite different. For this reason a Disaster Committee is needed with membership from major departments and ancillary services, including the hospital administrator or his designate.

The size and location of a hospital are fundamental considerations. A large city hospital must be prepared to accept large numbers of casualties from an external disaster, such as a public transportation accident, bad weather, or civil disturbance. On the other hand, if enemy action should be directed at a large city, the city hospital might be so badly damaged that it could not function. In this event, evacuation of patients would be the major consideration.

For a smaller hospital located in a suburban area, the Packaged Disaster Hospital, a prepackaged 200 bed hospital, may be most valuable. In our opinion, it requires a considerable amount of time to set up and become familiar with details of the various components of this hospital. Several individuals of the hospital staff must be prepared to initiate the setting up of this hospital on short notice.

Additional information may be obtained from the booklet "A Package Disaster Hospital, Improved Mass Casualty Care" issued by the Division of Health Mobilization, United States Public Health Service, Catalog #FS2.302:D-6. The acquisition of such a prepackaged hospital probably should be done in conjunction with the State Medical Society.

At the University of Illinois Hospital, in the West Side Medical Center of Chicago, our location is so close to the downtown complex that enemy action or an atomic attack would almost certainly render this hospital nonfunctional.

It is necessary for every hospital to run at least two disaster drills to retain accreditation by the Joint Committee on Accreditation. Fortunately, the Fire Department of the City of Chicago is most cooperative in providing casualties which are made up to simulate actual injuries.

The shortcomings of such a drill is that it is planned in advance and is no surprise to anyone. The advantages are that it does help to establish certain habit patterns and helps acquaint house officers and attending staff with various key areas and the basic problems attendant to the management of an influx of mass casualties.

The backbone of our disaster management is contained in what we call our "Red Packet." The contents of this Red Packet are simple; house officers and attending staff are not expected to remember their contents but merely to remember where the Packet is.

The following items are contained in the Red Packet:

1. A brief summary of the hospital plan for handling mass casualties resulting from a community disaster. In the summary is contained methods of alerting the hospital. Also contained in this outline is the location of the hospital Disaster Control Center. Some details are devoted to communications, personnel, supplies and equipment, internal coordination of transportation of casualties, external traffic and visitor control, medical records of hospital patients—both casualty victims and patients being evacuated.
2. Alert to staff and personnel that disaster conditions exist. This includes a mobilization or Chain Call system.
3. A section is devoted to the problems of the Department of Nursing. These include a Chain Call for obtaining additional help and assignments to key areas in the event of a disaster. Also listed is the Relatives Information Center, the Press Center, and a few sentences about ancillary services.
4. Chain Call. This begins with a call to the Hospital Administrator, since an administrator is present day and night. Should the administrator declare that disaster conditions exist then key personnel are notified and they in turn notify others down the Chain. As an example, the first individuals to be called are the Medical Director, Nursing Office, Chief of Surgery, and the Assistant Administrators. They, in turn, notify other key personnel who are usually heads of departments, and this goes down the line to other needed people.
5. General House Staff Assignments. This applies to hospitals with

house officers. In the event that a hospital does not have an intern and resident staff, then attending personnel must be assigned specific duties. These duties would include selecting patients who could be evacuated from the hospital with ease, such as those awaiting operation or those about to be discharged. Anesthesiologists would be mobilized and other subspecialty physicians must be notified.

Surgeons and surgical specialists should go to the main receiving area to assist in the initial diagnosis and sorting of injured patients.

6. Disaster Orientation Sheet. This contains a) the sorting procedure (triage) and lists priorities in treatment; b) the ultimate destination for these patients based upon their injuries; c) an area to which patients who are so badly injured that time cannot be spared to help them until the less critically injured are cared for; d) a clinic for treatment of ambulatory injuries; and e) the management of *radiation* casualties.

It is important that some thought be given to patients who are injured and are also radioactively contaminated, should there be factories or experiment stations using radioactive materials in the area (Fig. 1). These patients must have simultaneous treatment because they are decontaminated as well as having their injuries cared for, especially if the injuries are serious (Fig. 2).

Other portions of the Disaster Orientation Sheet show *the chain of command* of a hospital, *patient care areas* with telephone extensions, including *Blood Bank, Central Service, Physical Plant*, and so forth.

We have found it advisable to list the teams of doctors who would perform certain functions, such as treatment of shock, evacuation of the wards and formation of operating teams.

Because communications are so important another larger sheet is devoted simply to telephone numbers of various key areas. In this regard, communications are usually the first facility which becomes nonfunctional because of the influx of telephone calls.

For this reason, arrangements must be made for an intercom telephone system linking key areas such as the Emergency Service, the Holding Area (which is an area where patients can be given initial care while awaiting transport to ward or operating room), and Operating Rooms. All of these are linked with the Disaster Control Center.

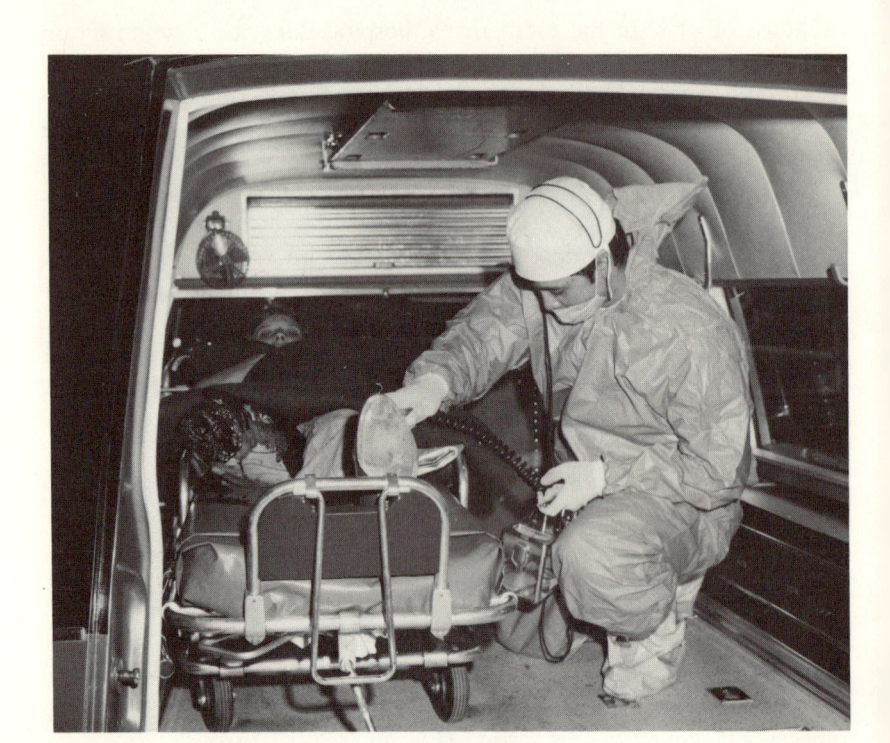

Fig. 1. Screening for radioactive contamination.

It is important that the telephone numbers of the physicians of the hospital be recorded in several places, including Nursing Office, Emergency Area, and Administrative Area, so that additional help can be summoned. Each department should have its own chain calling system so that additional help can be obtained rapidly.

It is implicit in the above discussion that all services are involved. Pediatric, obstetric and gynecologic problems, shock, burns, and various other patient conditions may all be a part of the influx.

Ancillary services, such as Social Service, are vital in receiving and disseminating information on individual patients to anxious relatives. It is necessary to provide a place for relatives to remain while a member of their family, or a close friend, is being treated and where they can obtain information.

On pages 14 and 15 of Chapter 2 is a minimum list of supplies

Ch. 3: Disaster Planning and Triage / 21

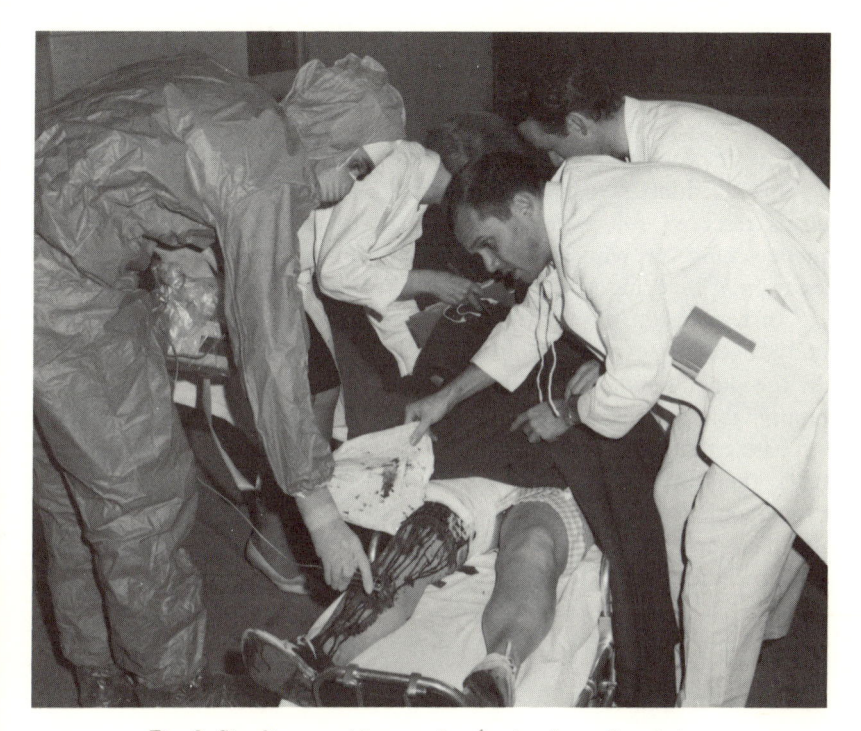

Fig. 2. Simultaneous triage and screening for radioactivity.

which should be kept in a First Aid Station. The Supplies in a Disaster Area should be similar and kept close to the Receiving Area so that a large number of patients may be received and recorded in orderly fashion. There should also be disaster tags, log sheets, and other items necessary to keep track of the patients. Containers holding supplies to protect personnel who may have to be exposed to radiation also should be close at hand.

The above implies that one area is designated as a Decontamination and Treatment Area. Waterproof uniforms are needed to protect the medical and nursing staff from radioactive material. Surgical supplies should also be stored in this decontamination area so that medical care as well as decontamination activity can be carried on simultaneously.

What is most important is that there must be adequate medical supplies kept in the Holding Area which ideally would be a rather large area containing hospital beds sufficient to care for the casualties upon initial arrival.

This area must contain water and various fundamental equipment which is necessary to clean and cover wounds, stop hemorrhage, treat shock, give blood transfusions, and treat other injuries such as fractures.

In our disaster plan the *Emergency Area* is *not* used primarily, but is reserved for patients who need life-saving measures such as tracheostomy, or who are bleeding severely and need rapid care for cessation of bleeding, treatment of shock, and resuscitation.

In conclusion, I should say that preparation for disaster is absolutely necessary from the standpoint of community responsibility. On the other hand, it is an endless and rather thankless job entailing innumerable details, all of which are rarely resolved. One should emphasize that the planned disaster drill is of value. However, surprise drills, the purpose of which is to assay the numbers of personnel which come to their appointed stations and how long it takes to assemble them, are of inestimable value and will serve to keep all hospital personnel on the alert for disaster from the outside.

4 / Anatomy and Physiology

CHARLES B. PUESTOW

For one to administer first aid intelligently he should have some knowledge of the structure of the human body and the functions of its component parts. Our body is a complicated mechanism, so constructed that it can exist, develop, and reproduce itself and also mend its own injuries, and combat enemy forces such as disease and often partial destruction. The chief value of most first aid care as well as the bulk of medical therapy is to render conditions most favorable for the body to recover from various types of diseases or injury. It is not our intention to present in detail human anatomy and physiology, but merely to review briefly those essentials which are important for the administration of sound first aid.

Anatomy is the study of the structure of the component parts of the body and their relationship to each other. *Physiology* deals with the activity or functions of these various parts. As a machine is built of various types of material so arranged and integrated as to perform as a single unit, so the living body is composed of various types of tissues each supporting and aiding the others. The smallest unit of the body is the *cell*, of which there are many types. A group of similar cells connected together and serving a definite purpose is spoken of as a *tissue*. A number of tissues which are grouped together and perform a definite function constitute an *organ*, as for example the heart. A group of organs which act together to perform a main function of the body are spoken of as a *system*. The main systems of the body are spoken of as a system. The main systems of the body are the skeletal, muscular, nervous, respiratory, circulatory, digestive, excretory, endocrine, and reproductive.

Structural Systems

Because the functions of the skeletal and muscular systems are so closely related, and injury to one so frequently involves the other, it is well to consider them together. The *skeleton* (see Fig. 1) consists of many *bones* joined together by ligaments and hinged in many places to permit motion. The functions of bones are to give form to the body, rigidity and strength to certain parts, and protection to many vital organs. In order to permit locomotion of the entire body as well as motion of one part upon another, many bones are connected by *joints*. A joint may permit movement and yet must have stability. As a general rule, the greater the range of motion of a joint, the less stable and more easily injured it will be. For example, the shoulder joint offers a great degree of motion but is easily dislocated. The elbow joint, in contrast, allows motion in one direction only, and that to a limited extent. It is so stable, however, that injury will more frequently break the bones than dislocate them at the joint. Where both stability and motion in various directions are needed, as in the wrists and ankles, we are provided with many small bones with joints between each.

The movement of one bone upon another is accomplished by the action of *skeletal muscles*. To produce motion in a joint a muscle must be attached to the bones on each side of it. To help support the joint and to produce motion in opposite directions, opposing muscles are present, one relaxing when the other contracts. Where the bulk of a muscle would interfere with the use of a part of the body, the main muscle body may be located at some distance and is connected to the bones by *tendons*. This is true in the hands and fingers, most of whose movements are produced by muscles in the forearm. There are no muscles in the fingers, but tendons from muscles located in the hand and forearm control their motion.

There are three types of muscle: 1, *skeletal muscle*, which produces all voluntary motion and is under control of the will; 2, *smooth muscle*, found chiefly in the walls of the stomach, intestines, blood vessels, and various ducts and organs in the body and not under voluntary control; and 3, *heart muscle*, which likewise functions involuntarily. The action of a muscle is initiated by a stimulation transmitted from the central nervous system through nerves.

EXTREMITIES. Although our arms and legs are not vital structures

Structural Systems / 25

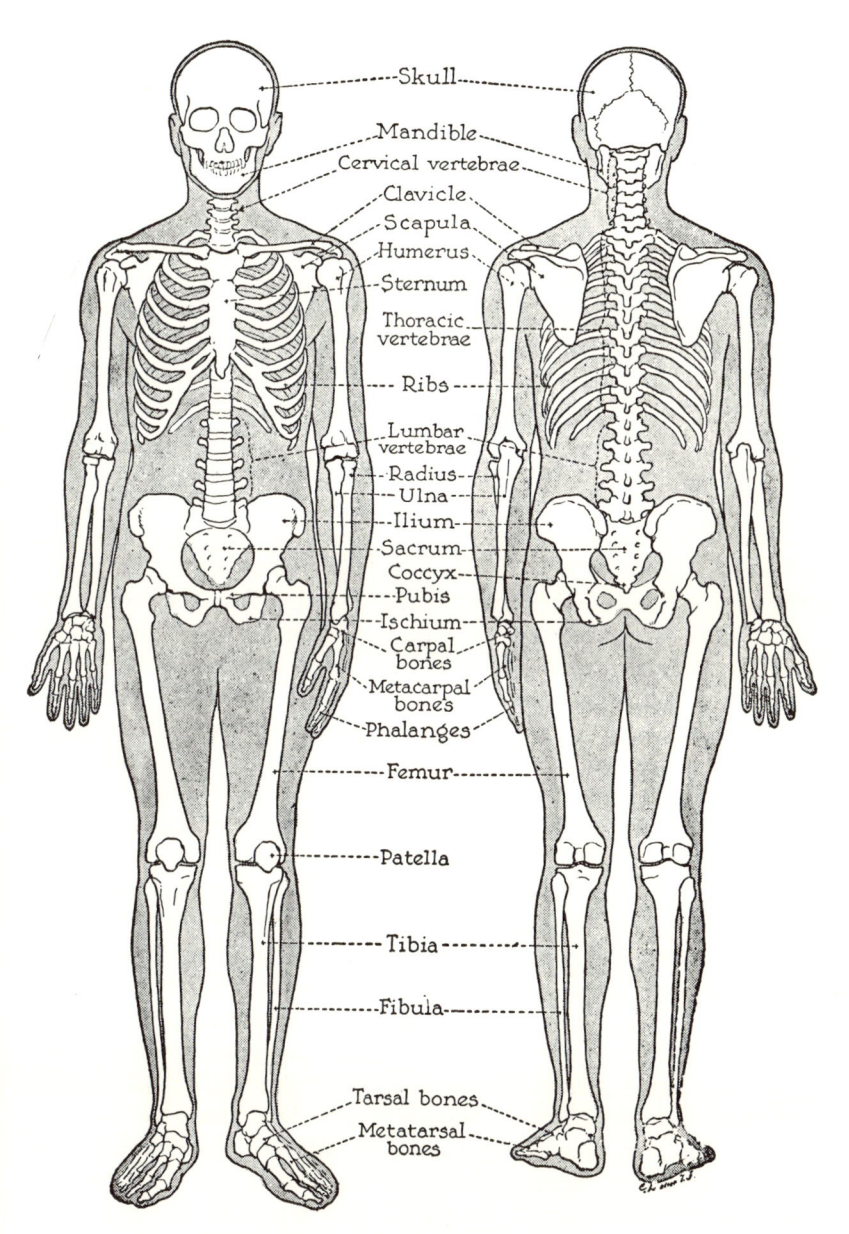

Fig. 1. Anterior and posterior views of skeleton.

and we can live with the loss of one or more, they are extremely important to our comfort, independence, and earning ability. A severe injury to a hand may not jeopardize one's life as much as a body injury, but it may be far more crippling and may cause much permanent unhappiness. For this reason injuries to the extremities demand the greatest care.

The *upper extremity* consists of the shoulder, arm, forearm, wrist, hand, and fingers. Two bones are present in the shoulder: 1, the *clavicle* (collarbone); and 2, the *scapula* (shoulder blade). The clavicle is attached at one end to the sternum (breastbone); at the other end near the tip of the shoulder it joins with the scapula. The scapula has no other bony attachment to the body, being fastened to the back of the chest by muscles, and, therefore, has a wide range of motion. It is triangular in shape with its upper edge comparatively horizontal. The lateral corner spreads out to form the acromion process (tip of shoulder), to which muscles are attached and which overhangs the shoulder joint. Because the collarbone is long and thin, is attached at both ends, and is close to the surface, it frequently is broken. As the scapula is firmly fixed at only one corner and as it is fairly well protected by muscle, it rarely is fractured. The nerves and vessels of the shoulder are well protected by bone and seldom are injured. The arm possesses only one bone, the *humerus*, one end of which is rounded and fits into the shoulder socket, the other end joining with the bones of the forearm to form the elbow joint. The shoulder joint permits a great range of motion and is quite weak. It is, therefore, frequently dislocated. The large amount of muscle tissue around the joint gives some added support to the joint capsule and ligaments. The shaft of the humerus is surrounded by muscles which protect the bone as well as the vessels and nerves which are located close to the bone. However, a bad fracture of the humerus may cause considerable muscle damage and also may injure the artery or nerve. The elbow joint is formed by the junction of the humerus and ulna, and is a strong hinge joint which permits motion in one direction only and that limited to 135 degrees. Most vessels and nerves pass anterior to the bones at the elbow where they are most protected. The ulnar nerve passes behind the medial part of the elbow and is easily bruised causing pain down the inner side of the arm (crazy bone).

The forearm possesses two parallel bones: the *radius* and the *ulna*. The ulna is on the medial side, is large at the elbow and small at the wrist. The radius lies on the thumb side, is small at the elbow and large at the wrist. Many of the arteries and nerves passing through the forearm lie between and are partially protected by these bones. Joint action of these bones on each other permits rotation of the forearm (pronation and supination), a very important motion. The distal end of the radius spreads out to form a broad surface to articulate with the bones of the wrist. When a person falls on his hand the impact is transmitted to the distal end of the radius, often fracturing it (Colles' fracture). In the wrist are eight small bones (*carpal bones*) arranged in two rows of four each. They articulate with one another as well as with the bones of the forearm and hand, and permit a wide range of motion. Many of the tendons extending from muscles in the forearm to bones of the hands and fingers pass down the front and back of the wrist close to the surface. Lacerations here may sever these tendons and thus cripple the fingers. Nerves are located close to the surface here and also may be severed. There are five *metacarpal* bones in the hand, each joining with the carpal bones at the wrist and the finger bones (*phalanges*) at the base of the fingers and thumb. The thumb has two phalanges whereas each of the other fingers has three. Too much emphasis cannot be placed upon the importance of the hands. The great majority of people are entirely dependent upon them for their livelihood. The loss of a hand may convert one from a self-supporting individual to a disabled, dependent, and unhappy invalid. The thumb is the most important digit. A good thumb and any one finger gives a very useful hand. Four fingers without a thumb is of much less value.

The *lower extremity* consists of the hip, thigh, knee, leg, ankle, foot, and toes. Because of its important weight-bearing function, the lower extremity has greater stability than the upper but has a smaller range of motion in most joints.

The hip forms the junction between the lower limb and the body. It contains the *innominate* bone, formed by the union of three bones: the *ilium*, *ischium*, and *pubis*. The hip joins with the spine posteriorly and with the other innominate bone anteriorly to form the bony pelvis. These joints are very solid and allow practically no motion. Joint strength is very important here, more so in man than in other animals, because in walking in the erect position the entire weight of the body is thrown upon these joints. Thus, in spite of their strength the joints between the innominate bones and the spine (sacroiliac joints) are often subjected to very great strain and may be injured. This is one of the common causes of low back pain. Within the bony pelvis, which is a funnel-shaped cavity, lie several important structures including the bladder and rectum. Crushing injuries to the pelvis may cause the bone to be fractured, and broken fragments may injure or tear the viscera within the pelvis.

On the lateral surface of the innominate bone is a cup-shaped cavity into which the rounded head of the thigh bone (femur) rests to form the hip joint. Although this is a ball-and-socket joint, it is quite stable in comparison to the shoulder joint and requires much more force to be dislocated. With its increased stability it permits a smaller range of motion. Because a great deal of strength is necessary to support and move the body when we are standing, walking, or running, powerful muscles are necessary to control the motion of the thigh and leg, especially those motions in which the hip joint is involved. To supply this power large muscles exist in the hip and in the thigh.

The *femur*, the only bone in the thigh, is the longest bone in the body. Although it is very strong, it is not infrequently broken because of the great stress which at times may be put upon it. In elderly persons, whose bones have become more brittle, fractures at the upper end (neck) frequently result from falls and other comparatively simple injuries. Fractures of the femur are serious accidents because of several anatomic and physiologic characteristics. The large amount of muscle around the bone makes it difficult to bring the fractured ends together and maintain them in good position. The great force necessary to break the bone often is transmitted through the jagged end into the surrounding muscles, causing extensive muscle damage. Enough bleeding from such injuries can occur into the muscles and the surrounding soft tissues to produce severe shock, which may be fatal.

Many essential motions are present in the hip joint and are controlled by opposing groups of muscles. Thus, one group of muscles swings the thigh forward (flexion), another posterior group swings it backward (extension); one group pulls it laterally (abduction) and another pulls it toward the midline (adduction). Still others permit rotation of the thigh to some degree. These are complicated and coordinated motions which are essential to normal locomotion. The lower end of the femur broadens out to form two rounded knobs, the medial and lateral condyles. These articulate with and rest upon the upper surface of the tibia to form the knee joint.

The knee joint is a very strong hinged joint which allows limited motion in one plane only, but which is strongly supported by ligaments. The joint is protected in front by a small disc-shaped bone, the *patella* (kneecap). This bone is embedded in the tendon of the powerful anterior group of muscles (quadriceps) which extends down the thigh, and by means of a tendon is fastened to (inserted on) the upper anterior surface of the tibia. As the kneecap receives the force of falls upon the knee, it frequently is injured and often fractured. If fracture is complete and the surrounding tendon divided, the fragments will separate and the patient will be unable to walk. Besides this protective function, the kneecap gives greater leverage to the muscle action which straightens the leg upon the thigh (extension). Most of the large vessels and nerves which extend down the thigh continue behind the knee joint where they are least likely to be injured.

The portion of the lower extremity extending from the knee to the ankle is called the leg. It contains two bones: the larger, which supports the weight of the body and is on the medial side, is the *tibia*. The *fibula* lies lateral to the tibia, and although it helps form the ankle joint at its lower end, it is not a weight-bearing bone. The upper surface of the tibia is broad and flattened, and articulates with the condyles of the femur. The shaft of the bone is somewhat triangular in shape with an edge extending down the anterior surface (shin). Its lower end has a flat surface which articulates with the ankle bone (*talus*) and has a bony prominence extending down the medial side (the *internal malleolus*) which supports the ankle on this side. The upper end of the fibula extends to the knee joint but does not form a part of it. The lower end extends down lateral to the talus and supports and protects the lateral portion of the ankle joint. The most powerful muscles of the leg are on the posterior portion and form the calf of the leg. The blood vessels and nerves lie largely between the two bones and are protected by them.

The ankle contains seven *tarsal* bones, which are larger than the corresponding eight carpal bones of the wrist. They also give greater support and have less mobility. They permit a fairly wide range of motion but are sufficiently strong to support the weight of the body. With the bones of the foot they form the arches which are very important in normal walking. In the foot are five *metatarsal* bones, which correspond to the metacarpal bones of the hand. One end of each of these bones articulates with bones of the ankle and the adjacent metatarsal bones. The other end articulates with the first phalanx of the corresponding toe. The first toe has two bones or phalanges correponding to the thumb, the other toes have three. Motion of the ankle, foot, and toes is produced largely by the action of muscles located in the leg. These muscles are connected with the respective bones by tendons.

HEAD. The bony portions of the head (skull) can be divided into two main divisions: 1, the cranium, which is the cavity containing the brain; and 2, the bones which make up the face. The cranium is composed of 8 bones and the face of 14. The bones of the cranium are so constructed that they have great strength in proportion to their weight. This is accomplished partially by their composition of an outer and inner firm table of bone between which there is a spongelike bony framework. This may be compared in principle to structural steel or corrugated paper. The rounded shape also gives added strength by transmitting to the entire cranium the force of a blow received in any one area. Although eight separate bones make up the cranium, they are so firmly united by irregular edges set together like jigsaw puzzles that no motion is permitted between them. The large bone in front underlying the forehead is called the *frontal* bone. The *occipital* bone forms the back and base of the head, and on each side are the *parietal* bones. Below these are the *temporal* bones, which contain the ear canals. Between the cranial cavity and the bones of the face are two other bones, the *sphenoid* and *ethmoid*. The occipital bone articulates with the uppermost bone of the spine and has a large opening in it through which the spinal cord passes.

A number of small openings in the floor and anterior portion of the cranium permit the passage of blood vessels and nerves, especially those dealing with our special senses and those controlling muscles of certain head organs such as the eyes and tongue. The brain and its coverings fill the cranial cavity except for a small amount of fluid which covers the brain and helps both to nourish it and to act as a protective cushion when the head is injured. Soft tissues of the body tend to swell when they are injured. Swelling of the brain likewise occurs when it is injured. However, as the size of the cranial cavity cannot enlarge to accommodate this swelling, increased pressure on the brain develops and may produce headaches, vomiting, disturbed vision, and mental confusion or unconsciousness (symptoms of concussion). Injuries which are sufficiently severe to fracture the skull most frequently produce a longitudinal fracture line without displacement of any fragments. This often occurs in the base of the skull and produces concussion of the brain, usually accompanied by bleeding from the ears and nose, and black and blue discoloration (ecchymosis) about the eyes (see Chap. 17).

Thirteen of the bones of the face are firmly attached to each other and to the cranium. They form protective cavities for the eyes and nasal passages. In some of these bones are cavities (sinuses) which increase vocal resonance and give a maximum amount of strength to the bones in proportion to their weight. The fourteenth bone forms the lower jaw (*mandible*) and is the only one with well-developed joints. The inner surface of this bone is closely covered by the mucous membrane lining the mouth. Nearly all fractures of the mandible tear the mucous membrane covering it, thus causing an open fracture and increasing the danger of infection.

TRUNK. The main supporting bony structure of the trunk of the body is the spine. This is made up of 33 bones called *vertebrae* fastened together to form a strong but somewhat flexible column. On the upper end rests the head; attached to the lower end are the bones of the pelvis. Each vertebra consists of a disc-shaped body behind which is a ring of bone which forms a canal for the spinal cord. A number of bony projections extend from this ring for the attachment of muscles and tendons and to partially lock the vertebrae together so that one cannot slide upon the next and thus encroach upon and injure the spinal cord. Firm pads of cartilage lie between the bodies of the vertebrae to serve as cushions and to permit some motion of the spine. Because the spine bears much strain it must be strongly supported. This is accomplished by strong tendons and ligaments and by powerful back muscles. Although little motion is permitted between any two vertebrae, the combined motion allowed by all of the joints of the spine gives a considerable range of motion. A pair of nerves passes from the spinal cord and between adjacent vertebrae on each side.

The spinal column is divided into five portions: 1, the cervical (neck) composed of seven vertebrae; 2, the thoracic (chest) composed of twelve; 3, the lumbar (abdominal) composed of five; 4, the sacral (pelvic) composed of five vertebrae which are fused together into one bone (sacrum); and 5, four coccygeal bones forming a rudimentary tail.

The bones of the neck permit a greater range of motion than other portions of the spine and enable us to turn our heads sideways (rotation) as well as to bend it forward and backward (flexion and extension). The neck contains many other important structures, including the larynx (voice box), trachea (windpipe), esophagus, thyroid gland, and the blood vessels supplying the head. Injuries to the neck which damage these structures usually are very serious.

The *thorax* is composed of a bony cage made up of the twelve thoracic vertebrae, twelve *ribs* on each side, and the *sternum* (breastbone). Joints exist between the ribs and spine which permit rotation of the ribs. The ribs are attached to the sternum by means of cartilage which also allows some motion. Muscles extend between the ribs and cover them. By their action the ribs are elevated and lowered, swinging on their hinged ends. This motion increases and decreases the capacity of the thoracic cavity. The lower surface of the thoracic cavity is covered by a dome-shaped muscle, the *diaphragm*, which separates the thoracic from the abdominal cavity. Contraction of this muscle also increases the air capacity of the chest. This change in volume of the thoracic cavity is essential to our breathing, as the increasing volume sucks air into the lungs and the diminishing capacity forces air out.

Within the chest cavity are the lungs, the right composed of three lobes, the left of two; the air passages; the heart and its connecting blood vessels; and the esophagus, which connects the mouth with the stomach.

The *abdomen* and *pelvis* are supported by the lumbar spine and bony pelvis. These are supported by powerful spinal and back muscles and by the abdominal muscles, which are arranged in layers running in different directions to give support to the abdominal organs and to aid in movements of the trunk. The abdominopelvic cavity contains a number of hollow organs including the stomach, intestines, gallbladder, and urinary bladder; it likewise contains such solid organs as the liver, spleen, pancreas, and kidneys. Because the diaphragm, which forms the upper limit of the abdominal cavity, arches up into the thoracic cavity, the lower ribs offer protection to some of the abdominal organs, especially the liver, spleen, stomach, and kidneys. These organs, however, are likely to be injured if a blow or crushing injury strikes or fractures the overlying ribs.

The entire body is covered by the *skin* and its appendages. This serves to protect and support the underlying tissues. It also serves as an excretory organ by means of the sweat glands. The regulation of body temperature is partially controlled by the skin, due to the dilatation or contraction of its blood vessel, thus regulating the amount of radiation of body heat.

Circulatory System

In discussing the anatomy of the body we have stated that the smallest unit is the cell. Each cell maintains itself to the extent of developing its own heat and energy, nourishing and repairing itself, and reproducing. To do this, it must have food and oxygen (fuel) and must be able to dispose of its waste products. The circulatory system is the transportation system of the body which brings supplies to the cells and carries away waste products. It consists of the heart, which pumps the blood and is thus the motivating force; a closed system of vessels, the arteries, capillaries, and veins; and the blood itself. The liquid portion of the blood is able to pass through the capillary walls and among the cells to deliver oxygen and food to them and to take away their waste products.

BLOOD. This is a very important body fluid (which really must be classified as a tissue) and constitutes about one thirteenth of our body weight. It may be divided roughly into the solid portion, which constitutes nearly half its volume, and the liquid portion. The solid portion consists mainly of *red blood cells* (erythrocytes), *white blood cells* (leukocytes), and blood *platelets*, all of which are microscopic in size. In each cubic millimeter (small drop) of blood there are normally about five million red blood cells, each cell being disc-shaped and concave on each side. They do not possess nuclei and consist chiefly of a limiting membrane containing hemoglobin, an iron protein compound. Hemoglobin readily combines with oxygen in the lungs and carries it to the cells of the body, where it gives it up in exchange for carbon dioxide, which is a waste product of the cells. It then carries the carbon dioxide to the lungs, where it is given off and expelled in our expired breath (see Chap. 15). The life of red blood cells is very short, and they are constantly replaced by new ones which develop in the bone marrow.

White blood cells (leukocytes) number from 6,000 to 8,000 in each cubic millimeter of blood. There are a number of kinds of leukocytes, but the chief functions of all are to defend the body against foreign bodies such as bacteria by engulfing and destroying them, and to aid in the repair of damaged body tissue. When infection occurs in the body the number of white blood cells rapidly increases (leukocytosis) to help combat it and may reach 20,000 or 30,000 or more in each cubic millimeter. Platelets are small bodies numbering about

250,000 to the cubic millimeter. They are important in the clotting of blood.

The liquid portion of the blood is called *plasma*. Nearly 90 percent of it is water. This is essential to make the blood sufficiently fluid to flow readily in the vascular system, to carry sufficient materials in solution to supply the body cells, and to carry away waste products through the excretory organs. Blood proteins, chiefly albumin and globulin, constitute about 7 percent of plasma and remain fairly constant in amount under healthy conditions. Another protein, fibrinogen, remains in solution in the blood vessels but solidifies in wounds and aids in clot formation. Sodium chloride (salt) and other inorganic salts constitute nearly 1 percent of blood plasma and are very important to life. They are essential to the chemistry of the body, helping to maintain a constant acid-base balance of the blood and preventing either acidosis or alkalosis from developing. They also aid in carrying carbon dioxide from the tissues to the lungs.

As body cells contain protein, they need material to build or synthesize protein within themselves. This material, the amino acids, is carried in the plasma from the intestinal tract, where it is obtained as a product of digestion, and is transported to the cells. Likewise, certain nitrogenous waste products as urea, uric acid, and creatinine are carried from the tissues to the organs of excretion, chiefly to the kidneys. The main source of heat and energy for the body is sugar. This is absorbed from the intestine in the form of glucose, stored in the liver as glycogen, and converted into glucose and returned to the blood as it is needed. Plasma contains about 0.1 percent glucose, varying somewhat with the time relationship to meals. Other substances contained in plasma are enzymes and hormones and certain protective antibodies which help to protect us from disease.

The clotting of blood is a complicated mechanism by which blood solidifies when it escapes from the vascular system. If this did not occur we would bleed to death from minor cuts or bruises. Clotting results chiefly from the conversion of fibrinogen (a liquid) into fibrin (a solid), which seals off the bleeding area. This conversion is due to the interaction of a number of agents from the blood (including fibrinogen, prothrombin, calcium, and platelets) and from the damaged tissues (including cephalin). If blood is allowed to stand in a tube, a clot will form which enmeshes the blood cells and leaves a yellowish clear fluid called *serum*. Thus blood serum is blood plasma minus fibrinogen.

THE HEART. This organ is the motor mechanism which supplies the power to force blood through the vascular system and plasma through the capillary walls to nourish the cells. As there are two essential vascular systems, the *pulmonary* (to the lungs) and the *systemic* (to the rest of the body), two pumps are provided, one for each system. Therefore, the heart is composed of two separate pumps, the one on the right forcing blood through the pulmonary arteries to the lungs, from which it is returned via the pulmonary veins to the left side of the heart. The left pump in turn forces the blood through the aorta and throughout the systemic circulation from which it returns into the right side of the heart (see Fig. 2). The heart is a muscular organ which lies in the mediastinum, the space between the lungs in the thoracic cavity. It is covered largely by the sternum (breastbone) with about one third to the right and two thirds to the left of the midline. It slants obliquely downward to the left, terminating in the apex, which usually can be felt with each heart beat below the fifth rib just medial to the nipple line. The top, or base, of the heart is in the midchest and connects with the large blood vessels. The heart is surrounded by a closely fitting sac (the pericardium), which contains a small amount of fluid which acts as a lubricant and permits the heart to beat with a minimum of friction. Each side of the heart is composed of two chambers, the *auricle* (atrium), which collects blood from the veins and helps fill the other chamber, and the *ventricle*, which is the real pump. A valve is present between the auricle and ventricle, which closes when the latter contracts and prevents the blood from regurgitating into the auricle and veins. The force exerted by the contracting heart is sufficiently strong to maintain movement of the blood, overcome resistance to it, and partially distend the elastic arteries. This force, with the resistance it meets, creates a pressure in the arteries called *blood pressure*. When the body is at rest the heart beats about 70 times per minute and pumps from one to two ounces of blood with each beat. The increased demand for blood products caused by exertion is partially met by an increased heart rate. Each heart beat consists of a contraction of the auricle followed very quickly by contraction of the ventricle; then both remain at rest until the next beat.

BLOOD VESSELS. There are three types of blood vessels: 1, arteries; 2, capillaries; and 3, veins. The *arteries*, which lead from the heart to the capillaries, have comparatively thick walls composed of three layers: the inner (intima) forming a lining, the media containing smooth

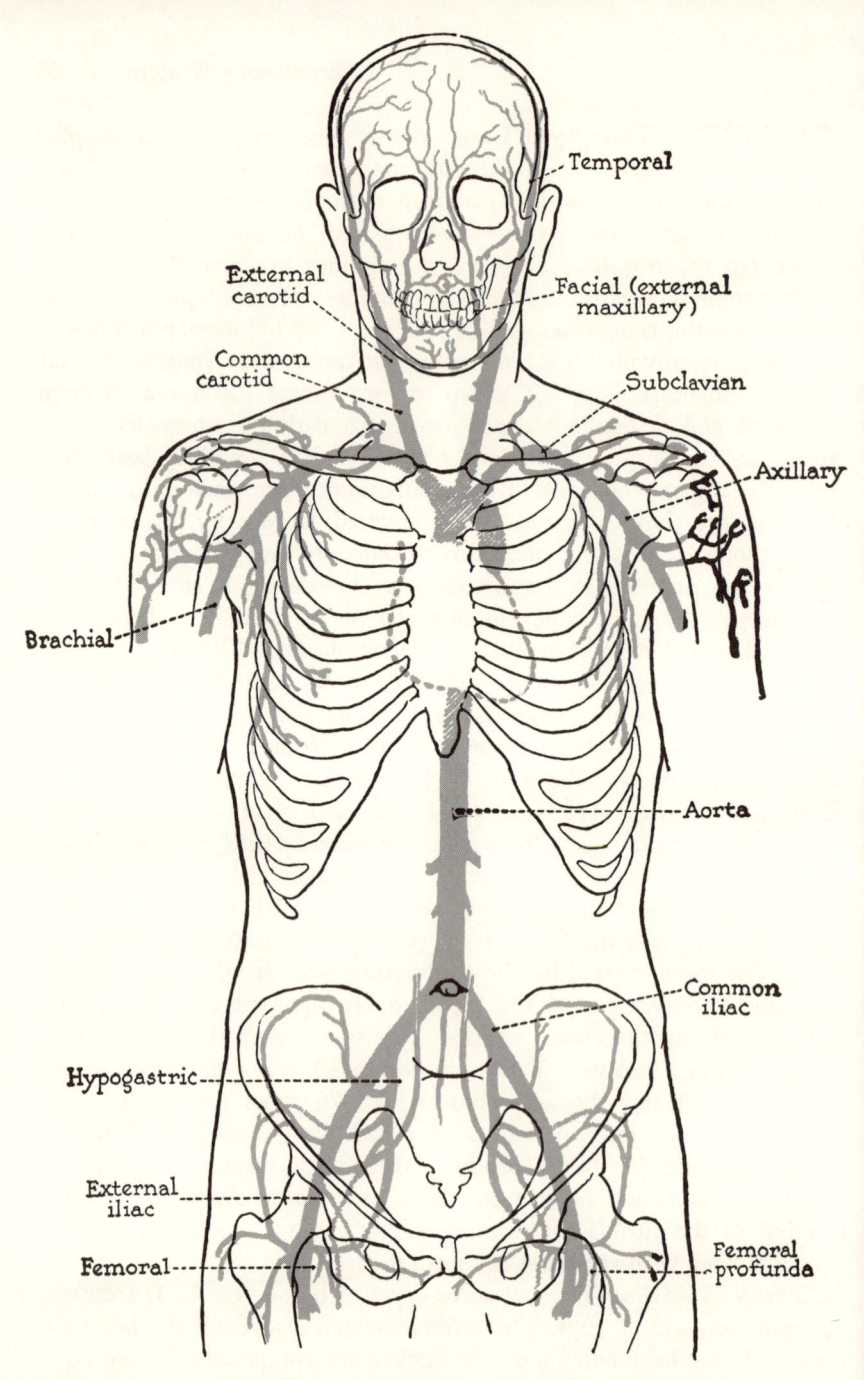

Fig. 2. Main arteries of the chest and abdomen.

muscle and elastic tissue, and the outer (adventitia) forming an elastic protective covering. Arteries diminish in size and repeatedly branch as they extend away from the heart and finally terminate in *capillaries*. These are very small vessels only slightly larger in diameter than a red blood cell and are made up of a single layer of cells. Between the cells, plasma can escape to nourish body cells and can return to the circulation to bring back waste material. The flow of blood through capillaries is very slow and is under very little pressure. Blood flows from the capillaries into small *veins* which gradually join with others to form larger veins which in turn empty into the vena cava leading to the heart. Veins have walls composed of three layers, but they are much thinner than the walls of arteries of corresponding size.

As the force of the heart beat is transmitted to the arteries, the pressure within them (blood pressure) is comparatively great. It is determined by the strength of the heart beat, the resistance offered by the walls of the vessels themselves, and the amount and viscosity of the blood. When the heart beats and pumps blood into arteries, the pressure rises, accelerating the flow of blood, dilating the arteries, and increasing the blood pressure to about that exerted by 120 mm of mercury. At the conclusion of the beat the heart relaxes and blood pressure falls but is held to a minimum of about 80 mm of mercury by contraction of the arterial walls. By the time blood reaches the capillaries, pressure from the heart is greatly diminished, and when it reaches the veins it is almost entirely spent. That is why bleeding from severed arteries is abundant and comes in spurts under pressure, whereas bleeding from veins occurs in a slow, steady ooze. Pressure in the veins alone is inadequate to return blood to the heart, and this return circulation is aided by action of skeletal muscles, negative pressure created in the chest with each inspiration, and dilatation of the heart after each beat.

The *pulmonary circulation* receives its pumping action from the right side of the heart, the right ventricle forcing blood through the pulmonary arteries into the capillaries, where carbon dioxide is given off and oxygen absorbed. The blood returns through the pulmonary veins to the left auricle to be pumped by the left ventricle through the systemic circulation.

The *systemic circulation* originates in the left ventricle and goes from there into the aorta. This arises from the top of the heart in the midportion of the chest, arches backward, and extends downward adjacent to and in front of the spine throughout the thoracic and abdominal cavities finally to divide into the two common iliac arteries (see Fig. 2). The first arteries given off from the aorta are the *coronary* arteries, which carry blood to nourish the heart muscle itself. These vessels are rarely injured accidentally, but an interference with their circulation by spasm or blood clots may cause sudden heart attacks, which frequently are met with by a first aid worker. From the arch of the aorta, blood vessels are given off which supply the head and upper extremities; on the right side the innominate artery arises from the aorta and divides into the *right common carotid* and *right subclavian* arteries. The *left common carotid* and *left subclavian* arteries arise separately from the aortic arch. The common carotid arteries pass up the neck on each side of the trachea (windpipe) where their pulsations can be readily felt. Fortunately, this artery lies deep enough so that the average cut or injury to the neck rarely penetrates it. When the common carotid artery is divided, fatal bleeding is likely to occur unless *immediate* first aid care is given. High in the neck, the common carotid divides into two branches: the *internal* and *external carotid*. The internal carotid artery passes into the skull where it helps to nourish the brain. The external carotid artery gives off branches which supply the face, head, and muscles of the scalp. It continues on upward in front of the ear where it can be felt as the *superficial temporal* artery. A branch, the *external maxillary (facial)* artery passes over the lower border of the jaw slightly in front of the angle to supply the lower portion of the face. The subclavian artery passes laterally behind and slightly below the collarbone. It can be felt at the base of the neck back of the collarbone where the artery passes over the first rib. Before reaching this position it gives off the *vertebral* artery, which passes up into the skull to help nourish the brain. The subclavian artery continues through the axilla as the *axillary* artery, then courses down the arm on the medial side of the humerus as the *brachial* artery, which passes in front of the elbow joint. Slightly below this it divides into the *radial* and *ulnar* arteries (see Fig. 3). These course downward on the forearm and can be readily felt on the anterior surface of the wrist. Both of these arteries supply branches which extend to the hand and fingers and unite with each other.

In the thoracic cavity the aorta gives off *intercostal* arteries, paired vessels which extend laterally under the border of each rib. They communicate in front with branches of the *internal mammary* arteries, which arise from the subclavian arteries and extend downward inside

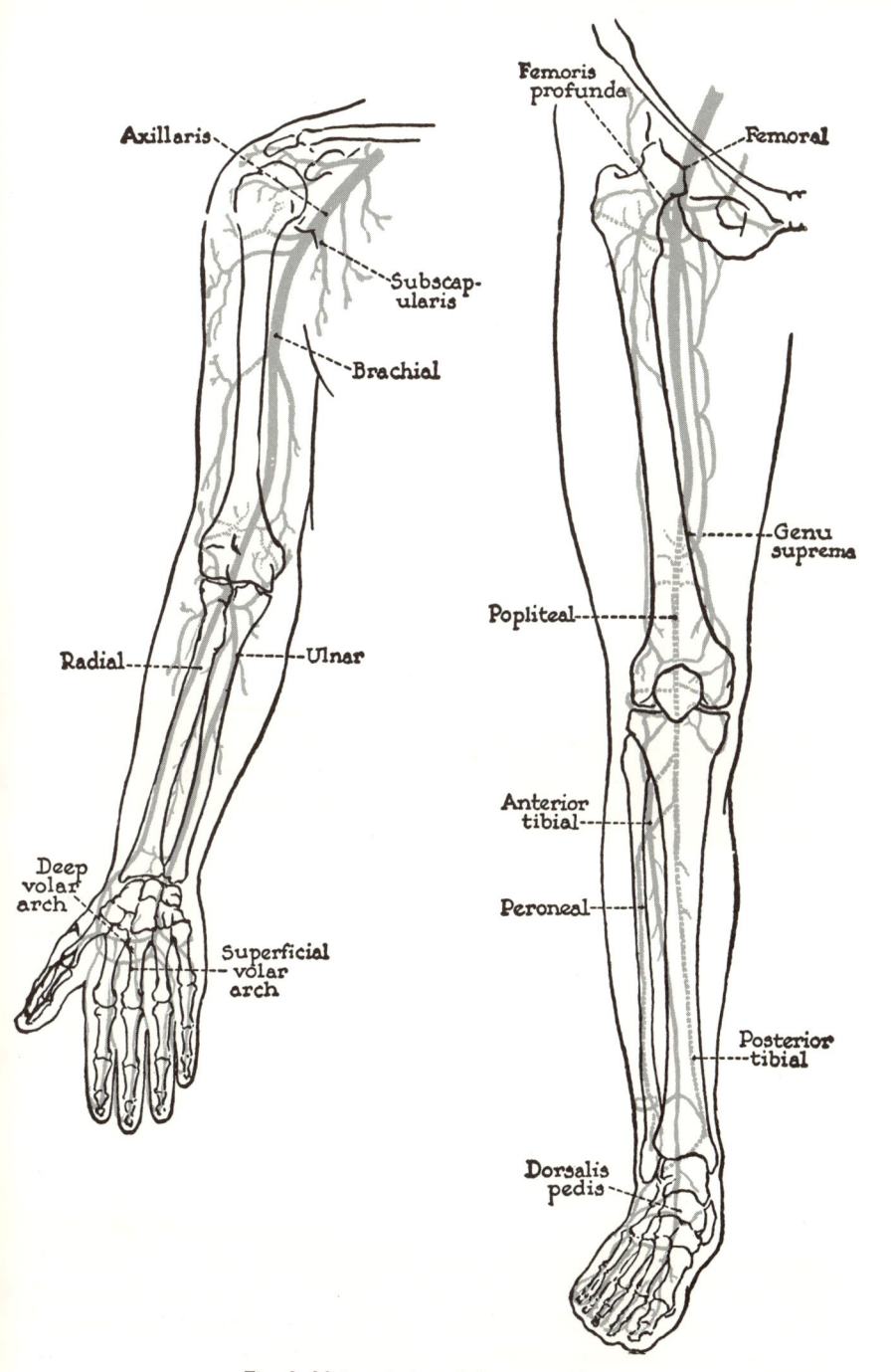

Fig. 3. Main arteries of the extremities.

the anterior chest wall. Penetrating wounds of the chest very frequently sever the intercostal arteries and produce bleeding to the surface or into the chest. Penetrating wounds in the front of the chest wall often sever the internal mammary arteries. Bleeding from these vessels may be serious, especially if blood flows into the chest cavity. The thoracic aorta sends arteries to the esophagus, bronchial tree, and diaphragm. In the abdomen, the aorta gives off arteries to the liver, spleen, stomach, intestines, kidneys, regenerative and other organs, and regional muscles. As these vessels are deeply placed in the abdominal cavity, being protected in front by the abdominal viscera and behind by the spine and spinal muscles, they rarely are injured. The abdominal aorta terminates by dividing into the right and left *common iliac* arteries at about the level of the fourth lumbar vertebra. The *hypogastric* (*internal iliac*) artery branches to supply blood to the pelvic organs including the regenerative organs, bladder, and rectum. The *external iliac* artery continues downward and passes over the anterior ramus of the pubis and under Poupart's ligament. The vessel is fairly superficial in the groin, and its pulsation can be readily felt. In this region and in the thigh it is called the *femoral* artery. It continues down the anteromedial portion of the thigh, becoming more deeply placed and giving off numerous branches to the muscles. It passes medial to the lower third of the femur and extends behind the knee in the popliteal space, where it becomes the *popliteal* artery. Slightly below the knee it divides into the *anterior* and *posterior tibial* arteries. The anterior tibial artery courses down between the tibia and fibula and becomes superficial over the anterior surface of the ankle, where its pulsation can be felt. The posterior tibial artery passes down the posterior surface of the leg, is deeply placed, and gives a number of branches to the muscles. It becomes superficial as it passes around the medial malleolus and gives branches to the foot and toes.

In general, arteries are accompanied by corresponding *veins*. In addition to these veins, however, there are many superficial veins which can be seen coursing under the skin. In the hand and forearm are many superficial veins (see Fig. 4) which unite near the elbow to form the *basilic* and *cephalic* veins of the arm. In the leg, superficial veins empty posteriorly into the *small saphenous* vein, which empties into the *popliteal* vein behind the knee. Anteriorly and on the medial surface, the *great saphenous* vein drains the superficial veins and

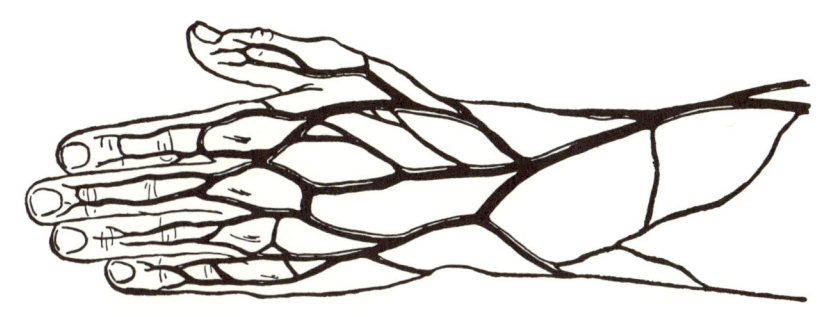

Fig. 4. Illustration showing the veins of the dorsum of the hand and distal forearm. The veins are more numerous and superficial than the arteries here as in other parts of the body.

empties into the *femoral* vein in the groin. Because of the superficial location of these veins, they are more easily divided than the arteries, and thus lacerations are more likely to produce venous than severe arterial bleeding.

Respiratory System

Respiration may be defined as the mechanism by which oxygen is supplied to the tissues and carbon dioxide is removed from them. That exchange which occurs between the blood stream and body cells is spoken of as *internal respiration*. The exchange between atmospheric air and the blood is spoken of as *external respiration*. This is carried on in the respiratory system, which consists of the nose and mouth, pharynx, larynx, trachea, bronchial tubes, and lungs. All but the latter are merely passageways for air to reach the lung tissue. In them, however, the air is cleaned, warmed, and moistened. The *nasal passages* contain protruding shelves of bone (turbinates), which are covered with mucous membrane and increase the surface available for moistening and warming the air. Hairs also are present to filter out the larger particles of dirt. The *pharynx*, the cavity back of the nose and mouth, connects these cavities with the esophagus, leading to the stomach, and the larynx, leading to the lungs. The *larynx* (voice box) has a valvelike cover (epiglottis) which opens when we breathe to let air into the lungs but closes when we swallow so that food and liquids will not enter. The larynx is very prominent in males and is spoken of as the "Adam's apple." It contains the vocal cords which assist in speaking. Below the larynx is the *trachea* (windpipe), which descends into the thoracic cavity and divides into the right and left main bronchial tubes leading to the corresponding lung. The *bronchial* tubes branch into smaller and smaller ones which finally lead to the *alveoli* and air sacs. These are honeycomblike spaces lined with a membrane which is in intimate contact with blood capillaries and which permits an exchange of gases between air and blood (see also Chaps. 14 and 15). As most of the oxygen in the lungs would soon be absorbed if the air were not replaced, the lungs are constantly emptied and refilled by breathing.

Breathing is accomplished by increasing and decreasing the volume capacity of the thoracic cavity. This in turn expands and contracts the lungs. The act of increasing thoracic volume is called *inspiration* and is accomplished by the contraction of muscles which elevate the ribs and also by contraction of the diaphragm, which depresses itself. Relaxation of the diaphragm and depression of the ribs forces air out of the lungs (*expiration*). There may be a difference in lung capacity of over four quarts between forced expiration and maximum inspiration. This is called vital capacity and is about eight times as great as the normal exchange during quiet breathing.

The *lungs* are located on each side of the mediastinum, the central area of the chest cavity containing the heart, great vessels, gullet, and bronchial tubes. Blood vessels and bronchi enter the medial surface of each lung in an area called the hilus. Each lung is surrounded by a closed sac invaginated into itself (*pleura*). One side of the sac covers the lung, the other covers the inside of the chest cavity. This pleural sac contains only a small quantity of fluid and is airtight. Thus when the chest wall expands, the negative pressure, or vacuum, expands the lung and air rushes into it through the air passages. If an accident makes an opening into the pleural cavity so that air can enter it either from the lung or through the chest wall, the vacuum will be broken and the lung will partially collapse. Until the vacuum is again established, that lung will receive little air to carry on the function of respiration. Bleeding into the pleural cavity also can compress the lung and disturb respiration.

Anything which will interfere with the exchange of gases between the blood and body cells will produce *asphyxia*. Many things may interfere with external respiration. Obstruction to the nose and mouth by gags or blockage of the larynx or trachea by a foreign body may cut off the supply of external air. Inspired gases devoid of oxygen or containing poisons which interfere with the proper exchange of gases will produce asphyxia. Filling the lungs with fluid (drowning) will have a similar effect. Paralysis of the nerves which initiate expansion of the chest as results from certain diseases, injuries, or poisons will disturb respiration. Diminished lung capacity from the presence of air, fluid, or blood in the pleural cavity, if sufficiently great, will cause partial asphyxia. The lung may also be compressed by herniation of abdominal viscera through tears in the diaphragm. Internal respiration may be interfered with by disturbances of the circulatory system. Thus heart failure, anemia, blood loss, shock, and altered blood chemistry, all can be factors in asphyxia.

Digestive System

Two essentials for the maintenance of life are oxygen and food. The digestive system of the body receives and prepares food, reducing it or converting it into products which can be utilized by the cells of the body for the production of heat and energy and for growth and repair. It includes the alimentary tract with the teeth, mouth, pharynx, esophagus, stomach, small and large intestines, and the associated organs of digestion, the salivary glands, liver, and pancreas. In the head we have the teeth, mouth, tongue, and salivary glands, all of which aid in the proper mastication of food, the breaking down of large food particles and their mixture with saliva to aid in some phases of digestion and to permit swallowing. The *esophagus,* which extends from the pharynx to the stomach, passes through the posterior portion of the mediastinum, directly behind the windpipe and in front of the spine, and then going slightly to the left passes through an opening in the left side of the diaphragm. The facial and neck portions of the alimentary canal generally are not of much concern to a person administering first aid, as they rarely are injured and, if so, more important considerations are met with. However, one must remember that injuries in these regions may interfere with swallowing, and in administering fluids care must be taken to avoid their passage into the trachea. The great bulk of the digestive system is located in the abdominal cavity. The *stomach* lies high under the left diaphragm and is protected by the lower left ribs (see Fig. 5). The lower portion of the stomach (pylorus) crosses in front of the spine to empty into the first portion of the small intestine, the duodenum. Severe blows to the upper abdomen or crushing injuries to the left lower chest may readily puncture the stomach, especially if

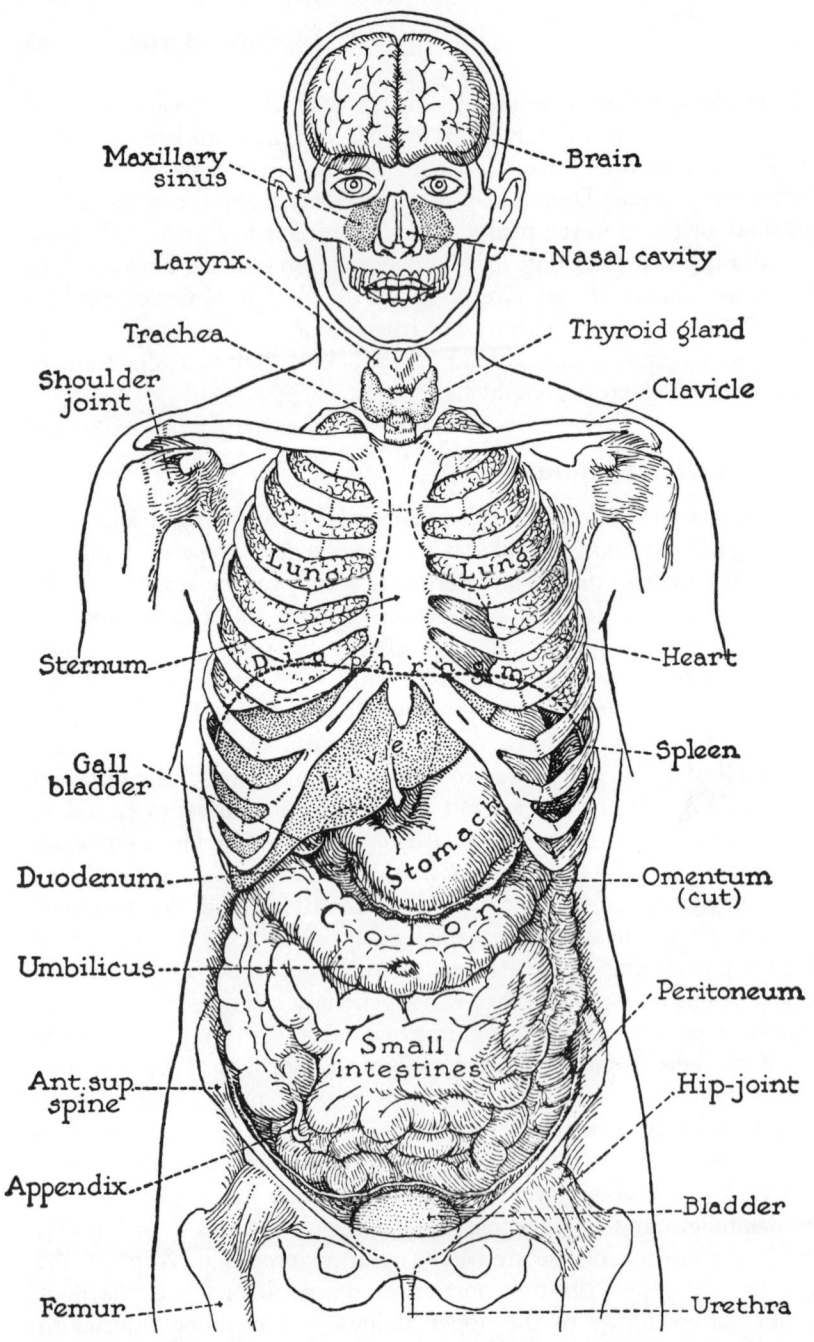

Fig. 5. Anterior view of torso and head, showing relationship of the organs.

it is filled with food or fluids. The *duodenum*, the first portion of the small intestine, lies partially behind the peritoneum and is relatively fixed. As it also lies in proximity to the spine, a severe blow in the upper portion of the abdomen may damage or rupture it. The remainder of the *small intestine*, which is about twenty feet in length, floats freely in the abdominal cavity suspended by a sheet of tissue, the mesentery, between the leaves of which run the blood vessels supplying it. Injury by blunt force to the abdomen is less likely to damage this portion of the small intestine. However, because it has no bony protection either in front or on the sides and because it occupies such a large part of the abdominal cavity, penetrating wounds of the abdomen usually will puncture the small intestine. The *large intestine* (colon), which is about five feet in length, extends up the right side of the abdomen, across the upper portion, and down the left side to enter the pelvic cavity and terminate at the anus. Most of it is less mobile than the small intestine, and it is partially protected by the pelvis, ribs, and back muscles. The *liver*, which is the largest single organ in the body, lies in the right upper abdomen filling the space under the diaphragm down to the lower level of the ribs. It has a left lobe which extends across the midline partially to underlie the left diaphragm (Fig. 5). This organ receives considerable protection from the ribs in front and the spine posteriorly. However, crushing injuries to the abdomen and lower chest are likely to rupture the liver, producing serious and frequently fatal results. The *pancreas*, an elongated digestive organ, lies directly in front of the spine crossing it transversely in the upper abdomen. It is partially surrounded by the duodenum, is covered by peritoneum, and lies behind the stomach. As a result, it is protected posteriorly by the spine and back muscles and is protected anteriorly by the overlying abdominal viscera and abdominal wall. Consequently it rarely is injured.

Another intraabdominal organ, which is not a part of the digestive system but which might be mentioned at this time because of its frequent injury, is the *spleen*. This organ, a part of the lymphatic system, lies under the left diaphragm laterally and posteriorly. It is close to the left lower ribs, and fractures of these ribs frequently injure the spleen. This organ also may be ruptured by a blow over it which does not fracture the ribs.

Food entering the stomach generally is retained for several hours to be mixed with gastric secretion, important to digestion. It then passes into the duodenum, where it is mixed with the highly active digestive juices produced in the pancreas, as well as with bile from the liver and duodenal secretion. Throughout the remainder of the small intestine food is propelled by peristaltic action and during this passage is gradually broken down by digestive ferments into suitable end products, which are absorbed by the intestinal wall and carried by the blood stream to their place of destination. These end products of digestion consist mainly of water, inorganic salts, sugar (glucose), amino acids (the end products of protein digestion), and fats. Inorganic salts are utilized to maintain the proper chemical balance of the body. Glucose is the main fuel for the production of heat and energy. It is carried from the intestines through a network of veins into the portal vein, which empties into the liver. Here it is stored in the form of glycogen until needed to maintain a proper level of sugar in the blood. As the body cells utilize the sugar in the blood, replacement takes place from the glycogen in the liver. In other words, the liver is an automatic stoker which furnishes a constant supply of fuel to the body cells by means of the blood. Glycogen is also stored in the muscles for their own use. The amino acids are very important for the growth and repair of body cells, and a prolonged shortage of them will prove serious to the patient. Fats are primarily a source of energy and generally are stored until needed. Their absorption from the intestinal tract is made possible by the action of bile salts manufactured in the liver.

The main function of the large intestine is the absorption of water from bowel contents, digestion and absorption of food products having been nearly completed in the small intestine. Some mucus is secreted by the colon and mixes with the bowel contents, which then are stored in the lower colon until the time of evacuation. The danger of damage to the gastrointestinal tract, as well as to any other hollow organ in the abdominal cavity when the abdomen is traumatized, is directly proportional to the degree of distention by food or fluid.

Urinary System

In order to regulate the chemistry and composition of the blood and body tissues certain products must be eliminated from the body. These include excesses of water and inorganic salts and waste products of cell metabolism. Water is given off in fairly large quantities by the lungs. This may amount to a quart or more a day. The skin gives off water and certain salts through the sweat glands. Some undesirable products such as poisons and heavy metals are removed from the blood by the liver. The main organs, however, which "purify" the blood are the *kidneys*. These organs are very important in the maintenance of a proper fluid and chemical balance of the blood. When excessive amounts of water are absorbed from the intestine into the blood the kidneys will rapidly remove it. When the body is depleted in water the kidneys will remove very little. They remove many inorganic salts when they are excessive but will not disturb them if they are needed for chemical balance. Certain nitrogenous waste products resulting from the utilization of amino acids are secreted by the kidneys. These include urea, uric acid, and creatinine. The amino acids which are not needed by the body cells are broken down in the liver into glucose, which is stored as glycogen, and urea, which is secreted by the kidneys.

We possess two kidneys, one lying on either side of the upper lumbar spine against the posterior wall of the abdomen. Each kidney is about four inches long and shaped like a kidney bean with its concave side toward the spine. The kidneys lie in front of the back muscles, which offer some protection, and are covered anteriorly by the parietal peritoneum (lining of the abdominal cavity). Each is supplied by an artery from the abdominal aorta and sends a vein to the inferior vena cava. The urine secreted by the kidneys is collected in a funnel-shaped sac (*kidney pelvis*) extending from the medial side of the organ. This empties into the *ureter*, a long tube leading to the bladder. The ureters extend downward on the posterior abdominal wall on each side of the spine, cross over the brim of the pelvis, course around the inside of the pelvis to empty into the bladder. The *bladder* is a muscular sac lined with mucous membrane and covered on the outside with peritoneum. When empty it lies entirely in the pelvis, directly behind the pubis (the front part of the pelvic bone). Behind it in men is the rectum, and in women, the uterus. When the bladder is distended with urine it extends up into the abdominal cavity and can be felt above the pubis.

Because of the deep location of the kidneys and their protection behind by the spine and heavy back muscles, injury to them is infrequent. Occasionally, severe trauma will rupture them, producing hemorrhage into the back and flank. The ureters are also well protected and seldom are injured. The bladder, however, because of its more vulnerable location and its exposure to trauma, especially when distended, frequently is ruptured. This often accompanies fracture of the pelvis.

The bladder is emptied through the *urethra.* This is a short duct in women but is much longer in males and is surrounded by the prostate gland and other structures. Straddle injuries, especially in males, frequently injure or rupture the urethra and result in extravasation of urine into the surrounding tissues.

Nervous System

Although each cell of the body carries on its own metabolism and each organ has its own function, these activities must be coordinated for the body to function as a unit. This is accomplished by the nervous system. We may divide the nervous system into the *central nervous system,* composed of the brain and spinal cord, and the *peripheral nervous system,* composed of the cranial, spinal, and autonomic nerves.

The *brain* fills the cranial cavity. Its function is to coordinate the activities of the entire body as well as to generate thinking power and direct much of our body activity according to our will. It is divided into a number of parts, each performing a definite function. Nourishment is supplied by arteries entering through the base of the skull. A clear fluid escapes from a plexus of arteries in the brain to fill spaces in the brain called ventricles and to cover the surface of the brain and pass down around the spinal cord. This *cerebrospinal fluid* aids in nourishing the brain and spinal cord and acts as a buffer medium between the bone and nerve tissue to disseminate the force of impact and diminish injury to nerve tissue. Brain tissue is easily injured and has little power of recovery. Impairment of its circulation for a short time will cause irreparable damage. For this reason it is supplied with an abundance of blood vessels, and its blood supply is maintained at the expense of all other parts of the body except the heart itself. The skull is so constructed as to offer a maximum of protection in proportion to its weight, and severe trauma is necessary to fracture the skull and injure the brain. Likewise, most of the blood vessels are well protected and rarely are ruptured. The middle meningeal artery, which runs for a short distance in the temporal bone, may be severed in fractures of this bone and produce a hemorrhage over the brain often causing paralysis of the opposite side of the body.

Twelve pairs of *cranial nerves* emerge from the brain. They supply chiefly the organs of special senses, such as the eyes, ears, nose, tongue, and vestibular apparatus (for equilibrium) and their associated muscles. They also control the muscles of the face and transmit sensations from the face to the brain. Some of these nerves may be damaged in skull injuries (see also Chap. 17).

The *spinal cord* extends down the spinal canal (within the vertebral column) to the level of the fifth lumbar vertebra (see Chap. 17, Fig. 5). It is surrounded by spinal fluid and by membranous coverings. It gives off 31 pairs of nerves which extend out between the vertebrae on each side to reach and supply all parts of the skeletal muscle system of the body and the skin. The *spinal nerves* control the action of these muscles (voluntary motion) and enable us to perform willful physical acts. They also receive all sensation, such as pain, temperature, touch, pressure, and vibration, and carry these impulses to the spinal cord and brain. Division of any nerve will cause loss of sensation in any part of the body from which it carries sensory fibers and will cause paralysis of all muscles to which it carries motor fibers. If the spinal cord is severed or severely damaged, as frequently occurs in fractures or dislocation of the spine, all nerves below the level of injury will be affected, and the body below that region will be paralyzed and insensitive. If the spinal cord is traumatized but not destroyed, partial and temporary paralysis may result, and disturbed sensations, often increased sensitivity, may occur.

The *autonomic nervous system* is not directly controlled by the will. It directs the activity of our viscera (organs), controlling and regulating such things as heart action, intestinal motion, and secretion of digestive juices. It also controls the smooth muscle in our vascular system, shunting the circulation to various parts of the body as needed. In accidents where hemorrhage occurs it helps to prevent or delay the development of shock by contracting the blood vessels, diminishing the capacity of the vascular system, and thus maintaining blood pressure.

5 / Bandaging

WARREN H. COLE

Bandages are very useful, in fact, necessary, in first aid work. Several types are available. The one most commonly used is the rolled gauze bandage. Two types of elastic bandages are available: 1, one in which elasticity is furnished by the type of weave and; 2, one in which rubber strands are woven into the bandage. These elastic bandages maintain pressure very effectively but in inexperi-

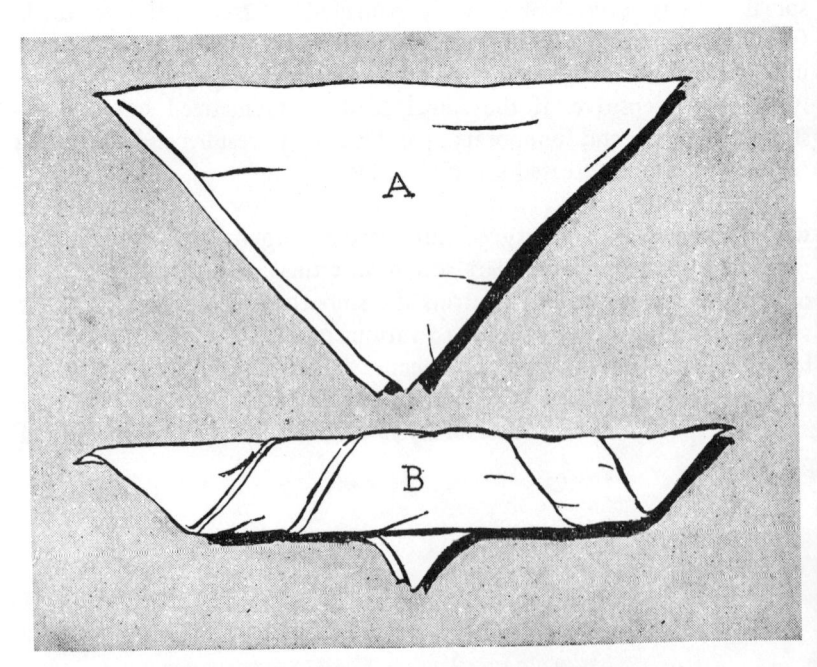

Fig. 1. A, triangular bandage; B, bandage folded several times making cravat.

enced hands are dangerous because there is a tendency to apply them too tightly.

The so-called triangular bandage made from any type of cloth and folded forming a cravat 2 to 4 inches wide (see Fig. 1) is rarely used in hospitals but may be very applicable to first aid work when roller bandages are not available. The triangular bandage can be made from almost any type of cloth; muslin is inexpensive, strong, and usually the material used.

A *sling* is very useful in first aid work and consists in reality of a triangular bandage. A square piece of cloth can be folded to make a triangle which can be applied as a sling to the upper extremity for immobilization of injuries of the hand, forearm, arm, and shoulder (see Fig. 2). The sling is applied by placing the base of the triangle under the wrist and the apex toward the elbow. The arms of the sling are then carried upward around the neck and tied.

FUNCTION OF BANDAGES. In general, bandages are applied for one or more of five purposes: 1, asepsis; 2, pressure to prevent bleeding; 3, fixation of dressing; 4, to increase the temperature of the part; and 5, to anchor splints. These points will be discussed later under Wounds.

GENERAL PRINCIPLES IN TECHNIQUE OF BANDAGING. A few decades ago, bandaging was considered an important and necessary art in medicine. In fact, a doctor's ability was commonly judged (erroneously) by the neatness of the bandages which he applied. Since then we have learned that it is not necessary for a bandaged extremity to resemble a work of art to perform the function desired. Naturally, neatness in the appearance of bandages is highly desired, but there are so many other things in medicine more important that the medical student is no longer given special classwork in bandaging. Since the need of attaining perfection in bandaging has been exaggerated, the average doctor may be content with developing a sufficiently refined technique during his internship.

Although a refined technique of bandaging can be acquired only by practice, certain prerequisites must be understood and utilized. *The most common error* in applying the ordinary type of bandage is that it *is applied too loosely*. The bandage must be applied rather snugly, since it stretches after a period of a few hours, particularly if there is motion of the part. It must be emphasized, however, that *if the bandage is applied too tightly, the blood supply to the parts distal may be seriously interfered with,* resulting in grave complica-

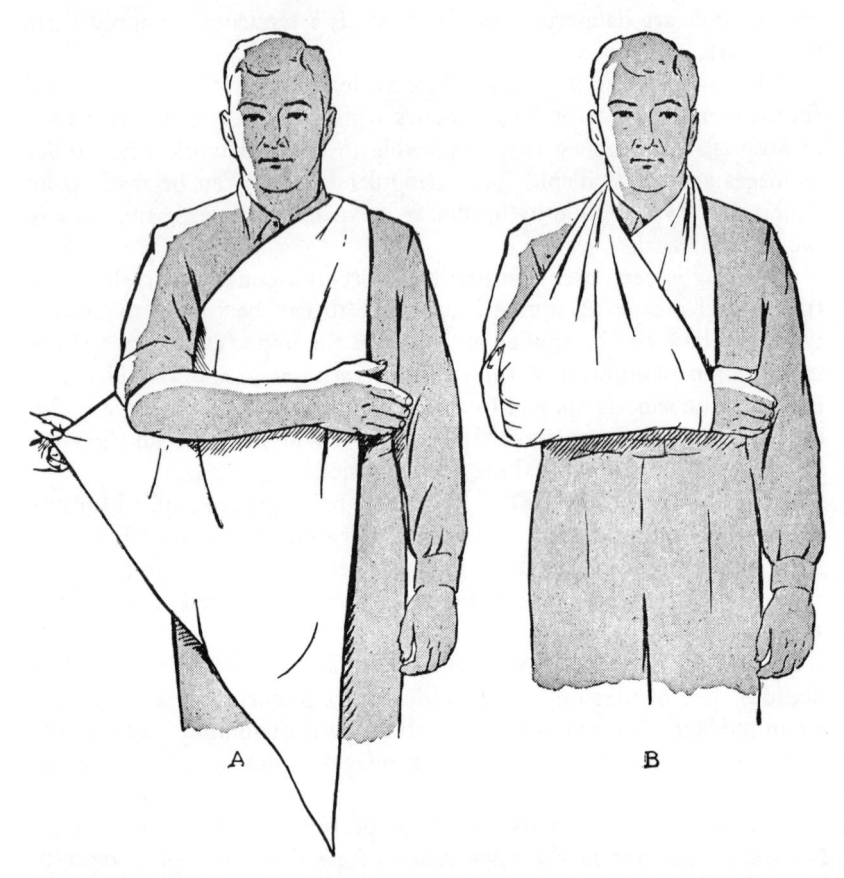

Fig. 2. Sling made from triangular piece of cloth. A, the forearm is held in the position desired for carriage and the sling carried under it as shown. B, the arms of the cloth are tied behind the neck and the apex pinned to the sling in front of the elbow.

tions including gangrene and paralysis. Most bandages should be reinforced with adhesive to prevent shredding of the edges and to prevent undue stretching of the gauze.

When an open wound is present on an extremity, a dressing will have been applied to the wound and fixation achieved with a bandage. The bandage is applied by holding the end of the bandage in one hand, the roll in the other, taking a couple of turns around the extremity to anchor it, and progressing upward or downward (preferably upward) in a gradual way in order to leave no gap, and yet distribute the bandage evenly. Use as few turns as possible. The bandage should be applied *with the limb in the position in which it is to be carried.* The tips of the fingers and toes should be left exposed wherever possible so that color changes may be observed. As mentioned previously, it is exceedingly important that the bandage not be applied too tightly. Fortunately, numerous manifestations exhibit themselves to warn the doctor or attendant of undue constriction. The color of the skin distal to the *bandage applied too tightly may be cyanotic (bluish) or pale.* Pain usually is experienced within a few minutes after the application of a tight bandage. A bandage which is too tight will produce *coldness of the extremity* and, within an hour or two, perhaps *numbness and tingling.* It should be emphasized, however, that after several hours, pain and discomfort produced by a tight bandage tend to disappear, but when this occurs, *severe damage has already been inflicted.* This decrease in sensation usually implies that constriction of the blood supply is complete and has been present for several hours or long enough to numb sensation. The resultant paralysis of muscles is apt to be permanent or nearly so, and in severe cases actual gangrene results. The consequences of a bandage applied too tightly, therefore, are expressions of negligence, and the doctor or attendant is held accordingly.

There are several *fundamental turns* available for bandaging. The *circular* turn is best adapted to cylindrical parts. The turns are applied at right angles to the axis of the extremity, and each turn directly overlies the previous one. A bandage is spoken of as *spiral* when it covers the part in a spiral manner (see Fig. 3B). It may be applied to cylindrical portions of an extremity and is applied in such a way that each turn overlaps the other, finally attaining coverage for a relatively large area. A *spiral reverse* bandage is particularly useful when the shape of the part to be bandaged is not cylindrical but slightly cone-shaped, for example, the forearm, as described later (see Fig. 5). *Figure-of-eight* turns are very commonly used and can be applied to almost any portion of the extremities. The bandage is anchored by one or two circular turns (Figs. 4, 6, and 7). *Recurrent turns* are useful in covering the scalp and ends of fingers (Fig. 3) or extremities.

TECHNIQUES OF INDIVIDUAL TYPES OF BANDAGES. One of the most common types of bandages used will be the *finger* bandage, since the hand is so frequently injured. If the lesion is small, application of a small sterile dressing which is covered with a few circular turns may be all that is required. If the injury affects the end of the finger, the tip naturally will have to be covered. This is done by

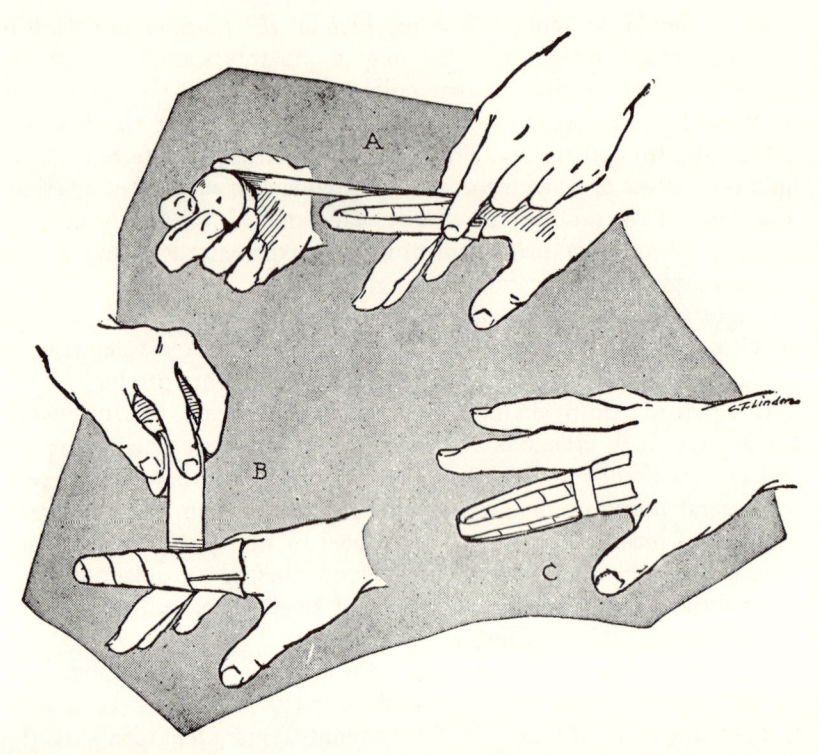

Fig. 3. Recurrent bandage to the finger. A, the bandage is anchored with a few circular turns and then extended across the tip of the finger. B, the recurrent folds of bandage are anchored by circular turns. C, the bandage is fixed by the application of narrow strips of adhesive.

utilizing a recurrent type of bandage after it is anchored at the base with a few circular turns (Fig. 3). The recurrent part of the bandage is accomplished by holding the bandage with the index finger of the left hand at the base where it has been anchored with the circular turns and bringing the bandage out over the tip of the finger to the other side. The thumb then holds the bandage on the other side as it is returned to the original side. Sufficient recurrent turns are taken to cover the fingertip as desired. The edges of these recurrent turns are then covered with a circular type of bandage to anchor the edges. The edge of the gauze must be anchored with a narrow strip of adhesive extending around the finger. It must be anchored further, however, to prevent it from slipping off the finger. This additional fixation is achieved by a piece of narrow adhesive about 6 inches long, starting on the medial side and extending over the tip across to the lateral side onto the skin for a distance of 2 to 3 cm (see Fig. 3). Application of such a strip on the anterior and posterior side of the finger will lend still more stability to the bandage. If the injury extends onto the base of the finger or thumb, a figure-of-eight type of bandage with one loop of the eight extending around the finger or thumb and the other loop extending across the palm of the hand or the wrist will be advisable (see Fig. 4). This type of bandage limits mobility of the finger and hand, and is applied therefore when immobility is desired.

The *spiral reverse* bandage is applicable chiefly to portions of extremity which are conical and not cylindrical, e.g., forearm, leg, and thigh. If the ordinary spiral bandage is applied to a conical portion of an extremity, it will be found that the edge of the bandage toward the smaller portion of the extremity will be loose, thereby making the bandage untidy and insecure. The use of the spiral reverse principle obliterates this looseness. Although the bulk of a dressing under

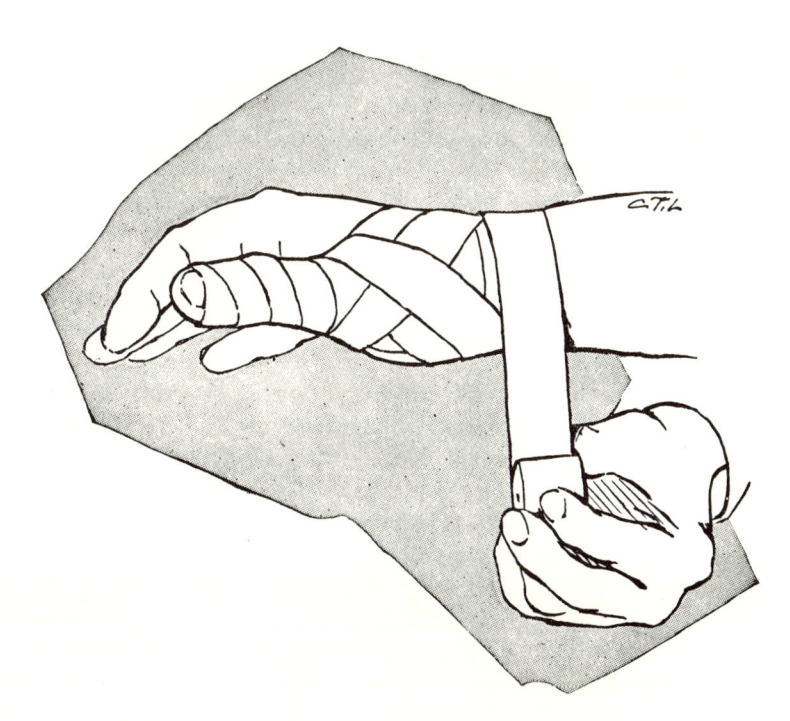

Fig. 4. Figure-of-eight bandage to the thumb and wrist.

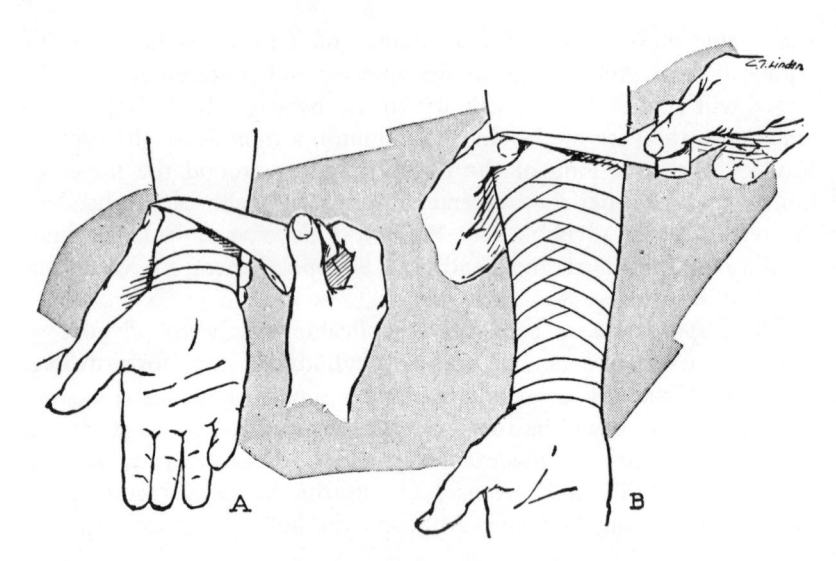

Fig. 5. Spiral reverse bandage to the forearm. The spiral reverse bandage as shown is used very little, but its application is of teaching value, since a reverse turn is needed now and then in many bandages to maintain neatness and even pressure.

the bandage will usually make use of the spiral reverse principle unnecessary all the way up the extremity, the principle must be utilized for an occasional turn on most bandages applied to cone-shaped structures. To apply it to the forearm the bandage is fixed at the wrist by two or three circular turns. The bandage is then carried upward with a few spiral turns until the distal edge of the bandage becomes loose; at this point the spiral reverse principle is utilized (see Fig. 5). The bandage is turned over one-half turn holding the thumb at the point where the reverse begins. Holding the thumb at this point or some point in the reverse fold will prevent the bandage from wrinkling and folding into untidy shapes. A reverse is made with each turn of the bandage, executing the turn at the same place with each turn so as to maintain consistency and neatness.

The *ankle* lends itself readily to a *figure-of-eight* type of bandage, which may be supplied to cover wounds or to lend support to a sprained ankle (see Fig. 6). If the bandage is being applied for a sprained ankle, the foot should be held about in a right angle position, the bandage anchored with one or two circular turns around the foot and continued upward across the anterior surface of the ankle, taking a turn or two around the distal part of the leg. These turns in a figure-of-

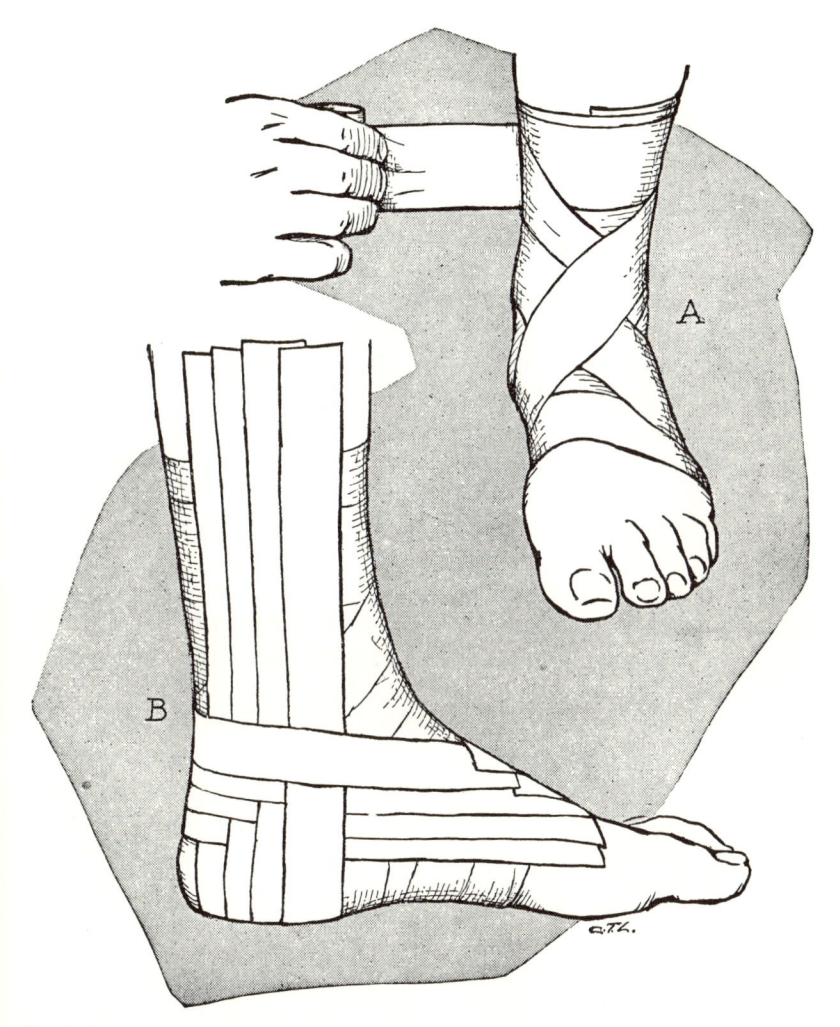

Fig. 6. Bandaging the ankle. A, figure-of-eight bandage. B, to obtain a splinting effect, as for example for a sprained ankle, strips of adhesive are applied over the bandage as described in the text.

eight fashion are taken in sufficient number to cover the skin of the foot, ankle, and distal half of the leg and to afford considerable immobility. The end of the bandage is anchored with a circular turn of adhesive. Since bandages tend to stretch to a degree largely proportionate to the length of time they have been on, such bandages must be reinforced with adhesive if they are applied for a sprained ankle. Strips of adhesive 1 inch wide and 12 to 18 inches long are utilized for this fixation. The adhesive is anchored on the medial side of the ankle, carried downward across the plantar surface of the foot, extended upward over the lateral and anterior surface of the ankle, crossing toward the medial side of the leg, and must be long enough to extend onto the skin for 2 to 3 inches. It is important to apply the first strip of adhesive in this direction when a sprained ankle is being treated in order to obtain eversion or external rotation of the foot. Fixing the ankle in eversion or external rotation puts the torn ligaments at rest and allows approximation of their edges, since the ligaments torn in a sprained ankle are usually those on the lateral surface. The second strip of adhesive starts on the lateral side of the ankle, extends across the plantar surface of the foot toward the medial side of the ankle and upward across its anterior surface to the lateral side of the leg, again extending 2 or 3 inches onto the skin. Three or four more strips are applied on each side, overlapping each other sufficiently to incase most of the bandage in an adhesive covering. Many doctors prefer to apply the adhesive directly to the skin when treating a sprained ankle. This procedure, however, results in wrinkling of the adhesive, which pinches the skin and becomes uncomfortable. It does afford slightly greater immobility, but not to a very significant extent if the adhesive placed over the gauze bandage is anchored to the skin of the leg. Unquestionably, the dressing with bandage underneath the adhesive is more comfortable and affords just about as much immobility of the ankle. Such dressings will need to be changed in four to six days, regardless of the type used. When a sprained ankle is sustained in the woods or areas where little material is available, and when it is necessary for the injured person to walk home or to a source of transportation, the cravat type of dressing may be utilized by applying it over the shoe. The cravat is formed by folding cloth of any type several times to attain a width of about 3 inches. If only short cloth is obtainable, pieces may be tied together. This cravat is applied very tightly over the shoe in a figure-of-eight fashion and affords remarkably effective immobilization.

    The *figure-of-eight bandage to the neck and axilla* will be found useful to bandage wounds on the lateral side of the lower portion of the neck and for wounds over the clavicle (collarbone) or shoulder. It is started by one or two circular turns around the neck for anchorage. The bandage is then carried across the clavicle, going under the arm (axilla) on either the anterior or posterior side (see Fig. 7).

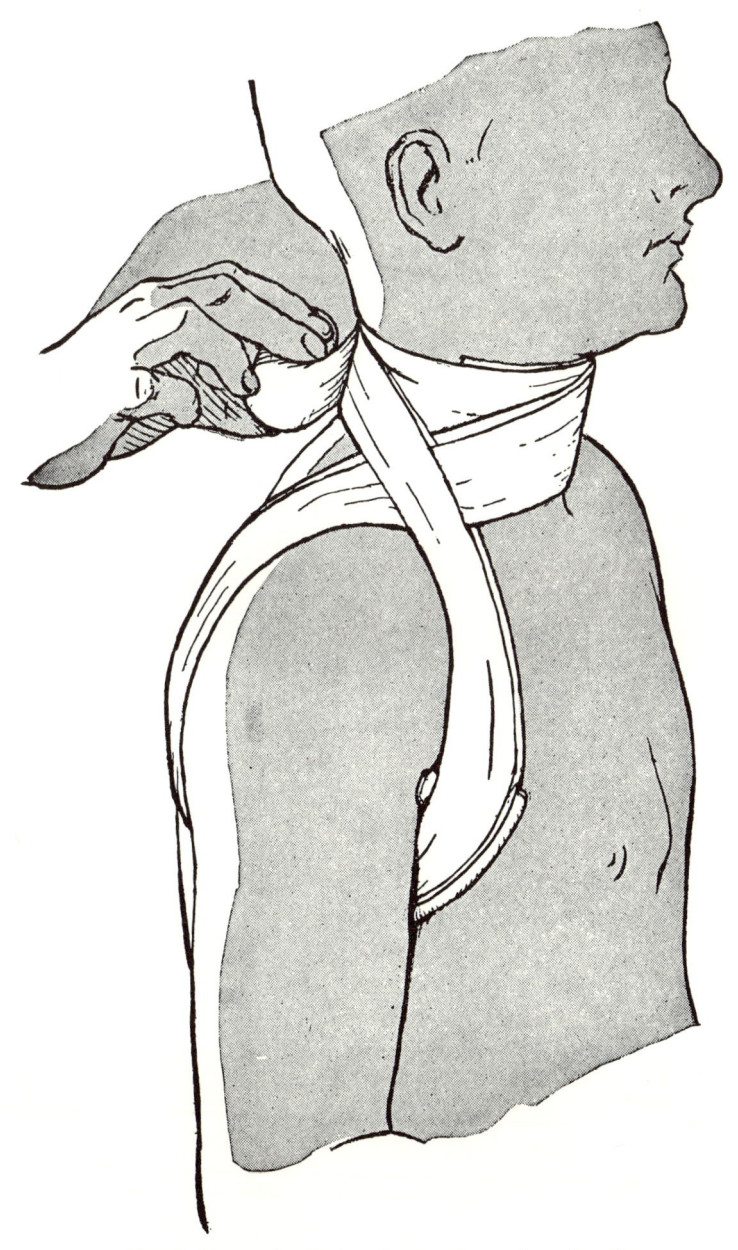

Fig. 7. Figure-of-eight bandage to the neck and axilla.

It is then carried up over the clavicle, crossing the bandage going to the axilla, and is extended around the neck. The figure-of-eight process is repeated as often as necessary and is overlapped sufficiently to cover the wound and its dressing. It can, of course, be extended to the opposite axilla, but need for doing so will probably be somewhat uncommon. The *figure-of-eight bandage to the neck and thorax* will be found very useful in injuries of the lower part of the anterior or posterior portions of the neck or in wounds of the anterior or posterior portion of the upper thorax. The bandage is anchored by a turn or two around the neck and carried across the wound in the anterior or posterior portion of the chest; it is then extended halfway around the upper chest and is brought back to the neck. The figure-of-eight

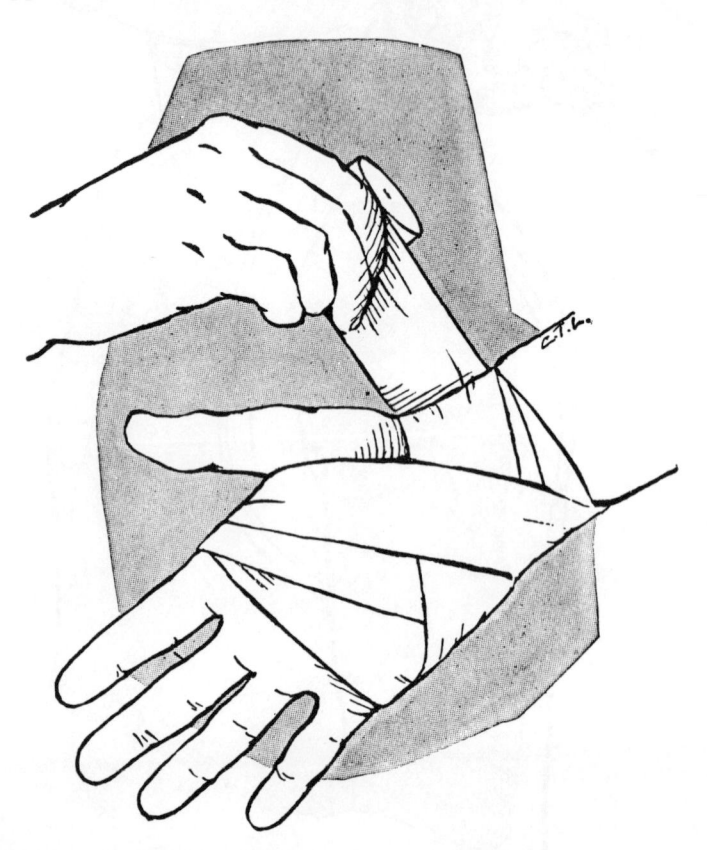

Fig. 8. Figure-of-eight bandage to the hand and wrist.

type of bandage in these areas will make the bandage more secure and lessen the danger of the bandage or dressing slipping away from the wound. The figure-of-eight bandage is likewise very applicable to wounds of the hand and wrist, areas where injuries are very commonly sustained (see Fig. 8).

When the side of the face or jaw is to be bandaged, the *oblique bandage of the jaw* is very applicable. If the right side of the jaw is to be bandaged, the end of the roller bandage is placed on the right temple and carried for two circular turns from before backward, around the head above the ears (see Fig. 9). As the third turn arrives over the ear, the bandage is extended under the back of the head, forward under the jaw, up the right side of the face, between the ear and eye. It is then extended over the dome of the head downward back of the left ear, under the jaw, and again up the right side of the face. This process of extending turns around the vertex of the head and jaw and across the occipital region is repeated four or five times until the purpose of the bandage is accomplished. This type of bandage can be used for a fracture of the jaw, but before it is applied, the lower jaw should be pulled forward as much as possible so that it may be fixed by the bandage with relatively little overlapping of bony fragments. This oblique bandage of the jaw is similar to the Barton bandage, which is *advised erroneously* for a fracture of the jaw by some surgeons. The serious *defect of the Barton bandage* is the combination of a turn around the anterior portion of the chin across the back of the neck with the oblique bandage. This turn across the chin and back of the neck tends to increase the overlapping of bony fragments and pushes the tongue backward against the pharynx, thereby impinging on the air passage of the posterior pharynx. If the patient is unconscious, such an error of bandaging the jaw backward may actually result in suffocation and death.

The *recurrent bandage of the scalp* is particularly useful in fixing dressings to wounds over the vertex of the head. After a sterile dressing is placed over the wound, a 2-inch bandage is started around the forehead and back of the head just above the ears, requiring two or three turns for fixation (see Fig. 10). When the bandage reaches the midline anteriorly, it is held in position by the patient or an assistant. It is then extended directly posterior to the suboccipital region, where the physician himself anchors it with his own left hand. It is then carried back to the forehead, held in the position by the patient or

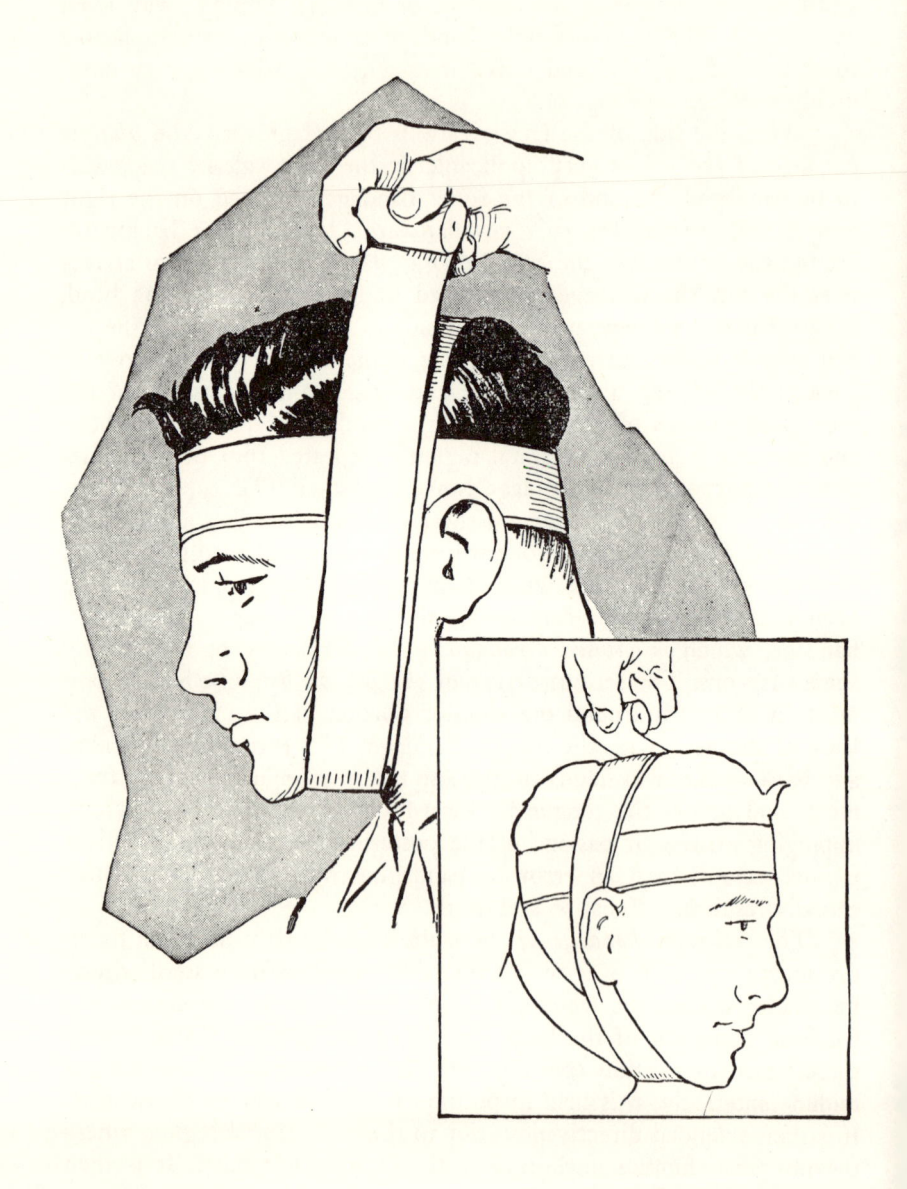

Fig. 9. Oblique bandage to the jaw showing appearance of the bandage on each side.

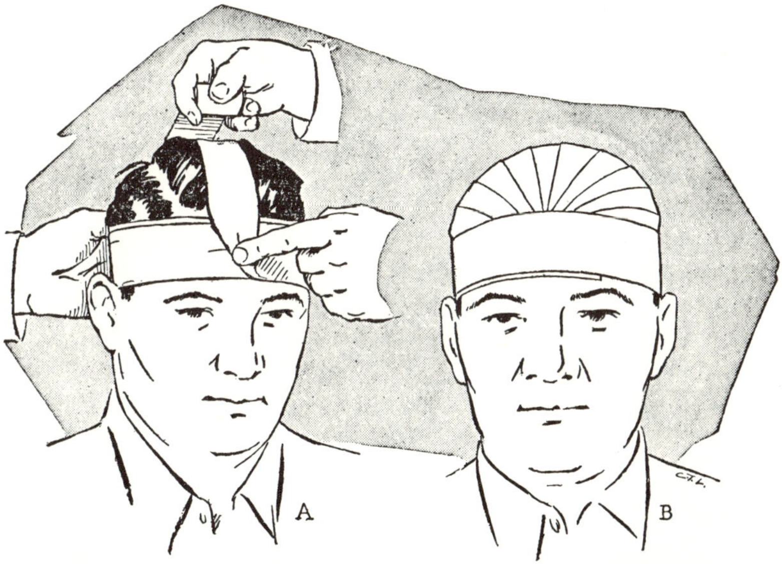

Fig. 10. Recurrent bandage to the scalp and head.

an assistant, and returned again to the occiput. Each strip extends across the vertex and overlaps the preceding one laterally so that the entire scalp region can be covered. The loose ends at the front and back of the head then are anchored by two or three additional circular turns. This bandage must be reinforced by a circular turn of 1-inch adhesive extending all the way around the forehead and occipital region. If it is not fixed with adhesive, it will stretch and slip off the top of the head. Usually it is advisable to put several strips of adhesive across the top of the head to prevent ruffling of the edges of the bandage. In the absence of a roller bandage, the triangular bandage serves well to fix dressings to the head and prevent contamination to wounds of the scalp (see Fig. 11).

The *figure-of-eight bandage to the eye* is useful in anchoring dressing over wounds about the eye and in protecting the eye from light. It may, of course, be applied to either eye or both. To bandage the left eye, the bandage should be started on the forehead, carried over the left ear, across the occiput (back of the head) to the starting point for anchorage. It is then carried again back above the left ear, around the occiput, across the left eye and cheek, under the left ear

64 / Ch. 5: Bandaging

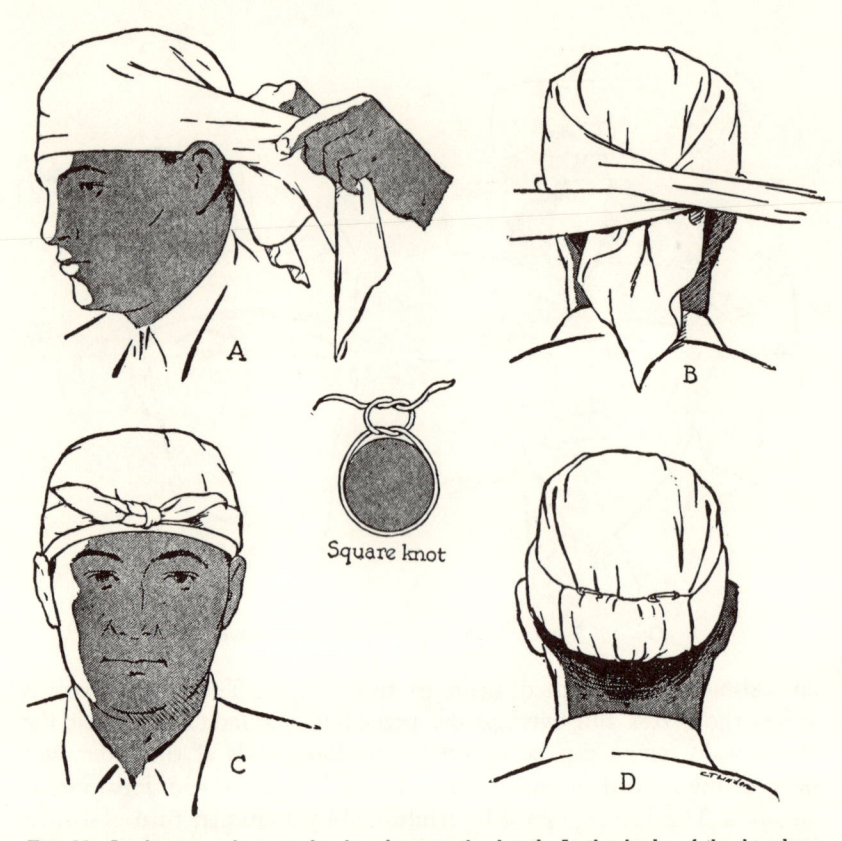

Fig. 11. Application of triangular bandage to the head. A, the body of the bandage is placed over the forehead, and the arms extended posteriorly crossing over the occiput, as shown in B. C, the arms are tied over the forehead. D, the apex of the bandage is folded over the crossed arms.

(see Fig. 12). Another complete circular turn around the forehead and occiput is made, followed by an oblique turn under the left ear, across the face and eye. This procedure is repeated as often as necessary to fix the bandage; overlapping of the turns will add to the coverage of the bandage. The oblique turn across the eye should be fairly loose to prevent discomfort. It frequently adds to comfort to place a piece of cotton or bandage behind as well as over the ear and to carry one or two turns across the ear, not under it.

The *spica bandage of the hip* is useful in wounds of the groin, especially when pressure is required to stop hemorrhage (see Fig. 13).

Techniques of Individual Types of Bandages / 65

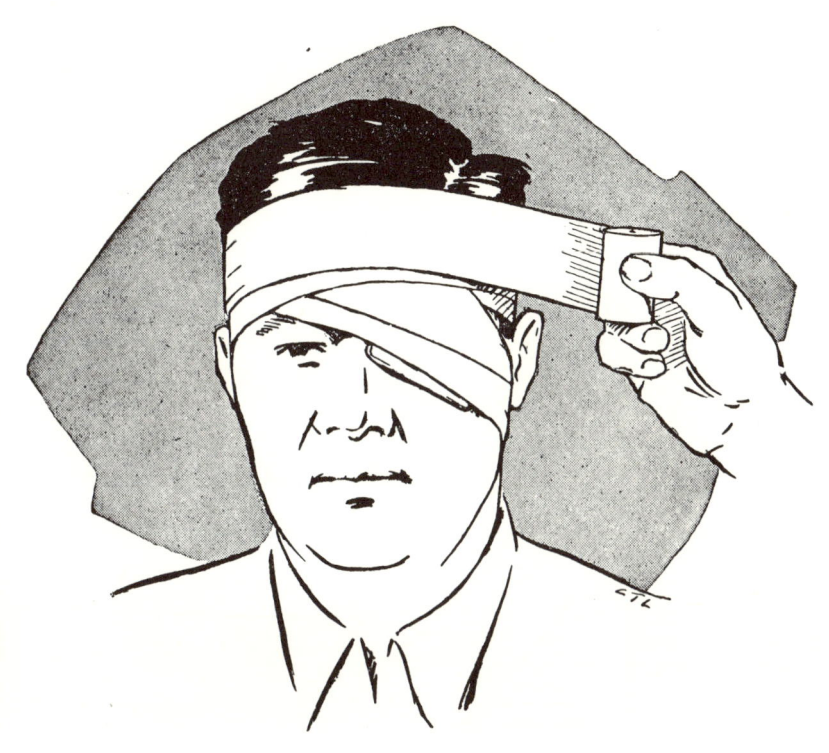

Fig. 12. Figure-of-eight bandage to eye.

This spica bandage is in reality a figure-of-eight bandage, one loop of the eight extending around the upper thigh and the other loop around the lower part of the abdomen, crossing in the groin. By applying a bulky dressing in the groin, considerable pressure against a bleeding point can be achieved. This pressure can be maintained and actually increased by applying strips of adhesive in somewhat the same direction as the turns of bandage. Such a dressing may be utilized for wounds in the upper thigh and lower abdomen. It should control hemorrhage from all veins and most small arteries. It will not control bleeding from the femoral artery. If hemorrhage arises from this vessel, cessation of bleeding may be attained only by direct pressure (see Chap. 9). This direct pressure may have to be maintained until the patient is transported to an operating room.

When bandages are not available numerous substitutes may be

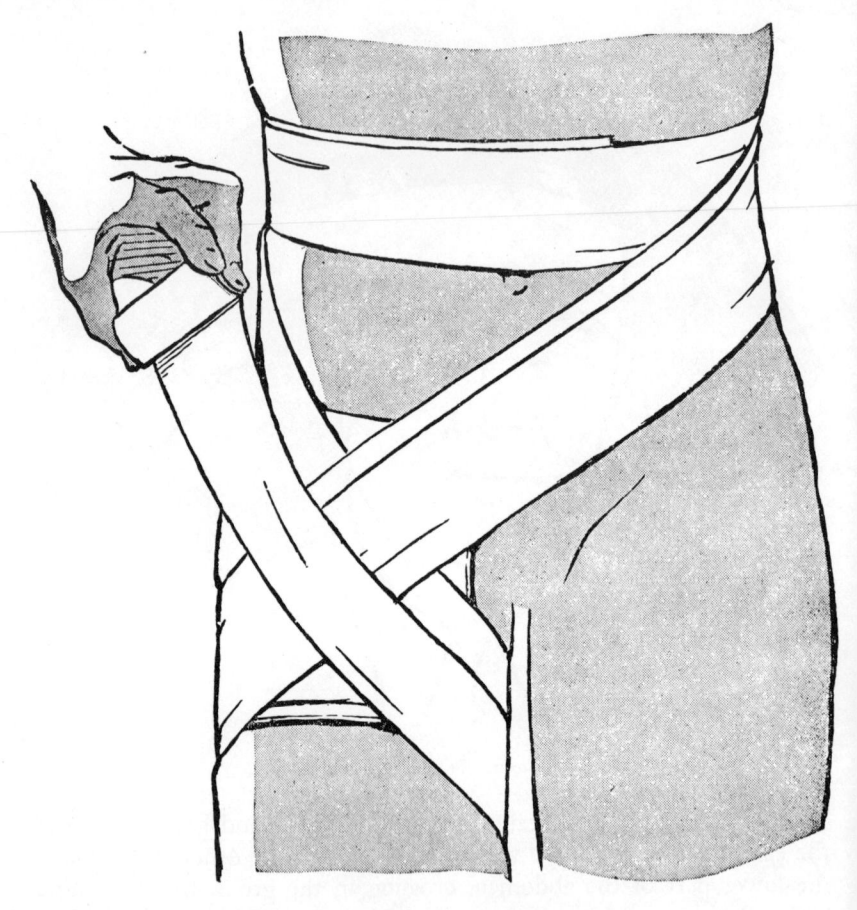

Fig. 13. Spica bandage to the thigh and groin.

employed. Sheets, pillow cases, shirts, and so on, may be torn into strips of desired width and used as bandages. Figure 14 illustrates the numerous uses which may be made of a substitute material, e.g., a stocking.

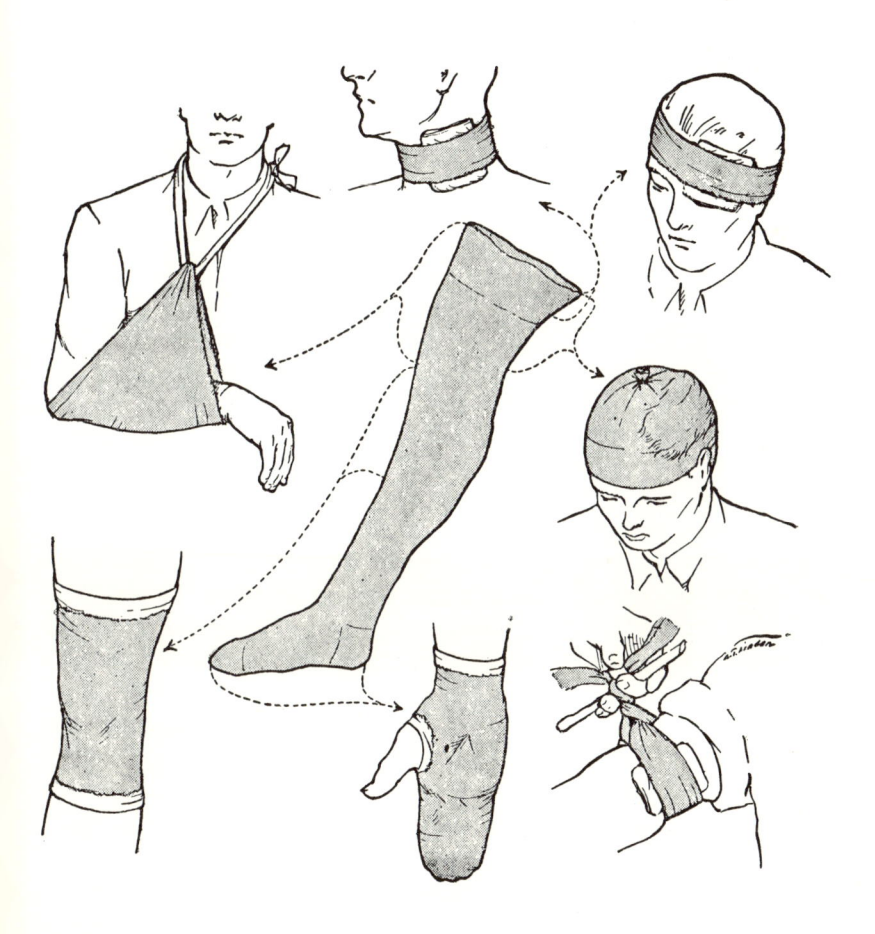

Fig. 14. In the absence of complete availability of medical supplies numerous types of material may be utilized. Illustration shows methods in which a stocking may be used to reinforce bandages and dressings.

6 / Wounds

RUDOLF J. NOER

Wounds may be defined as injuries to the body produced by external agents. They may be open, i.e., with a break in the skin, or closed. Open wounds introduce additional obligations in first aid care because of contamination and possible infection and the frequency of hemorrhage. The problems in closed wounds more often relate to injury of the underlying structures, such as fractures of bones.

The type of wound will be determined by many factors, including primarily the mechanism by which the wound was inflicted and the degree of violence. In general, wounds incurred out-of-doors, e.g., farm accidents, auto accidents, will be grossly contaminated with a variable amount of dirt or grease. Wounds sustained indoors are apt to be relatively clean.

First aid care of wounds discussed in this chapter will be limited to those produced in civil life; the care of military wounds is discussed in Chapters 12 and 26. Burns, because of the special problems they present in treatment, are separately considered in Chapter 10.

Definitions or Types of Wounds

(Fig. 1) *Contused wounds* result from the impact of blunt objects and although the skin is not penetrated, there may be much crushing of tissues beneath the skin. There is always a variable amount of hemorrhage which takes place at the time of injury and frequently for a few hours after. The soft tissues may be lacerated (torn) to a marked degree, so that vital structures may be damaged frequently. Some swelling develops 24 to 28 hours after infliction of the injury. This swelling is due to hemorrhage and edema (extravasation of serum). The blood clot which forms at the site of a contusion is

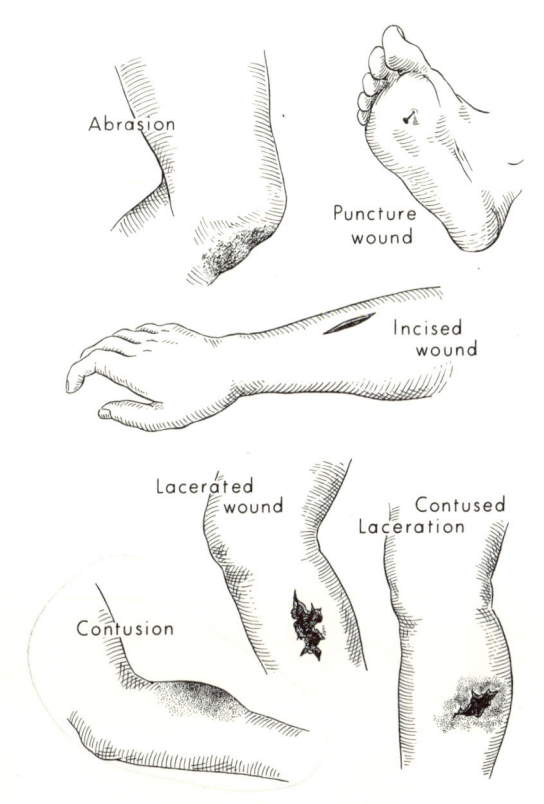

Fig. 1. Types of wounds.

spoken of as a *hematoma*. The blood in the hematoma escapes from broken blood vessels into surrounding tissues, including the skin, and produces the bluish discoloration spoken of as a bruise. Within a few days, this blue or blue-black color changes to a green or yellow color because of oxidation of the blood pigment.

An *open wound* may be defined as one in which the skin is incised or torn, thus exposing the tissues beneath. There are four major types of open wounds. 1) An *abrasion* is the most superficial and least serious of the open wounds, usually consisting of rubbing off of only the skin surface without penetrating through the entire skin. The familiar "brush burn" of the athlete and the "skinned knee" of the active boy are good examples. There may be some bleeding of the abraded surface, but rarely more than a few drops. Much dirt may be ground into the abrasion and in street accidents coal dust so introduced may result in a permanent tattoo unless care is taken to remove it by scrubbing following injury. 2) An *incised wound* is one made by a sharp object. The edges of the skin or mucous membrane and underlying tissues severed will be smooth because of the sharpness of the object inflicting it. Obviously, if such a wound is deep, important structures such as large blood vessels and nerves may be severed. Such wounds bleed freely, the amount of blood determined by the location and number and size of blood vessels severed. 3) A *lacerated wound* is inflicted by a rather blunt object, but sufficiently sharp to tear the tissues. As in an incised wound, important structures beneath the skin may be damaged. By looking at the exterior of the wound, it is usually impossible to determine what important structures may have been injured, since the edges of the wound will fall together obstructing vision of the depth of the wound. Obviously, if important blood vessels are severed, the resultant hemorrhage will be ample evidence of vascular injury. Usually the amount of hemorrhage in a lacerated wound is less than that produced by an incised wound. This is true because the tearing and stretching of the tissues allow curling and folding of the blood vessel wall, thereby obstructing the lumen and resulting in more rapid and extensive blood clot formation. 4) *Penetrating* or *punctured wounds* result from penetration of the skin or mucous membranes with a sharp object. It will obviously be impossible from the appearance of the external wound to determine just how far the object penetrated. A wound inflicted by a dagger may make a wound of entry no longer than 0.5 to 1 inch, but may penetrate 3 or 4 inches, cutting intestine, lung, liver, or other organs, depending upon the site of injury. Nails or other sharp objects may penetrate quite deeply and frequently carry bits of clothing, dirt, or other foreign materials into the deeper tissues.

The Ill Effects of Wounds

CONTUSED WOUNDS. Since contused wounds are not associated with superficial laceration, they are not subject to the serious effects accompanying open wounds. However, if the contusion is extensive, there may be crushing of important structures, which may even result in death. Intestinal loops may be crushed so severely as to be severed completely, thereby requiring an immediate operation to save life. The spleen and liver are frequently ruptured in blunt injury to the abdomen. Contused wounds involving the heart may seriously affect the conduction system, thereby altering the heart beat and perhaps even stopping it. Blunt injuries to the chest may constitute one of the most lethal of the situations often encountered in automobile crashes. The jagged ends of broken ribs may puncture the pleura and/or the underlying lung with grave consequences. Special considerations of these and related types of chest contusions are described in Chapter 15. Since the brain is protected on all sides by bone, it would appear that contusion of the brain would be infrequent or even impossible. However, contusion of the brain accompanied by laceration and hemorrhage is quite common. The brain is soft and can be seriously injured by impact transmitted from the skull itself, or it may be damaged when the motion of the skull is suddenly arrested, inertia driving the brain against its containing skull. Peculiar to the brain is the so-called "contre-coup" injury in which a blow on the skull causes the contained brain to be driven against the opposite side of the skull thus producing contusion on the side of the brain opposite to that of the blow.

A rather frequent and serious complication or ill effect of contusions is a fracture, which may be located in any bone depending upon the site of injury. Fractures may be sustained even though very little evidence of soft-tissue injury is manifest. Considerable injury to adjacent tissue may be inflicted by the jagged bare ends of bone. Blood vessels may be severed, resulting in a variable amount of hemorrhage, depending upon the size of the vessel and type of therapy, if any, rendered immediately after the accident. Since fractures usually require reduction and always require more time for healing than does disruption of most soft tissues, an x-ray is indicated if there is even suggestive evidence of a fracture (see Chap. 13).

OPEN WOUNDS. Many effects and complications may result from open wounds. On many occasions these secondary effects will be more serious than the primary effects of the accident and may result in the patient's death. Infection is a constant and serious hazard resulting from the contamination sustained at the time of injury.

HEMORRHAGE. As already mentioned, hemorrhage is one of the most serious effects of wounds, and although of most significance at the time of injury, secondary hemorrhage may take place many hours after the injury. When hemorrhage is secondary it is usually due to infection or to dislodgment of a clot by a second injury. Obviously, arterial hemorrhage is more serious than venous. Arterial blood is bright red, contrasted to the dark red or bluish-red color of the venous blood. As will be discussed later in detail, massive hemorrhage results in the development of shock, which requires immediate therapy to save life. About 8 percent of the body weight is blood. Loss of one half of this blood at one time without any replacement is usually fatal.

OPEN FRACTURES. When the skin and subcutaneous tissues over a fracture are broken so that the fracture site connects with the exterior, the fracture is spoken of as *open* or *compound* (Fig. 2). This situation complicates tremendously the treatment of the fracture and likewise increases the difficulties from numerous aspects, including increase in complications, particularly infection of both soft tissue and bone. The patient must be taken to the operating room immediately and the wound debrided (see Chap. 13).

INJURY TO SPECIAL STRUCTURES. There is much more chance of injury to vital deep structures in open wounds than in closed ones. Injury to blood vessels has already been discussed. Injuries to nerves and tendons are common and require careful repair. Laceration through a joint capsule requires repair of the wound as soon as possible. As previously mentioned, it is difficult to determine from the external appearance of a wound just how deep it is. For example, a foreign body may make only a small open wound penetrating the abdominal wall; but if it penetrates the intestine or severs a large vessel, an abdominal operation will be necessary. Omission of repair of such injuries leads to a needless fatality. For the most part, however, diagnosis and treatment of these deeper injuries is beyond the scope of first aid and must await hospitalization.

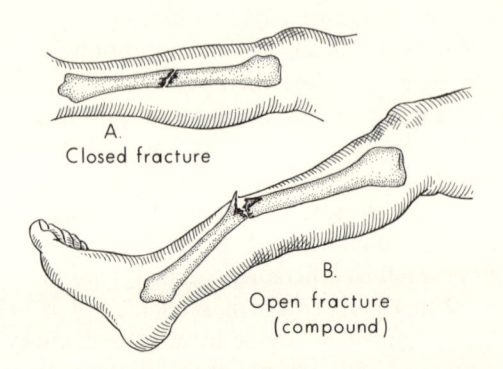

Fig. 2. Two common types of bony fractures: A, closed (no breaks in the skin) and B, open or compound (break in the skin poses danger of infection).

INFECTION. Infections are produced by bacteria, which are present everywhere except where sterilization has taken place. The world owes this knowledge of the relationship of bacteria to infection to the noted French scientist, Pasteur, whose first discoveries, made no earlier than the middle of the last century, were based upon the demonstration of bacteria in the air. This can be corroborated readily by exposure of an agar plate (for culturing bacteria) to the air for an hour or so and incubating for 24 to 48 hours. Even in rooms which are kept clean, as many as 50 to 200 colonies will grow, indicating that this many bacteria dropped on a plate from the air. It should be emphasized, however, that air is a relatively minor source of bacteria, more being introduced by or from the various solid objects (clean or dirty) which surround us.

In spite of cleanliness, the human skin is teeming with bacteria. The mouth contains even more, many of which are very pathogenic, i.e., produce active serious infection. Fortunately, the skin and mucous membranes offer a splendid protection against the invasions of organisms. Only occasionally do bacteria penetrate these structures. Tonsillitis, furuncles, and carbuncles may be mentioned as examples of spontaneous penetration of bacteria through the mucous membrane of skin. Many bacteria are not harmful to the human body and in fact are helpful to certain bodily functions such as digestion.

The most virulent common organisms affecting man are the *streptococci* and *staphylococci*. The streptococcus is not as prevalent as the staphylococcus but tends to produce a more serious infection, invading more rapidly, and is more apt to be fatal. It can be found in the mouth of most people, frequently in large numbers; some strains such as the hemolytic streptococcus are exceedingly virulent. The staphylococcus is very prevalent over the skin of the body, and infection produced by it is not rapidly invasive, although serious.

The *colon bacillus*, which is a constant inhabitant of the intestinal tract, is likewise pathogenic to man if it enters body cavities or subcutaneous tissues. The *tetanus bacillus*, which produces tetanus (lockjaw), and the *gas bacillus* (several strains), which produces gas gangrene, are spore-bearing organisms not readily killed by heat, such as boiling water, and are very serious when they obtain a foothold in the body. The latter two organisms are frequently present in the intestinal tract of man, but they are much more prevalent (particularly *tetanus bacillus*) in the intestinal tract of animals, thus accounting for a high incidence of development of tetanus (lockjaw) when wounds are inflicted about barnyards. The *tetanus bacillus* and *gas bacillus* (Welch bacillus) are anaerobic, growing without the presence of oxygen, whereas aerobic organisms require oxygen for growth. Because of these factors punctured wounds, apt to seal themselves off, are subject to the development of tetanus, since oxygen does not have access to the depths of such a wound. A simple punctured wound is not apt to result in gas gangrene because these organisms grow best in necrotic tissue, especially dead muscle, resulting from massive tissue destruction. Unquestionably, the presence of aerobic organisms using up oxygen accelerates the development of either of the anaerobic infections mentioned.

All wounds except those made in the operating room under aseptic conditions are contaminated with a variable number of bacteria. Such wounds are spoken of as contaminated wounds. After six to eight hours, the bacteria may begin to multiply profusely and penetrate the tissues beneath the surface. At the end of 24 hours an obvious infection will have become manifest. The wound is then spoken of as an *infected wound*. Naturally, when wounds are inflicted by a skin by a clean sharp object, little contamination results. Examples of this trivial contamination would be an incised wound inflicted by a razor in shaving or by broken glass while washing dishes. Such wounds will heal readily if given proper rest and antiseptic care. On the contrary, wounds which are inflicted by contact with the ground and which contain many foreign bodies, such as dirt and bits of clothing, contain numerous organisms. In other words, they are severely contaminated and require expert care to prevent development of infection.

Dressings

Dressings must be differentiated from bandages, since the former are applied to the wounds to control hemorrhage and prevent bacterial contamination, and the latter are used to anchor dressings, cover injured parts, and support them (Fig. 3) (see Chap. 5). On rare occasions must a bandage be sterile, whereas on all occasions when a dressing is applied to an open wound, the dressing must be sterile or as nearly so as possible. Some of the functions of a dressing are similar to those of a bandage and may be listed as follows: 1) In the presence of actual bleeding the most important function of a dressing is control of hemorrhage. Light pressure will not control

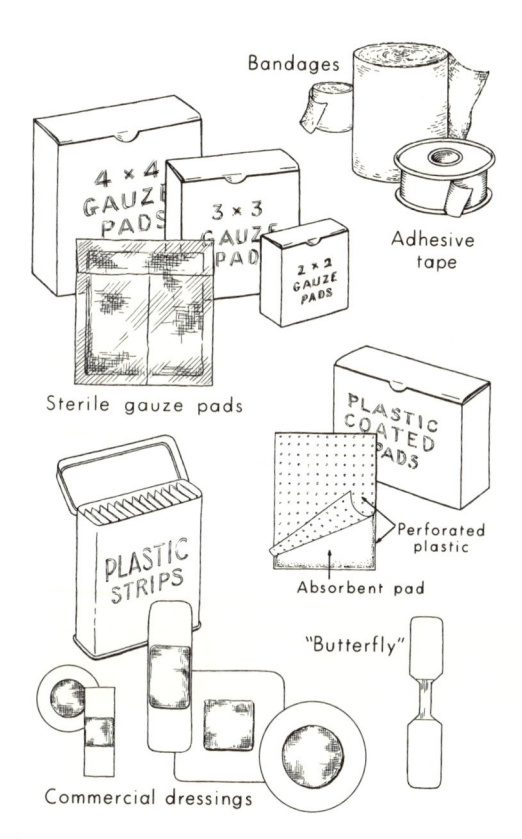

Fig. 3. Various types of prepared dressings commercially available.

severe hemorrhage; active pressure with the hand over the dressing must be used in many such instances. 2) Almost equally important in the function of a dressing is the protection of the wound from contamination by bacteria. 3) Dressings promote absorption of fluids, which consist chiefly of exudate containing bacteria and their toxins. It is important that this exudate, particularly if it develops into pus, not be allowed to accumulate in pockets in the wound. Removal of purulent material facilitates healing. 4) A dressing increases the temperature about the wound and of the tissues in the wound, thereby increasing vascularity and the reparative processes. 5) Dressings may aid the application of medicinal agents, although relatively few such agents should be applied directly into a wound.

Treatment of Wounds

CONTUSED WOUNDS. The treatment of contused wounds consists of cold applications to discourage continuation of bleeding and the application of a pressure bandage. Rest is likewise important, since activity would encourage continuation of hemorrhage and increase in size of the hematoma. A day or so after the injury when all bleeding has stopped, the application of heat, which produces a dilation of the blood vessels and an increased blood supply, will facilitate absorption of the blood clot.

OPEN WOUNDS. *Abrasions* might be classified as open wounds, but in reality the scratch or tear does not involve all the layers of the skin; accordingly, there is only slight danger of deep infection, i.e.,

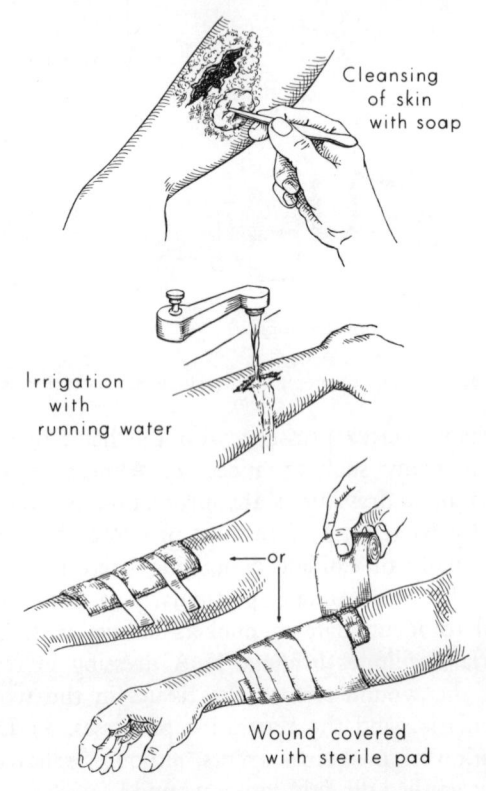

Fig. 4. Emergency care of a fresh wound.

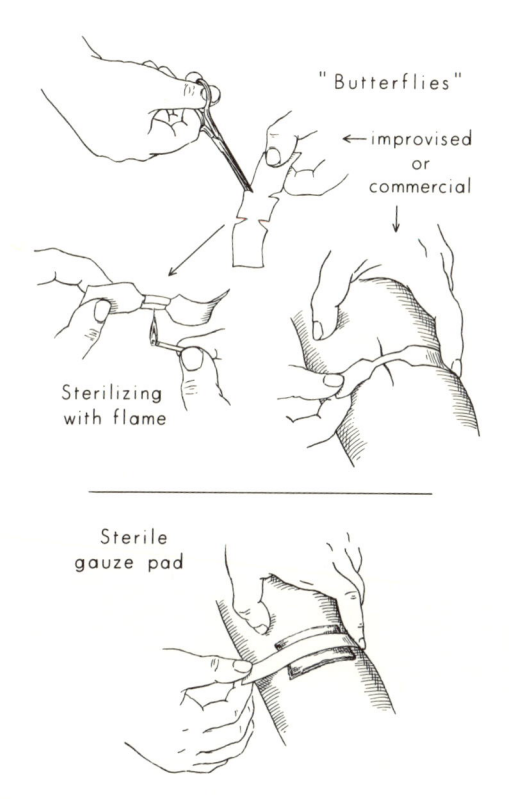

Fig. 5. Closure of wounds with sterile or sterilized tape.

beneath the skin. If they are sustained under fairly clean circumstances no treatment other than the application of a sterile dressing will be necessary. If they are sustained under unclean circumstances it will be preferable to wash the area gently with soap, water, and a clean cloth or sterile gauze sponge before application of a sterile dressing, which can be purchased at most drugstores (Figs. 4-6). There are several soaps containing hexachlorophene now commercially available and there is good evidence that gentle scrubbing of fresh wounds with these soaps will aid in preventing infection. Since all antiseptics are usually injurious to body cells (even in the skin), they cannot be recommended as routine therapy in abrasions; simple mechanical cleansing, as described, will suffice. Antibiotics such as penicillin or tetracycline should only be given later, if found necessary, by a physician.

78 / Ch. 6: Wounds

Commercial dressings

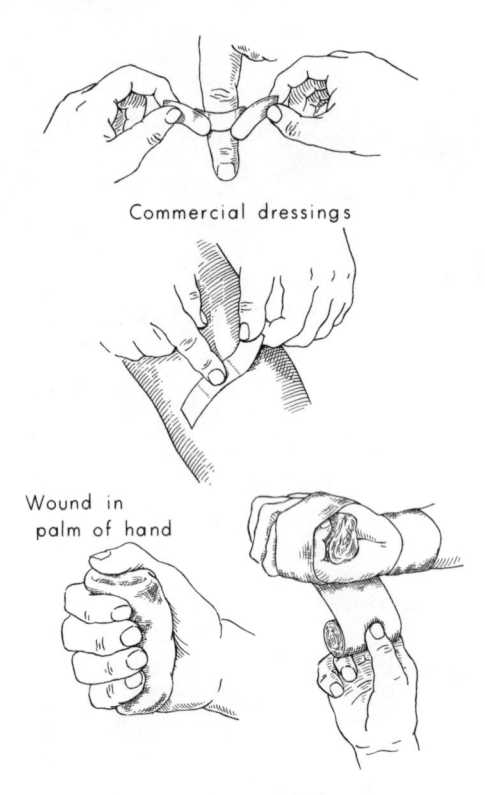

Wound in palm of hand

Fig. 6. Application of dressings.

The treatment of *deep wounds* is much more complicated than the treatment of contused wounds or abrasions. As already discussed, the most important immediate act in therapy of a deep wound is to stop hemorrhage. Three procedures are available for the control of hemorrhage: 1, application of a pressure dressing to the wound, which may require sustained pressure by the hand or finger for several minutes; 2, compression of the artery above the wound; 3, application of a tourniquet; and 4, simple elevation of the part, e.g., holding a bleeding arm above the head; in venous bleeding, this alone will often do much to help stop the flow of blood. If possible, dressings used in the packing of a wound should be sterile; otherwise a freshly ironed handkerchief or towel, which is unfolded to obtain an unexposed surface, may be used. The unsterile hand should not be inserted into the wound. Only on the rare occasion when no type of dressing is available may the hand be plunged into the wound for the purpose of stopping a serious hemorrhage; it is obviously preferable to have a live patient with an infected wound than a dead patient with a clean wound. Usually, the application of a pressure dressing combined perhaps with compression of the artery proximal to the wound will be sufficient to stop bleeding. Rarely will there be indications for the application of a tourniquet. We wish to emphasize this point, particularly because *the indiscriminate use of tourniquets by amateurs in accident work will do more harm than good* (see also Chap. 9).

If bleeding has ceased by the time the first aid attendant arrives, he should *by no means disturb any blood clots* present, since their removal usually results in reactivation of the hemorrhage. Sterile dressings should be applied, assuming they may be obtained within a few minutes. While awaiting sterile dressings someone must watch the patient lest he contaminate his own wound with his hand, and must likewise protect the wound (in summer) from insects of various types. *No attempts should be made by the first aid attendant to wash out deep wounds,* lest bleeding be reactivated or contamination be increased by lack of aseptic conditions. If it is obvious that sterile dressings will not be available without a lot of delay, a freshly ironed handkerchief or towel may be used for a dressing, unfolding it so that an unexposed surface may be applied to the wound.

One of the major functions of first aid care is the prevention of additional contamination beyond that produced by the injury. As stated above, any dressings used to control hemorrhage should be as nearly sterile as possible. Likewise, dressings used to prevent additional contamination should be as nearly sterile as possible, e.g., freshly ironed sheets, towels, or pillow cases. The dressing must be anchored by adhesive or a bandage, depending on availability of supplies and the location of the laceration. If the wound is badly contaminated, chemotherapy may be instituted at once, but this decision should be made by a physician.

The suturing of lacerations is beyond the scope of the usual first aid procedure. It should not be attempted by anyone who has not had special instruction in the particular techniques involved. It is possible, however, to draw lacerations of various sizes together temporarily with adhesive strips, preferably with the portion to lie over the wound infolded and sterilized by passing that portion of the tape through a flame. There are now on the market "butterflies," pieces of tape so prepared for application directly to wounds, presterilized and packaged ready for use. Either is acceptable and larger gaping lacerations are probably better treated by lightly pulling them together without dislodging the clot in the manner described than left open. However, if a large gaping wound is filled with clot and not bleeding, it is probably safer not to disturb it but simply to apply a large sterile dressing and refer the patient to a surgeon for definitive treatment.

Finally, the importance of support for the injured part must not be forgotten. Motion of large lacerations may restart bleeding which has once stopped. Motion at a fracture site will almost invariably produce increased damage to the soft tissues surrounding the jagged bone ends. Splinting is of the greatest benefit, not only for fractures, but for soft tissue injuries as well. Adequate first aid splinting as described in Chapter 13 should be used wherever possible not only for fractures but also for severe soft tissue injuries as well, if the patient is to be transported to another site.

INFECTION. Although it takes at least a few hours before infection is apparent, it is well for first aid workers to know the signs and symptoms of this problem so that they may be recognized in patients who cannot be immediately brought to medical attention. Increasing pain in the injured area, discomfort, loss of appetite, and weakness may indicate infection and this diagnosis can be confirmed by observing the development of increasing swelling and redness together with extreme tenderness in the injured part. If it appears that infection of the wound is developing, and the wound has been pulled together with adhesive straps, it would be well to loosen them to allow drainage. Absolute rest of the injured part is essential to aid the body's efforts to combat infection. The patient should not be allowed to use or exercise either an upper or lower extremity which appears to be suffering from infection. The wound should not be further traumatized or irritated by undue local attention. Be gentle in all movements and see that the patient is brought to a physician's care as soon as reasonably possible. The physician will undoubtedly need to assure himself of adequate drainage and probably institute large doses of a chemotherapeutic agent such as penicillin or tetracycline. If the patient is not vomiting or sick to his stomach, the administration of ample fluids will be of benefit; hospitalization may be necessary (see also Chap. 7).

Foreign Bodies

Perhaps the most common foreign body with which the first aid attendant will be confronted is a *splinter*. If the area about the splinter is exceedingly dirty, it should be first cleansed with a solvent such as benzene or "lighter fluid" followed by soap and water or alcohol, taking care not to break off the splinter. A needle is then sterilized, perhaps by heating it over the flame of a match, and the splinter is removed. To prevent dirt being introduced into the depths of the wound after removal of the splinter it is advisable to apply a small sterile dressing.

Broken needles constitute a fairly common type of foreign body and usually will be encountered in the feet or hands. Obviously, if the broken end of the needle is visible outside the skin, it may be removed. If the patient felt the impact of a sharp object and the attendant can find a source of entry, the needle or foreign body should be searched for on the floor to ascertain whether or not it was broken and a part missing. Naturally, if the needle is whole and found at the site of injury, the probability is that no foreign body is present in the wound. If the needle is broken and an end not found, it is likely that the broken end is in the tissues. The presence of the broken end will appear more likely if pressure over the wound of entry produces significant pain. Occasionally, the fragment may actually be palpated. However, palpation should be minimal, since such pressure may drive the needle deeply into the tissues and actually encourage it to migrate. Since operative removal will therefore be necessary, the patient should be immobilized until a physician's aid may be obtained. If the wound of entry is on the foot he must not walk, since walking will produce migration of the foreign body and make removal much more difficult. The physician will localize the needle with the x-ray before removing it.

Bullets are much more common as foreign bodies in war than in civilian life. Contrary to the information extended to the public by movies, books, and so on, it is seldom necessary to remove bullets. In general, only those lying in joints, bone, or similar vital tissues need be removed. If an abscess develops several days after infliction of the wound, the bullet would have to be removed before the infection will clear. If an abscess does not develop within the few days following injury, the bullet tends to become surrounded with fibrous tissue, isolating it to some extent from the adjacent tissues. The ill effects of its presence are then limited to practically mechanical disturbance of function. Obviously, if a bullet is impacted against a tendon or in a tendon, movement of the tendon will be seriously interfered with, and removal of the foreign body would be required.

Wounds inflicted by shotguns are entirely different from those inflicted by a rifle. A shotgun discharged at close range produces massive destruction of tissue and carries with it large quantities of clothing, and so on. The anaerobic infections previously mentioned are prone to develop in these wounds not only because of the extensive tissue destruction but also because the tetanus organisms are often found in the wadding of the shotgun shell, made from felt of animal origin. Such wounds require expert debridement (i.e., excision of devitalized tissue, removal of foreign bodies, and so on), and the patient must be brought to the expert care of a physician without delay.

Wounds inflicted by *knives* and *daggers* may or may not be associated with a foreign body. Any foreign body present is usually the broken tip of the blade. If the sharp tip is of any size, its presence is apt to be detrimental; migration is apt to take place, and during migration, vital structures may be damaged. There is, therefore, a slightly greater indication for removal of the sharp ends of knife blades, particularly if vital structures are adjacent. The possibility of hemorrhage in the deeper tissue from a deeply penetrating agent must be kept in mind.

Paper wadding, burned powder, and other foreign bodies embedded in a wound produced by a *blank cartridge* contribute to the seriousness of the wound because of the possible development of tetanus. Although the skin about the wound of entry may be burned and discolored with burned powder, the actual wound of entry is usually small but may be multiple. A surprisingly large amount of foreign bodies, including bits of clothing and burned powder, can be carried into the subcutaneous tissue through a relatively small wound. This fact accounts for the high incidence of development of tetanus in such wounds unless antitetanic serum is given. The presence of foreign bodies associated with the absence of oxygen favors the growth of tetanus bacteria, which may have been carried in with the patient's clothing or with the paper wad.

Foreign bodies in the eye are extremely frequent and are remarkably disabling while the foreign body is present. Most of those which are not rapidly extracted spontaneously are under the lid. The space under the upper lid is so extensive that the patient himself will rarely be able to extract the foreign body. Solid, sharp objects, such as pieces of cinders, constitute most of the foreign bodies in the eye which produce symptoms. The attendant may remove the foreign body by clasping the lash between the thumb and first finger of one hand, pulling gently, and depressing the cartilaginous portion of the upper lid with a toothpick held in the other hand, while the patient is being instructed to look down. This everts the lid and allows the attendant to hold the lid in place with one hand while he removes the foreign body with the tip of a clean handkerchief, preferably first moistened in running water, held in the other hand. The everted lid stays in place, in fact requires a little traction on the lash to return it to its original position (see Chap. 18).

Foreign bodies in the nose (i.e., nasal cavity) are usually encountered only in children, who insert various types of foreign bodies, such as pebbles and corn, into their noses somewhat in an experimental way. Symptoms would consist of blockage of the air passage and perhaps the discharge of bloody mucus. Removal may be very difficult and can usually await transportation of the patient to a physician's care. The type of foreign body present and its location must be ascertained. If it is still located near the exit, it may be seen by shining a strong light into the nose and retracting the alae of the nose with some sort of makeshift instruments such as two bent hairpins. If the foreign body is located near the exit, a hook may be made by bending the end of a hairpin and inserting the hooked end behind the foreign body, *without pushing it farther back*, and pulling it forward. If the foreign body is far back or cannot be seen, it is usually preferable to delay treatment until a physician's services are obtained, lest the arduous efforts of the first aid attendant result in harm to the mucosa of the nose with consequent infection.

Foreign bodies in the ear are likewise usually encountered in children and are the result of misdirected play. Vision into the ear canal can be facilitated by pulling upward and outward on the upper lobe of the ear. If a foreign body is visible and near the exit, the bent end of a hairpin (forming a hook) may possibly be inserted behind the object by gentle and skillful manipulation; the foreign body can then be extracted. If preliminary attempts to remove it are unsuccessful it is indeed preferable to seek a physician's assistance, since unskilled attempts to remove the foreign body may produce trauma and infection, and may even result in perforation of the eardrum, a serious complication. The application of one or two drops of a bland clean oil, such as mineral oil, is permissible and may allay the discomfort until a physician's services can be obtained.

Wounds Inflicted by Animals

DOG BITES. Injuries inflicted by the bite of a dog are extremely common. The most serious phase of a dog bite is the possibility of the development of *rabies*. Fortunately, relatively few of the dogs inflicting injury by bite have rabies, but the disease is prevalent throughout the entire country. Rabies also has not infrequently resulted from the bites of foxes, bats, and other wild animals. The subject is extremely important, since the disease in the human being is 100 percent fatal. Fortunately, it can be prevented by the injection of appropriate immunizing agents (e.g., rabies vaccine).

Perhaps the most important duty of the physician or first aid attendant is to try to ascertain whether or not the animal is rabid. If the bite was inflicted by a pet dog which notoriously is cross and was being tormented, there should be no need for administration of the attenuated virus. On the other hand, if a patient is bitten by a strange dog on the streets, the chance of rabies becomes more prominent. Characteristically, the rabid dog, during the stage of development of the disease, when he is in a biting mood, has a desire to wander far and wide. He proceeds at a running gait, biting at everyone near him, and in fact goes out of his way to find his subject to satiate his desire for biting. Attempts must be made to *find this animal*. The police will cooperate in this problem. When the animal is found he should be locked up and observed *but not killed*. If the animal is rabid he will show unmistakable signs of the disease within 48 hours of inflicting the bite. For safety's sake, all animals responsible for such bites must be kept under observation for eight or ten days after the bite. Immunizing agents properly given at any time up to four to six days following the bite offer protection in at least 95 percent of cases. Treatment must not be delayed beyond this time. If the dog dies, the brain should be examined by the city or state health department to ascertain whether or not any Negri bodies are present.

The immediate treatment of a dog bite in which rabies is not suspected is relatively simple and does not differ greatly from that already described. Since there are relatively few pathogenic bacteria in the dog's mouth, compared for example with the human mouth, the chance of development of pyogenic infection is relatively trivial. Most dog bites will be penetrative with short areas of laceration not requiring suture. If the laceration is long, gentle irrigation and scrubbing of the wound should be carried out as already described. When the bite is inflicted on the face there will naturally be greater indication for suture of small lacerations in order to minimize the amount of scar. The judgment of a physician is important in treatment of all animal bites. Protection against tetanus with immune globulin is usually in order if the individual has not been previously immunized.

CAT BITES. Bites inflicted by cats are more serious than those inflicted by dogs, largely because the bacteria in the cat's mouth are more pathogenic to the human being. In this respect, the cat bite resembles the human bite in severity. Another reason that the cat bite is prone to develop serious infection is because the bite is usually penetrating with little laceration, thereby not allowing adequate drainage. Little can be done in the first aid way except to wash the area surrounding the bite and apply sterile dressings. Since infection is so prone to develop, it is essential that the wounded part be immobilized very effectively to aid the body in combating the infection. Chemotherapy is strongly indicated under direction of a physician.

SNAKE BITES.* Four types of poisonous snakes are found in the United States—the rattlesnake (several species), the copperhead, the cottonmouth moccasin, and the coral snake. Some feel that the seriousness of snakebite has been exaggerated since not over fifteen or twenty percent of adults bitten by rattlesnakes would die, even though untreated. These data may be misleading however. It should be emphasized that the size of the snake and the size of the person bitten largely determine the seriousness of the bite. A young child two or three years old bitten by a large rattlesnake would be confronted with at least a fifty percent possibility of fatality if untreated. People should be educated to be on the lookout for snakes, particularly in areas of the country where the poisonous species are common. Walking about in infested areas without protective boots or clothing and reaching for objects out of sight in bushes and other snake-infested areas are re-

---

* Detailed information on snakebites and their treatment is admirably set forth in a special issue of the Journal of the Florida Medical Association, 55 (No. 4): 317-50, April, 1968. Much of the information herein has been derived from that source, and is reproduced with permission of the editors of that journal.

sponsible for many of the bites. It has been pointed out that during heavy rain storms and in times of hurricanes, the elevated water level frequently causes humans, animals, and snakes to seek high ground; hence, bites are likely to occur with greater frequency at such times.

In snakebites much depends up the quality of first aid care and the effectiveness of definitive treatment. Identification of the snake is important since the antivenins are species specific; those effective against the pit vipers are not effective against coral snakes and vice versa. It is important to determine at the outset whether the bite is actually that of a poisonous snake. The finding of fangs within the mouth of the snake is proof, since nonpoisonous snakes do not carry fangs. Fang marks are often apparent at the site of the bite, and these indicate a poisonous species is responsible for the injury. It is characteristic of the poisonous snakebite that there is immediate, prolonged, and excruciating pain in the bitten area; such is not the case with the harmless snakebite. Prompt treatment is of the greatest importance and should include the following sequence:

1. Apply a tourniquet between the bite and the heart. It should be loose enough to permit insertion of a finger between the skin and the tourniquet. Such a tourniquet can remain in place for an hour or more; frequent release and reapplication should be avoided since this helps to spread the venom.
2. Wash the site of the bite thoroughly with soap and water to remove the venom on the skin about the fang marks. The skin should be prepared with iodine or other antiseptic after which incisions should be through the fang marks with a sterilized sharp knife or razor blade. These incisions should be parallel with the long axis of the extremity to avoid inadvertent transection of tendons, vessels, or nerves. Suction should then be applied with as little trauma as possible. "Snakebite kits," usually available in drugstores, should be carried in areas where poisonous snakes are found. They contain a suction device which is most effective. If no such device is available, the mouth can be used, spitting out the toxin and frequently washing out the mouth with water. It is suggested that suction be applied for fifteen minutes of every hour, and that, if available, hypertonic or strong salt solution be applied between suction periods.
3. Remember that muscular action produces a milking effect, which tends to spread the venom. The patient should use the bitten extremity as little as possible and should remain quiet. He should be transported to the nearest physician at once; if close, he should walk, not run, and, in any case, he should avoid as much excitement as possible. Alcohol and stimulants are contraindicated.

4. Packing the extremity in ice has been advocated but does far more harm than good. It should never be used. Properly controlled cooling may have some place in therapy but only in the hands of physicians experienced in its use.
5. If a physician and appropriate facilities are available within one half hour of the bite (or two hours, if a tourniquet has been applied as in paragraph 1) elliptical excision of the bite one inch from the fang marks is the most effective way to remove the venom before its absorption has taken place. The depth of excision should include the entire involved area. Usually this will mean down to the muscle fascia; if the fangs have penetrated that, some excision of muscle tissue will also be required.
6. The physician responsible for definitive treatment must be concerned with: 1) excision of the bite area as in paragraph 5 if this has not already been done and if seen early enough; (2) administration of the appropriate antivenin after skin testing for sensitivity;* (3) supportive treatment based upon the needs of the patient as observed clinically and by laboratory determinations.

INSECT AND ARACHNOID BITES. The most common of the serious bites is that inflicted by the *black widow spider*. This spider, which is relatively large, measuring 1 to 2 cm in diameter, is identified by the hourglass-shaped red spot on its under surface. However, very few bites inflicted by this spider particularly in adults are fatal. This spider is widely distributed and is found in practically all parts of the United States. The toxic condition created by the bite of the spider is called arachnoidism because of the fact that it belongs to the class Arachnida. The most important features of the toxic effects produced are abdominal pain and diffuse spasm of the abdominal muscles, thereby simulating other conditions which might require immediate surgical care. This abdominal condition may be differentiated from most other conditions requiring immediate operation because of the presence of only slight tenderness and usually because nausea and vomiting are absent. Muscle spasm may be overcome by the administration of calcium gluconate; in fact, this reaction of calcium gluconate is very effective in differentiating the condition from surgical conditions within the peritoneal cavity. If the victim is a baby and the bite is detected soon after infliction, a tourniquet should be applied above

---

* Identification of the snake is of great importance for the antivenins are species specific. Wyeth Laboratories supply a polyvalent antivenin for pit viper bites: Antivenin (Crotalidae) Polyvalent. Coral snakes (usually found only in nine southern states) require another type of antivenin; requests for information on coral snake antivenin should be referred to the National Communicable Disease Center, 1600 N.E. Clifton Road, Atlanta, Georgia, 30307; telephone (404) 633-3311.

the bite, and the area incised. Suction may be applied if a suction cup or pump is available. Antivenin should be given if available.

The *brown spider*, Loxosceles Reclusa, ("brown recluse spider") has recently been receiving much attention because of indications that its range is spreading from the Central and Southern United States in a westerly direction. This spider is easily identified by a dark brown violin-shaped mark extending from its eyes onto the back. There is no appropriate first aid treatment, but if the bite is suspected of having been inflicted by the brown recluse spider, it is important to consult with a physician at once to obtain treatment which may prevent serious complications which sometimes result in marked extensive destruction of tissue in the region of the bite (Hershey, Falls B. and Aulenbacher, Carl E. Ann. Surg., 170:300-308, 1969).

Scorpions are feared by most people, but the sting is practically never fatal except in infants stung by large scorpions. These injuries are extremely painful; a small amount of a local anesthetic agent injected into the site will bring welcome relief.

Much more serious are *bee* or *hornet* stings when the victim is stung by a large number of the insects. If this happens, toxic effects develop rapidly and are serious and even fatal. Local application of ointments containing cooling drugs, such as menthol or thick paste made of water and sodium bicarbonate, will relieve the local pain to a great extent. Ice packs may be applied to the areas involved, producing vascular constriction, thereby slowing up absorption of the toxins injected by the insects. Injection of serum or blood obtained from a well-immunized apiarist may be effective in neutralizing the toxins from numerous bee stings, although bee antivenin is more desirable and effective if available (Beck).

Occasionally, a person is allergic (sensitive) to the poison of the insect or arachnoid bite, and serious reactions may appear with alarming rapidity, sometimes even leading to death (anaphylaxis). Under such circumstances epinephrine and antihistamine compounds will be indicated as soon as they can be obtained and given.

Chiggers are very troublesome in certain localities, particularly in the South. They are red in color and barely visible to the eye. They do not burrow into the skin but attach themselves to the integument. Commonly they attack the skin at points of constriction, e.g., near a belt or garter. Prophylactic treatment, consisting of the application of 5 percent sulfur in talc as a dusting powder, is quite effective when applied before exposure. Several preventive aerosol sprays are commercially available for application to legs and clothing before entering areas infected with chiggers. Thorough scrubbing of the exposed parts with soap and water and a brush will do much to eliminate the parasites if carried out reasonably soon after exposure. A fairly effective solution in eliminating the itching and irritation is calamine lotion to which menthol and camphor have been added in sufficient quantities to make a 0.5 percent solution of each. Rotenone (2 percent solution) has been recommended for elimination of the parasites.

HUMAN BITES. Although human bites are relatively uncommon, they are extremely important because of the severity of infection which so frequently develops in the wound. The tissue itself may be badly lacerated; the wound usually is a punctured one, thereby explaining in part the tendency for the development of severe infection. The massive contamination produced by contact with the human mouth is the other important factor in the severity of the infection. The bacteria most prominent in this type of infection are staphylococci, streptococci, fusiform bacilli, and spirochetes, the latter of which are anaerobic (i.e., grow without oxygen). Because of the tendency toward development of a serious infection, immediate treatment is important. Prompt, thorough irrigation under running water is indicated. A sterile dressing should be applied and the patient sent immediately to a doctor for definitive treatment. If there is much laceration, debridement is strongly indicated; the wound must not be closed. This procedure is advised by almost all surgeons, even though the wound is small and of puncture type. Large doses of penicillin intramuscularly or by mouth are advisable for a few days in an endeavor to keep the subsequent infection down to a minimum. The wounded part should be put at rest, particularly because of the tendency toward development of severe infection.

Crush Injuries

Various types of accidents may lead to crushing injuries. Obviously, if the chest and abdomen are crushed with some heavy object, the patient may die before help arrives. However, crushing injuries to the extremities are not immediately serious but become serious later because of *shock* and *kidney* complications. Crushing injuries are common in wartime, but also occur in civil life when walls of burning buildings collapse.

When the patient is extricated from the fallen debris he may show surprisingly few manifestations of shock. The blood pressure and pulse may be nearly normal, and in fact there will usually be little or no swelling of the injured parts. However, within a few hours, swelling of marked degree may develop. This swelling is caused by the extravasation of plasma or blood (or both) into the injured tissues. This loss of fluid tends to produce shock, which must be treated promptly, as discussed in Chapter 8. A day or so after the accident there commonly develops a serious disease of the kidney which often results in death. Blood, albumin, and casts appear in the urine; and the excretory mechanism is thereby interfered with.

First aid treatment can be very helpful indeed if properly carried out. Enough information is now available to prove that the shock is due to the loss of fluid into the injured tissue. As originally shown by Patey and Robertson (Brit. Med J., 2:212, August, 1942; Lancet, 1:780, 1941), immediate compression of the injured tissue by an elastic bandage will prevent the swelling and thereby minimize the shock. An elastic web bandage is superior to the other types. Naturally, care and experience are necessary in the application of the bandage. If it is too tight, severe obstruction to the blood vessels may develop and actual gangrene be produced. It should be applied from the distal part of the extremity proximally. Pain may develop shortly after extrication of the victim; morphine or a similar drug will then be indicated. The patient should have care equivalent to the prophylactic treatment of shock. For example, he should be subjected to complete immobility and not be allowed to get up or move about. Obviously, any open wound should receive care as has been described elsewhere. The application of cold to the crushed extremity is helpful, but only if it is applied immediately after the injury. Local heat may be of value later.

If the extremity is crushed so badly that the blood supply has been destroyed, amputation will be necessary. The patient should be observed closely during the convalescence, since the development of gangrene usually demands early treatment in the form of excision of that portion of the extremity. Penicillin or some other antibiotic will be indicated if an open wound has been sustained. The consequences of these extensive crushing injuries are so serious that the patients should be seen by a physician as early as possible. They will usually require hospitalization.

7 / Surgical Infections

WILLIAM A. ALTEMEIER AND EDWARD J. BERKICH

In this chapter will be included numerous conditions related to infections which in themselves are not strictly emergencies but may be urgent and at times may require first aid care, particularly when a physician is not immediately available. Perhaps these conditions do not belong in a first aid book for emergencies, but they are included because of their frequency and their associated symptoms. They may produce considerable discomfort, and first aid care may be useful in providing relief of pain and permitting rest until the care of a physician can be obtained for the patient.

GENERAL CONSIDERATIONS. To understand the principles involved in the first aid management of infections, one must first have some knowledge of what constitutes an infection and what reactions it produces locally and generally in patients. When tissues are injured by physical or chemical agents, a certain amount of local inflammation is normal as an integral part of the process of wound healing. Under ideal circumstances the degree of inflammation is minimal and not obvious. If bacterial growth develops as a complication in the wound, further inflammation will develop, the nature of which will be largely determined by the microorganisms growing within the wound and the adjacent tissues. Inflammation secondary to invading microorganisms is known as infection. As a consequence, healing of the wound or area of infection is delayed, further destruction of tissue may develop, and defects may become sequelae.

Many of the infections described in this chapter are relatively minor at the start, but all have the potential of becoming serious if neglected or untreated.

The bacteria which cause infection gain access to the physiologic interior of the body through breaks in the skin, through natural openings in the skin and body, by spread through lymph vessels, or by direct invasion of the blood stream from a local or regional infection. The type and degree of inflammatory response in a given case depend upon many factors, chief of which are the resistance of the host and the type of infecting microorganism. *Cellulitis* is a general term which refers to inflammation in tissues. *Suppuration* has occurred when visible pus develops in an area of infection. An *abscess* is a collection of pus confined within tissue or a space.

When an infection has occurred, there are cardinal signs of inflammation that usually can be observed. These are redness, heat, swelling, and pain. *Redness* is the result of dilation of regional blood vessels and of the congestion of previously collapsed capillaries. Local *heat* is the result of the same mechanism. *Swelling* develops in part from the increased blood supply and in part from the exudation of plasma and cells. *Pain* is caused by tension secondary to the swelling in the tissues and by the action of products of injured cells upon sensory nerve endings.

The primary purposes of first aid treatment of surgical infections are to provide comfort to the patient and to control his infection. In regard to the latter, first aid therapy should assist the body's normal defense mechanisms.

GENERAL PRINCIPLES. The general principles involved in the effective first aid treatment of many surgical infections consist of the following:

1) physiologic rest and, when feasible, intelligent immobilization; 2) elevation of the involved area when possible; 3) application of localized heat; 4) prevention of secondary infection by application of sterile dressings; 5) tetanus prophylaxis; and 6) utilization of the proper chemotherapeutic agents, topical and/or systemic, but only after consultation with a physician.

Whenever possible, discussion of a case with a physician by telephone is recommended until he can personally attend the patient.

The application of these principles varies necessarily with the type and location of the individual infection. *Rest* of an infected area aids in the localization of the infection and minimizes the tendency for its spread. In the ambulatory patient, *immobilization* of the involved area may be secured by the use of slings, splints, or dressings when practicable. It is important to apply the concept of rest and immobilization in their proper perspectives to their total advantage in the control of the infection and to discontinue them when these advantages are outweighed by any possible detrimental effects.

Elevation of an infected part may be helpful in reducing pain and decreasing swelling. When much swelling is present, the process of healing and repair of tissues is greatly retarded or even inhibited, particularly in the lower extremities.

The application of *local heat* for the purpose of inducing hyperemia and increasing the local blood supply is generally useful. It may also provide comfort. Local heat may be applied as warm dry or wet dressings which are changed at regular intervals. This therapy may also be valuable in dealing with infected areas containing nonviable or sloughing tissue, which must be separated from the wound before satisfactory healing can be obtained. In instances of cellulitis or lymphangitis, the application of a dry dressing insulates the part and retains the local heat generated in the infected areas, thus securing increased local temperature without the possible complications of maceration of the skin and spread of the infection. If wet dressings are used over open infected wounds, the solutions may act as vehicles for dissemination of bacteria in wound exudates and may cause maceration and infection of the surrounding skin.

Particular care is important in the *preparation of the skin* whenever any dressing is to be applied over an area of infection. The surrounding skin is carefully shaved over an adequate area, after which it is cleansed with soap and water and then painted with a suitable antiseptic solution. The meticulous care in preparation of the skin and the application of a good dressing will provide comfort and decrease the likelihood of secondary bacterial contamination and infection.

Drainage of abscesses by adequate incision is a fundamental objective of surgical treatment, and it is as important now as it was before the days of antibiotics and other antibacterial agents. This form of treatment should be done by the physician. The sooner the presence of suppuration is recognized and proper drainage carried out, the less local damage of tissues and the speedier the recovery.

All patients with fresh wounds, whether abrasions, avulsions, lacerations, or puncture wounds, need thorough cleansing and debridement (removal of damaged tissue and foreign material). This will require the services of a physician.

Prophylaxis against the development of tetanus is important either by a booster dose of tetanus toxoid in previously immunized patients or passive immunization with human tetanus antitoxin if the patient has not had prior tetanus immunization. In the latter instance, human tetanus antitoxin (Hypertet) will avoid the danger of anaphylaxis and provide a longer safe protective level than animal serum (T.A.T.-horse serum).

The selection of the proper *antibiotic agent* may also be of considerable importance, and a physician should be consulted in this regard. The topical use of antibiotics in the treatment of infected wounds should be reserved for specific indications. Their indiscriminate local use may increase the incidence of secondary infection by resistant bacteria and the possibility of drug sensitivity.

First Aid Treatment of Various Types of Surgical Infections

Minor surgical infections may be acute or chronic and localized, progressive, or invasive. They may be primary or secondary and monomicrobic (caused by one invading microorganism) or polymicrobic (caused by more than one invading microorganism).

WOUND INFECTIONS. The great majority of wounds which become infected do so either because of delay in proper treatment or because some principle of surgical care has been violated. Infected wounds are treated promptly by removal of any skin sutures, adequate opening of the wound with a sterile instrument, and the establishment of free drainage. This should be done by a surgeon who would be able to look for the presence of foreign bodies, such as pieces of wood or clothing, which may have been driven into the wound with the initial injury. He would then drain the wound with fine gauze to insure adequate external drainage. A dry dressing is usually applied to prevent secondary infection and, as advocated above, provide immobilization, rest, and elevation of the infected part. Antibiotic therapy, topical or systemic, is started only after consultation with a physician. Dressings are usually changed every one to seven days, depending upon the condition of the wound, the type of infection, and the progress of healing.

Abrasions are superficial wounds caused by friction, such as "floor burns," "grass burns," or "skin burns." Foreign bodies may be ground into the skin surface. The most important part of the treatment is the cleansing of the area with soap and water and, if necessary, a sterile brush or the tip of a sterile instrument is used to remove completely the foreign material which has been ground into the skin. Leaving foreign material in the skin may result in later pigmentation and disfigurement. This is especially important in abrasions on the exposed areas of the body, such as face, hands, and arms. A dry sterile dressing after application of a topical antiseptic solution usually suffices. When abrasions are seen late, they are usually infected and covered with crusts. Warm moist dressings with frequent changes may be necessary to remove the adherent material. Once the wound is clean, a dry sterile dressing is usually all that is necessary. Painting with a solution of 5 percent aqueous mercurochrome is sometimes recommended. Exposure to the air may be helpful in controlling low grade infections and to promote healing.

Avulsions are deeper injuries arising from tearing of tissues involving the full thickness of the skin. If the area is small, i.e., smaller than an inch or so in diameter, healing may occur without noticeable scarring. Often full thickness avulsion injuries require skin grafting to get a good cosmetic result. Initially the wound should be cleansed with soap and water and all foreign material removed. A dry sterile dressing is all that is necessary until a physician is consulted.

Lacerations are deeper wounds produced by tearing and cutting injuries in which the edges are jagged or irregular, and here a simple cleansing with soap and water is the first step in successful management. The excision of damaged tissue is necessary, and this must be done by a physician. The wound edges can then be approximated with sutures or in some instances by steri-strip adhesive tapes. If a lacerated wound is seen after six to ten hours, it should be considered to be infected and should not be closed, primarily since infection and suppuration will progress. Such late or infected wounds should be cleansed adequately, dressed, and permitted to remain unapproximated for proper drainage.

Puncture wounds are those made with a sharp pointed instrument, such as an ice pick or nail. If foreign material such as clothing or soil has been carried into the wound, it may be necessary for the physician to incise the wound through the point of puncture and under local anesthesia. Most puncture wounds, however, simply require thorough washing with soap and water followed by the application of a sterile dressing. It is very important that these patients receive tetanus prophylaxis as described earlier in this chapter under *General Principles.*

Clean puncture wounds, such as may occur with sewing needle

puncture, and so on, may be washed, left alone, and watched carefully for signs of infection. When infection develops, local treatment with warm compresses, rest, elevation of the part, and antibiotic therapy should be instituted.

ABSCESSES. Superficial or deep abscesses are the result of wounds, or they are residual complications of infections such as lymphadenitis, lymphangitis, cellulitis, infected wounds, and suppurative thrombophlebitis. As soon as localization and abscess formation have occurred, adequate incision and drainage by a physician is the only satisfactory treatment. If skin sutures are present, their removal should be considered. The direction and location of the incision should be chosen carefully by the physician to prevent injury to important adjacent structures and to avoid disabling or disfiguring scars. After incision and drainage, the necrotic material is removed, and the cavity irrigated with physiologic saline solution. The cavity may then be packed loosely with sterile fine gauze to insure proper drainage, and the entire area should be covered with an occlusive sterile dressing. Antibiotics may be used as directed by a physician.

INFECTED SEBACEOUS CYSTS. Sebaceous cysts or wens are found most frequently on the scalp, face, ear, and neck, and they are frequently complicated by infection. When the cyst is acutely inflamed and filled with pus, simple incision and drainage is all that is necessary. The abscess cavity should then be irrigated and cleansed. Attempts to dissect out the cyst wall should not be made by the physician in the presence of active infection. Occasionally, infection may result in a cure of the cyst after incision and drainage, but usually complete excision of the cyst wall is necessary in six or more weeks after the infection has been completely controlled.

CELLULITIS. Cellulitis is a diffuse inflammation of the skin and subcutaneous tissue due to invasion of pyogenic bacteria. It usually arises from an infected superficial wound, such as a laceration, infected ulcers, calluses, vesicles, or invisible puncture wounds produced by a needle or insect bites. The etiologic agents are usually either the hemolytic *Streptococcus* or the *Staphylococcus aureus*. The diagnosis is made on the basis of the diffuse redness, increased local heat, slight pain and tenderness limited to the superficial aspects of the area, and swelling of the involved skin and subcutaneous tissues. If extensive necrosis of the overlying skin, suppuration of the subcutaneous tissues, or undermining of the margins occur in neglected cases of cellulitis, the patient should be hospitalized immediately for treatment.

Surgical treatment is usually delayed unless and until abscess formation occurs and requires drainage. First aid treatment consists of rest, elevation of the part of the extremity involved, application of local heat, and antibiotic therapy. With the use of the latter, rapid control of the infection within 24 to 48 hours is often accomplished. If antibiotics are started while the infection is in the diffuse inflammatory phase, the chances are greater for spontaneous resolution of the process without development of cutaneous gangrene or localized abscess.

Erysipelas is also an acute cellulitis which is caused by the hemolytic *Streptococcus* and which deserves special consideration. The disease is characterized by an abrupt onset of chills, headache, severe malaise, and fever. The local lesion is characteristic, being manifest by the skin becoming red, hot, and indurated with a well-defined, raised, and sharply demarcated margin. The redness and the induration spread by direct continuity from the periphery, and vesicles or even large blebs may form as the infection progresses. Antistreptococcal chemotherapy with penicillin or sulfadiazine is the most important phase of treatment, penicillin being the drug of choice. Strict isolation technique should be used by those caring for these patients. Early hospitalization is advisable.

ACUTE LYMPHANGITIS AND LYMPHADENITIS. Acute lymphangitis and lymphadenitis are inflammatory processes of the regional lymph drainage systems caused by the extension of the infection from a neighboring focus. These infections appear either at the height of the local infection or within 7 to 10 days. The hemolytic *Streptococcus* is the most common causative organism. It is a spreading infection with little tendency to localize or produce tissue necrosis. A hemorrhagic vesicle may develop at the portal of entry, and red lines of spreading infection along the superficial lymphatics of the extremity may become visible, swollen, and tender. Chills and fever are usually present.

Involvement of the regional lymph nodes may occur with the development of lymphadenitis, either at the height of the infection or within 7 to 10 days. Lymphadenitis usually subsides spontaneously under conservative treatment, but the process may proceed to necrosis and abscess formation. Treatment is directed toward the control of the original portal of infection and the areas of lymphangitis and lymphadenitis. When suppuration occurs, incision and drainage become necessary. Antibiotics are often of considerable value in the control of this type of infection before abscess formation occurs.

FURUNCLES. A furuncle or boil is a localized staphylococcal infection of the skin and subcutaneous tissue which originates as an infection of a hair follicle or sebaceous gland. It develops gradually and, within two or three days, becomes an indurated, tender, red, conical area. A hair will be seen in the center. After several days, a yellow point will become visible as it "points." It may occur anywhere on the surface of the body, but usually is found where friction or irritation is common, such as the back of the neck, arms, axillae, hands and wrists, back and face. It continues to extend more deeply to produce a larger area of swelling and cellulitis. Secondary infection of adjacent or neighboring hair follicles, with a series of furuncles following one another, may occur.

First aid treatment includes immobilization of the infected part and application of warm dressings. Steps should be taken to determine whether or not the patient has diabetes. Incision may be necessary and should be done by a physician. Every effort should be made to keep the area dry to minimize spread of the infection to adjacent hair follicles. Warm compresses may be very beneficial. Antibacterial soaps and systemic antibiotic therapy with penicillin or one of the broad-spectrum agents may also be useful.

CARBUNCLES. A carbuncle, like a furuncle, is a spreading staphylococcal infection of the deeper layers of the skin and subcutaneous tissue but is larger and more serious. It produces local necrosis and liquefaction of larger areas of tissue. It is prone to occur on the back of the neck and face, and multiple yellow areas of drainage may be seen. They frequently occur in diabetic patients, and arrangements for hospitalization should be made. Temporarily, first aid treatment is similar to that described above for furuncles. Antibiotic therapy is very useful in the overall management. Local heat and rest are important and very often incision and drainage are necessary before the progress of the infection is halted. A core of necrotic material often makes this lesion one slow to heal unless properly treated. If diabetes is present, treatment of this disease must also be considered.

PARONYCHIA. Paronychia is the simplest type of infection that appears along the edge of the nail near the base of the distal phalanx of the fingers or toes. Hangnails and nail biting can cause minor trauma at the nail edge, with the result that microorganisms can invade the tissues and set up a local infection. As time goes on, the infection may spread from one side of the fingernail, under the eponychium and across the fingernail, to the opposite side, leading to the common name of "run around."

Treatment should include the application of warm compresses and the administration of antibiotics. If abscess formation occurs, incision and drainage may become necessary. The fingernail may have to be removed, especially if the infection becomes chronic or recurrent.

HUMAN BITE INFECTIONS. This infection is relatively uncommon, and it occurs when a human being sustains a puncture wound or other wound as a result of a human bite. The infection is usually a mixed infection caused by more than one invading organism. It may be associated with severe pain, disability, and marked fever. Destruction of the adjacent joint may occur. The part becomes swollen, red, painful, and temporarily useless. The granulation tissue developing in the wound becomes gray, edematous and soggy; and it exudes a thick, foul-smelling, purulent fluid. Progressive necrosis of tendons and joint capsule may follow. Many human bite infections are sufficiently serious to require immediate hospitalization and treatment.

Treatment should be prompt and consists of putting the injured part to rest in a sling or splint and penicillin or another antibiotic administered under the direction of the physician. If grossly infected, incision and drainage are necessary, following which the wound is left open and packed loosely with fine gauze. The injured part is immobilized in the position of rest and function. Warm soaks may be beneficial. If underlying injury to the joint capsule or tendons has occurred, repair of these structures is delayed until control of the infection and healing of the subcutaneous tissue and skin occurs.

INFECTED ULCERATIONS. Ulcers of the skin may occur at any location on the body where a chronic superficial infection persists. They are seen commonly in the lower legs. The base of the ulcer may become extremely thick and fibrous with poor healing qualities.

Stasis ulcers of the leg can generally be classified into two groups, varicose ulcers and postphlebitic ulcers. Varicose ulcers may occur in patients who are troubled with large varicose veins. The incompetent veins lead to dependent stasis and edema of the leg, with resultant fibrosis of the subcutaneous tissue and skin which then is very prone to breakdown and infection. Postphlebitic ulcers occur in patients with previous history of phlebitis, and here the leg is often fat and swollen without obvious varicosities. An incompetent deep venous system in the legs in these cases leads to swelling and breakdown of the overlying skin.

The treatment for both of these ulcers consists of elevation, rest, gentle cleansing with soap and water, and application of topical antibiotic agents. The use of elastic bandages or stockings to compress the varicosities, support the venous circulation, and reduce swelling is advantageous. When infection has been controlled and healing has occurred, surgical removal of the varicose veins may be necessary. Commercial two-way stretch hose, measured for the patient, are also available. Varicose ulcers are very difficult to manage and tend to be very indolent. Hospitalization may be required for complete healing, and skin grafting and removal of "feeding" incompetent veins may be necessary to insure a good result.

ACUTE THROMBOPHLEBITIS. Acute thrombophlebitis of the veins may occur, and the location is usually in the superficial or deep veins of the legs. This inflammation results in a red, firm, hard, painful cord along the involved vein. A wide area of tender edematous subcutaneous tissue may be evident along the thrombosed vein. In some patients fever and chills may be present, but in most there is only a low grade fever.

Treatment consists of bed rest, elevation of the leg slightly above the level of the heart, and warm compresses. These usually are serious inflammations and hospitalization is advisable. Anticoagulants ("blood thinners") are usually used in patients with thrombophlebitis but only under the careful supervision and responsibility of a physician, since these drugs are potentially dangerous.

Thrombophlebitis of the deep veins of the leg is a much more serious condition than that of the superficial veins. It frequently requires hospitalization and more intensive initial treatment.

INFECTED THROMBOSED HEMORRHOIDS. Hemorrhoids refer to protruding masses of tissue in the anal canal and at the anal surface. In essence they are dilated hemorrhoidal veins which become enlarged and may become ulcerated, thrombosed, or infected. *External* hemorrhoids are distal to the pectinate line and are covered with modified skin tissue. *Internal* hemorrhoids lie above the pectinate line and are covered by mucous membrane. Mixed hemorrhoids refer to the combination of these two types.

Thrombosis of a hemorrhoid usually occurs fairly rapidly and commonly without obvious cause. Severe pain develops and an indurated area, represented by the thrombosed hemorrhoid, may be palpated. The pain is usually so severe as to cause complete or at least partial disability. The recumbent position with applications of an ice bag to the affected area affords relief but, with conservative treatment of this type, it will usually require three or four days for the pain to subside. A much more effective method of irradicating the symptoms and the condition is for a physician to incise over the thrombosed hemorrhoid and express the blood clot. Invariably, this affords complete relief. A small dressing consisting of cotton and gauze is applied and the patient is allowed up as usual. Stool softeners, such as mineral oil, may be helpful in lubricating the stools and minimizing pain at the time of bowel movements.

Prolapsed hemorrhoids usually occur only in the severe cases in which there is a redundancy of the mucosa. This prolapse occurs during a bowel movement, but usually it is reduced spontaneously. At other times, the patient obtains reduction by pressure with a padded finger. On certain occasions, reduction by the patient may be unsuccessful. In this case, the patient should be put to bed with the buttocks elevated and an ice bag applied to the perineum. The administration of sedatives, such as aspirin, 10 grains, and phenobarbital, ½ grain, should be given in an attempt to obliterate spasm of the rectal sphincter which so commonly prevents reduction of the mass. This spasm also contributes to the pain through its pressure on the inflamed prolapsed hemorrhoid. Ordinarily it is advisable to have the mass reduced early by a physician before it becomes edematous and irreducible. In either event, ordinarily an operation will be necessary ultimately.

EARACHE. Pain in the ears is more common during childhood than in adult life. It is usually produced by an infection in the middle ear which causes pressure to be exerted on the tympanic membrane (ear drum). This infection frequently obtains access to the middle ear through the eustachian tube which connects with the pharynx or throat. Blowing the nose vigorously, particularly when the individual has a cold, tends to force infected material up the eustachian tube and thus instigate an infection.

First aid treatment consists of application of a hot water bottle covered with a towel to the affected ear. Instilling a drop or two of warm oil (e.g., mineral or olive) almost always affords relief unless the infection is progressing to actual suppuration (pus formation). When this occurs, it may be necessary for the physician to incise the eardrum for drainage of the pus to the outside. Nose drops may be used in an attempt to decrease the swelling in the eustachian tube and provide for drainage of the middle ear into the back of the throat. Sedatives and aspirin may also be given but, if the pain is not relieved after several hours, a physician should be called.

TOOTHACHE. Toothache is usually caused by a cavity in a tooth or by an abscess developing at the root. Obviously, preventive measures will minimize the incidence of toothache; regular observation and care by a dentist will result in the discovery of small cavities which can be filled, thus preventing toothache and further decay.

First aid treatment of toothache caused by a cavity consists in cleaning out food particles from the cavity and packing it with a small bit of cotton saturated with oil of cloves. A dentist should be consulted for further care of the cavity. When toothache is secondary to infection and abscess formation at the root of the tooth, relief is much more difficult to obtain. Sedatives, aspirin, and an ice pack may be helpful. If redness and swelling of the cheek develop, indicating progression of the infection, a hot water bottle may offer more relief. In these cases, a dentist or physician should be consulted, and possible incision and drainage of a developing abscess and antibiotic therapy should be considered.

8 / Shock and Hemorrhage; Electric Injury

WILLIAM T. FITTS, JR.

Introduction

The rescue worker who can recognize and treat shock effectively will save many lives. Few conditions are more important than shock in causing death after injury. If the causes of shock are learned, and if they can be forestalled by the careful early management of the patient, the full-blown picture of shock will not develop. Hemorrhage causes shock in many patients who are injured; therefore, the recognition and control of hemorrhage will be considered briefly in this chapter, although it is more fully covered in Chapter 9. Electric injury is also considered in this chapter because it so often causes shock that must be treated immediately if the patient is to be saved.

The Definition of Shock

A precise definition of shock is not agreed on by physicians and the word means many different things to different laymen. Consequently, some time will be spent in explaining how the term will be used in this chapter. According to the *Oxford English Dictionary*, the medical use of the word was derived from the French military word *choc*, a sudden or violent blow between two armed forces or warriors. By 1804 shock was used in the medical sense to describe the debilitating effect on the body produced by a sudden blow, and one reads of the "shock of a surgical operation." Shock then, in this sense, describes the effect that a blow or other trauma has on the human body—the effect of violence, rather than the violence itself. In 1850, Samuel Gross, an American surgeon, described shock as "a manifestation of a rude unhinging of the machinery of life."

Although one often reads of "the *shock* of bad news," emotional blows or shocks are not the subject of this chapter, although emotional factors may contribute to the production of physical shock. When the newspaper describes a mother as being in a state of *shock* because of the loss of her child in a fire, the mother is probably not suffering from the physical *shock* we are describing, but is suffering rather from extreme grief or mental suffering. Shock to us is a condition that can be measured by physical means.

In its broadest sense shock is a state in which the transport mechanisms serving the body cells, especially with their supply of oxygen, progressively fail. Shock is a discrepancy between the demand of the cells for oxygen and the oxygen supply. The vital processes of the cells are depressed and unless the condition is corrected the cells will die. The mechanisms by which oxygen reaches the cells are the airways, including the lungs, heart, systemic circulation, and interstitial fluid. If any of these mechanisms are faulty shock may result. Depending on which of the mechanisms fails, different types of shock are produced.

Types of Shock

Shock may be conveniently divided into the following types (although in a given patient more than one type may be present): 1, neurogenic shock; 2, anoxic shock; 3, cardiac shock; 4, hypovolemic shock; and 5, septic shock.

Neurogenic shock is due to dilation of the blood vessels from diminished tone by loss of nervous control. An example of this type of shock is seen in the common "fainting spell," due to changes in the sympathetic nerve regulation. This type of shock may also be seen in spinal cord injuries and in spinal anesthesia, in which the anesthetic agent paralyzes the nerves that control the tone of the blood vessels.

If shock is due to blockage of the transport of oxygen to the cells because of trouble in the respiratory tract, then *anoxic* shock is present. If a patient's windpipe is obstructed by aspiration of a piece of meat, oxygen cannot get to the lungs, and anoxic shock results. It can also develop with a sucking wound of the chest or with a crushed chest.

The circulatory system may be divided into three main parts: the heart, which pumps the blood; the arteries, capillaries, and veins, which form a closed system of tubes through which the blood flows;

and the blood itself. If the heart itself fails, the pumping mechanism stops and *cardiac* shock ensues. In this type of shock the circulatory failure is of central, rather than peripheral origin. This type of shock is often seen in myocardial infarction, the common "heart attack."

If the failure of supply of oxygen to the cells is due to a deficiency of fluid in the circulatory system, then *hypovolemic* shock results. This is the type of shock most frequently seen in the injured patient, because of loss of blood. This type of shock is easy to diagnose if the bleeding is obvious. Yet a large volume of blood can be lost in certain tissues of the body without being recognized. Such occult bleeding may occur, for example, in closed fractures of the thigh bone, the femur, when as much as three or four pints of blood may leave the circulation and be hidden in the tight fascial envelope of the thigh. A ruptured spleen from injury to the abdomen will produce shock by loss of several pints of blood into the abdominal cavity, which may not be easily recognized. In the shock from burns the plasma of the blood and electrolytes are lost into the burned tissues.

Septic shock is due to severe infection, and is also called bacteremic or endotoxic shock. Because it usually develops several days after injury, septic shock will not be seen in the patient requiring first aid unless the injury or disease process had gone unrecognized and untreated. In septic shock the exact mechanism that interferes with the cellular supply of oxygen is not completely understood at this time. Paradoxically, the circulation of the blood cells may be actually increased in this type of shock but a deficiency in the proper utilization of oxygen exists.

It is important for the first aid worker to realize that more than one type of shock may be contributing to the problem of a given patient. For example, a patient may have suffered a blow to the chest, and an open fracture of his femur. The chest blow may have produced cardiac contusion giving *cardiac* shock, and the loss of blood from the open fracture of the femur giving *hypovolemic* shock. If the chest injury had caused bleeding into the lungs, *anoxic* shock may have been added.

The Pathology of Shock: How Shock Kills

The common denominators of most shock states are inadequate peripheral circulation, inadequate perfusion of the tissues, and inadequate oxygen to the cells. With the progressive fall of an effective blood volume, the full-blown picture of shock develops. In extreme cases of blood loss, e.g., the laceration of a major artery like the aorta, shock may occur in a few seconds and death in a few minutes. If the brain is deprived of oxygen for four minutes or so, vital functions of the brain are destroyed and cannot be returned. The function of other vital organs—the kidney, heart, liver, and lungs—will tolerate longer periods of anoxia, but these too will be destroyed if the shock state continues.

If a patient's blood volume is reduced by hemorrhage by about 15 to 20 percent of the normal blood volume, mild shock will develop. The average male of 150 pounds has about 11 pints of blood. Loss of 2 pints of blood, therefore, will produce mild shock and loss of 3 or 4 pints may produce severe shock. In mild shock the blood pressure may be reduced, especially if the patient is in an upright position. The blood pressure can be defined as the pressure exerted by the blood against the surrounding walls of the blood vessels, and is usually measured in the large arteries of the arm. In man, during the cycle of a heart beat the highest pressure is about 120 mm of mercury (systolic pressure), and the lowest is about 80 mm of mercury (diastolic pressure). Although the severity of shock cannot always be correlated with blood pressure, the blood pressure is usually lowered in shock.

As shock progresses, recovery is impossible beyond a point even though death has not yet occurred and consciousness has not necessarily been lost. This point has been termed irreversibility and has been defined much more exactly in the experimental animal (especially the dog) than in man. The problem in management of the injured patient is to institute treatment that will prevent the patient from reaching the point of irreversibility.

The Diagnosis of Shock: Symptoms and Signs

Those responsible for emergency care must be alert to recognize the signs of impending shock and the earliest signs of shock that is full-blown. A delay in treatment may allow shock to become irreversible. Consider that any person who has been injured may be in incipient shock or may soon develop frank shock. How can such states be recognized?

A great deal may be learned from the type of injury suffered by the patient. Automobile accidents are particularly apt to produce serious injuries, to both the occupants of the car and to pedestrians. Blows to the chest and abdomen often seriously injure vital structures. If the thigh is deformed, suggesting a fracture of the femur, as much as three or four pints of blood may have been lost in the soft tissues about the bone. If a patient is burned over more than 25 to 30 percent of his body surface, burn shock may develop. Patients with injuries like those described above may be in frank shock or may be expected to develop shock unless it is prevented by early active treatment.

Many of the symptoms and signs of shock develop as the circulation fails. The patient appears anxious, is pale, may be sweaty, and may complain of being cold and thirsty. Other complaints may be weakness, nausea, faintness in the upright position, and apprehension. The pulse feels weak, its rate increases, and the blood pressure falls. The respiratory rate increases and breathing becomes more labored. The coolness of the body is usually more pronounced in the distal parts of the extremities, and as shock progresses this coolness spreads towards the center of the body. The pupils in late shock may become dilated and the eyes may have a vacant stare. As the shock state continues the brain becomes progressively depressed until complete unconsciousness ensues. Head injuries themselves, although accounting for many of the deaths following trauma, do not usually produce shock. If shock is found to be present in a patient with a head injury, it is probably coming from injury to another part of the body, e.g., a ruptured spleen; under these circumstances a search for injuries to other parts of the body must be made.

The symptoms and signs of shock may be influenced greatly by the position in which the patient is examined. If a patient is lying down, and especially if the head is lower than the feet, the symptoms and signs of shock may not be obvious; however, if the patient stands, he may become pale, dizzy and sweaty, and the pulse becomes weak and the blood pressure falls. Mild shock due to the loss of two to three pints of blood may be obvious only if the patient is in the upright position.

Patients who are injured or otherwise in need of emergency care may be under the influence of drugs, and this may affect their symptoms and signs. Probably one half or more of those injured in automobile accidents are either drunk or have taken drugs. If a patient's pupils are found to be contracted down to a small size, the patient may have taken a drug such as morphine. Patients taking heroin may show the puncture marks of multiple injections into the veins of the arms and forearms.

Since shock is so often caused by hemorrhage, examine the body carefully for any signs of bleeding. Remember that bleeding may be masked, especially if it is within the abdominal cavity, e.g., a ruptured spleen, or behind the peritoneum (retroperitoneal), e.g., a fractured pelvis.

If shock is due to anoxia, e.g., obstruction of the windpipe (trachea), the patient may appear blue (cyanotic). This is best noted by observing the skin and mucous membranes.

In recent years study of shock states has been improved by the use of central venous pressure determinations and the measurement of the amount of oxygen and carbon dioxide in the arterial blood.

The determination of central venous pressure (see Fig. 1, part 4), now recognized as adding certain information that measurement of peripheral arterial pressure and pulse rate do not provide, should be considered as an addition to the physician's armamentarium. The term central signifies that the catheter tip must be in the true central venous system. This location is such that peripheral venous constriction and intervening venous valves cannot interfere with transmission of the right atrial pressure directly to the venous catheter. The normal central venous pressure is from 6 to 18 cm of water. An important value of its determination is that a rise in central venous pressure with intravenous treatment may indicate a danger of fluid "overload." In the patient with shock with an associated low arterial blood pressure the central venous pressure is usually low (0 to 6 cm of water). This suggests hypovolemia and indicates vigorous intravenous therapy. However, if the central venous pressure becomes sharply elevated with transfusion, the delivery of blood is slowed or discontinued. A significantly elevated and rising central venous pressure indicates "overload." In this latter instance attention should more properly be directed to other causes of persisting low arterial blood pressure, and use of appropriate treatment, possibly including digitalization for heart failure. At times such a condition may be due to pericardial tamponade from bleeding into the envelope about the heart.

Treatment of Shock and Hemorrhage

The best treatment of shock is its prevention. In the injured patient, shock is best prevented by recognizing and correcting those conditions which by summation lead to shock. Cold, fatigue, pain, and anxiety may set the stage for the shock cycle. Management that precludes the development of these conditions will prevent or minimize shock.

If you are called upon to administer first aid to an injured patient, try to obtain quickly some history of the nature and the cause of the accident. If the patient is conscious, speak to him in a quiet and reassuring manner and learn not only the details of the accident, but also carefully evaluate the patient's mental reactions.

In the treatment of an injured patient, one must constantly keep priorities in mind. We will illustrate these priorities by considering a patient with multiple injuries (Fig. 1). This man has had a head injury without signs or symptoms of increased intracranial pressure, a fracture of the mandible with some obstruction of the airway, an open, sucking wound of the chest, and an open fracture of the femur. The patient has bled considerably and is in shock, as manifested by a fast, weak pulse, paleness, and low blood pressure. Immediately establish an adequate airway perhaps by an endotracheal tube, and close the open thoracic wound by an occlusive dressing. Remember that first priority must always be the establishment of an adequate airway and the stabilization of breathing. The rescuer may be able to accomplish this by turning the patient's head to the side and freeing the mouth and pharynx of foreign matter. During these procedures intravenous fluids consisting of balanced salt solution have been started as therapy for shock (Fig. 1, part 4) and arrangements for whole blood transfusion are made as rapidly as possible. In the illustration, one notes that a catheter has been inserted into the superior vena cava through the subclavian vein to monitor central venous pressure. Although utilization of this new technique may not be possible under emergency conditions, it should be accomplished as quickly as feasible to help in determining the safe amount of blood to give to a patient who is in shock, as well as in diagnosing whether shock is due to failure of the heart or hypovolemia. Without signs and symptoms of increasing intracranial pressure, the head injury needs only close observation for changing neurologic signs. The open fracture of the femur should receive a sterile dressing to the wound and adequate emergency splinting which, incidentally, is further therapy for the shock. Definitive treatment of the fracture of the femoral shaft must be postponed until the life-endangering injuries have been brought under control.

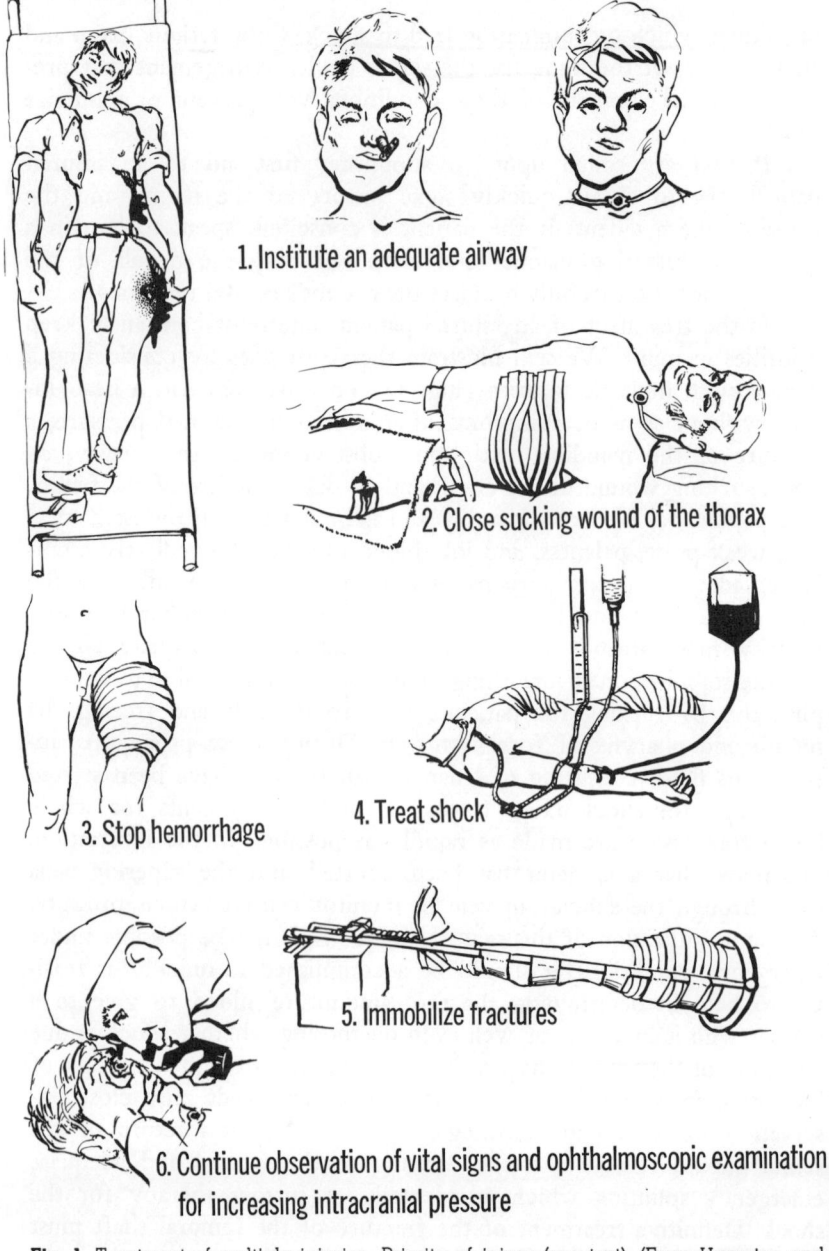

Fig. 1. Treatment of multiple injuries. Priority of injury (see text). (From Hampton and Fitts. **In** Rhoads et al., eds. **Surgery, Principles and Practice,** 4th ed., 1970. Courtesy of J. B. Lippincott Company.)

1. Institute an adequate airway
2. Close sucking wound of the thorax
3. Stop hemorrhage
4. Treat shock
5. Immobilize fractures
6. Continue observation of vital signs and ophthalmoscopic examination for increasing intracranial pressure

Active bleeding requires immediate treatment. There are two types of bleeding, arterial and venous. Arterial bleeding spurts intermittently, and the blood is bright red. Common locations of arterial bleeding following injuries are behind the knee, in front of the elbow, and on the inner aspect of the arm. Venous blood is darker in color, and it flows rather than spurts.

Of all the methods that can be used to stop bleeding, the best is direct hand pressure over sterile dry gauze. When the bleeding has been controlled, a large pressure dressing should be applied over the wound and the part elevated. Arterial pressure points proximal to a bleeding artery should be learned, but pressure on the wound itself will usually control bleeding. The two arterial pressure points that are most useful are the brachial on the inside of the arm and the femoral on the anteromedial side of the thigh.

A tourniquet should almost never be used. In this author's opinion it has usually done more harm than good. Not infrequently it is applied too loosely; therefore, it does not stop arterial bleeding, and makes venous bleeding worse by obstructing the blood flow back to the heart. If a tourniquet is applied, one must realize that it can only be effective if it is tight enough to obstruct the major artery beneath it. It must be left on until it can be removed by a physician in the operating room with good facilities available to him for controlling the bleeding and treating shock. Since such facilities may not be available for some time, a touniquet may have to be left on until the extremity distal to the tourniquet will have died (developed gangrene) from lack of blood supply and have to be amputated. Another danger of tourniquets is that they may be forgotten, especially if they happen to be covered with bandages. If a tourniquet has been applied tightly enough to stop the bleeding and has to be left on for a prolonged time, the limb will usually have to be amputated.

Replacement therapy for hypovolemic shock must be begun as soon as possible. This consists of balanced salt solution (0.9 percent sodium chloride if balanced salt solution is not available) and properly matched and prepared whole blood. If the injured patient has lost blood, nothing is more important than replacing the lost blood. Plasma, dextran, and gelatin prepared for intravenous use have all been advocated as "blood substitutes." They are often helpful in amplifying blood volume while whole blood is being obtained, but they add almost nothing to oxygen carrying capacity. They are more expensive than balanced salt solution. Pooled plasma is not recommended because of the danger of causing liver infection (hepatitis).

The overriding importance of an adequate airway, efficient ventilation, and replacement of fluids is highlighted in a recent study of Frey, Huelke, and Gikas.[1] They studied 159 deaths from automobile accidents to determine if ideal care could have prevented death. They carefully assessed the adequacy of the immediate care and transportation of these victims. Ideal emergency care in a large number of their patients would have necessitated the earlier establishment of an adequate airway and the earlier recognition and treatment of shock. Frey and his associates thought that 28 out of the 159 patients could have been saved by optimal resuscitative treatment. Had they survived, their injuries were of such a nature as to allow their return to the same mental and physical health they had enjoyed prior to the accidents. The majority of these 28 patients could have been saved if two things had been accomplished: 1, adequate airway; and 2, the early institution of intravenous fluid therapy. Accordingly, the emergency care of the severely injured should place establishment of an adequate airway, ventilation, and replacement of blood and other fluids as the highest priorities.

The best position for the patient in shock is for the head and body to be level and the legs elevated. The head should not be placed lower than the trunk because this position forces the abdominal contents against the diaphragm and diminishes effective respiration.

Patients should be protected from cold, and the patient's body heat should be conserved. Do not add heat to the patient in shock.

Pain must be treated, but too large a dose of an analgesic may be lethal for a shock patient. Morphine is not a corrective for shock and should not be given as a routine. It is indicated for pain only and is contraindicated for patients with head injuries. If it is needed it is probably best given intravenously to insure its rapid absorption. If given subcutaneously or intramuscularly to a patient in shock, the blood flow may be so deficient that the drug will not be absorbed until the blood flow to the tissues returns.

Supplemental oxygen may be tried and should be continued if it improves the color, lowers the pulse rate, and otherwise benefits the patient in shock. One of the great recent advances in the care of the injured patient has been the increasing availability of blood gas determinations in which arterial samples of blood are analyzed for the amount of oxygen and carbon dioxide that are present. In this way effectiveness of oxygenation can be estimated. The use of endotracheal tubes attached to respirators may be required to oxygenate the tissues properly.

Electric Injury

The widespread use of electricity throughout the country and the extensive network of electrically charged wires everywhere have resulted in frequent injuries due to electric currents. Too often these are the result of carelessness, but some are unavoidable. These accidents usually occur when medical aid is not readily available and when emergency care often must be administered quickly to save the victim. Many factors influence the severity of electric injuries. The voltage and amperage of the current are important, but death can follow contact with low voltage as well as high tension wires. Moisture from perspiration will increase the severity of injury whereas partial insulation by clothing will diminish it. The part of the body through which the electric current passes affects the results. If one leg contacts a wire while the other is on the ground and thus the current passes from one leg to the other, the danger of severe shock is less than if the current passes through the entire body. Often falls, as from poles, will follow electric injury and may produce additional severe trauma. Injury from electric current is seldom limited to the skin and often destroys deep tissues of the body. This tissue destruction may require amputation of entire extremities.

Electric injuries consist of tissue damage, muscular contraction, and ventricular fibrillation, the last causing heart stoppage. Damage to the nervous system may cause respiratory paralysis.

In rendering immediate treatment to a person who has received an electric shock and who usually is unconscious, the rescuer must remove the victim from contact with the current at once without endangering himself. Too often, in attempting to extricate the victim, the rescuer becomes injured himself. Extrication may be done safely by throwing a switch if one is handy or by cutting the wire with an axe having a wooden handle to protect the user. If the rescuer does cut the wire he should turn his head away so that the flash does not injure his eyes. The injured person may be separated from the live wire by the use of a dry stick, rope, or leather belt.

When the victim is freed he may be mentally confused or unconscious. If he is breathing regularly and his pulse can be felt, it is most important to keep him lying down quietly. Loosen the clothing about his neck so that he can breath freely and then leave him alone. He must be kept at rest where he is and carefully watched. Patients with electric injuries may attempt to get up and run when they regain consciousness. This should be prevented as it may be followed by death due to heart failure. After the victim has been at rest with normal respirations for an hour or more he should be moved to a hospital, preferably by ambulance or litter.

Severe electric shock may paralyze the respiratory center in the brain, causing a cessation of breathing; or it may cause ventricular fibrillation, a form of irregularity of the heart which almost always is fatal. If the victim is not breathing, he must be given artificial respiration. If he has no pulse, closed-chest compression must be carried out continuously at the same time as artificial respiration (see Chaps. 14 and 15). One must not stop until adequate help has arrived and it has been determined that the patient is dead. There are now available small closed-chest defibrillators that can easily and quickly stop fibrillation. They should ideally be available where large quantities of electric equipment are in use.

When the victim has been revived and is breathing regularly, keep him quiet and examine him gently for other injuries which may need immediate attention. Remember that he may go into secondary shock several hours after apparent recovery, especially if he is permitted to get up and exert himself. This secondary shock may prove fatal. Do not feel free to leave him alone until he is under adequate medical supervision, preferably in a hospital.

Reference

1. Frey, C. F., Huelke, D. F., and Gikas, P. W. Resuscitation and survival in motor vehicle accidents. J. Trauma, 9:292-310, 1969.

9 / Injury to Large Blood Vessels

WILLIAM H. HARRIDGE

Blood loss following injury is a major cause of succeeding complications and/or death. Shock and the loss of consciousness may be produced by the sudden loss of one quart or more of blood. Signs and symptoms preceding loss of consciousness may include pallor, rapid weak pulse, rapid shallow respirations, dizziness, nausea and vomiting, and uncontrollable restlessness.

Control of profuse bleeding should immediately follow the establishment of an adequate airway and efficient respirations. Bleeding may be either directly visible from a laceration or severed extremity or masked by extravasation into the soft tissues or a body cavity. Where no skin is broken, signs of bleeding are progressive swelling or discoloration of soft-tissue parts. The physiologic effect is the same, however, in that both types of bleeding cause a loss in circulating blood volume leading to shock.

If not contraindicated by obvious injuries, the victim should be placed flat on his back, as this position minimizes fainting, facilitates examination, and improves observation of the airway and respiratory excursions. An obviously bleeding site must be widely exposed prior to control. However if no open wound is evident and shock is present, all portions of the body are examined for the swelling and purplish discoloration produced by a hematoma. Soft tissue injury rarely causes enough bleeding to produce shock. Since "internal" injuries (e.g., laceration of the spleen or liver, or intrathoracic or intraabdominal arterial trauma) and brain injury are common causes of shock, these must be considered.

Types of Bleeding

ARTERIAL. Bleeding from an artery is characterized by a pulsating flow of bright red blood which usually accumulates rapidly. If this occurs from deep within a wound, pulsations may be absent but the volume is large and the color bright. This is the most serious type of bleeding and unless controlled rapidly may be fatal. The following hints may be of assistance in gauging the severity of arterial bleeding: 1, large spurts of blood indicate a serious condition and require direct pressure over a major arterial pressure point (to be described) or a circular compression bandage; 2, a small steady stream of blood requires either pressure over an arterial pressure point or a snug, padded, pressure bandage; and 3, a slow dripping of blood from the wound is the least serious and may usually be stopped by pressure directly over the wound.

VENOUS. Venous blood is dark red in color and flows with a steady slow stream and no pulsations. If venous bleeding occurs in an arm or leg, elevation of that extremity will slow the flow. Then manual pressure over a gauze compress, if one is available, will permit a clot to form. Steady pressure for a minimum of two minutes and preferably for five minutes, is usually adequate. If bleeding continues, a tight compression bandage is applied. Only a major vein injury will require a tourniquet and this should be avoided if at all possible.

CAPILLARY. A slow ooze as from a porous surface characterizes capillary bleeding. This is most frequent in a superficial injury such as an abrasion or scraped area. A sterile bandage or, if none is present, a clean towel or pillow case is placed over the wound and then secured with a bandage or hand pressure for several minutes. This usually suffices. In the occasional patient with a blood clotting defect, bleeding will continue but capillary oozing is usually not profuse enough to be dangerous.

Methods of Controlling Hemorrhage

The rate and volume of blood flow plus the facilities at hand will determine the method employed. A tourniquet is a hazardous implement which must be applied with care and then continuously observed. Thus, a tourniquet is used only when other methods have failed.

PRESSURE DRESSING. When bleeding is moderate the application of a bulky dressing which initially is held by hand against the wound and later maintained by a snug bandage will usually be adequate to control blood loss. Although sterile dressings are preferable to minimize wound infection, circumstances may prevent their use. Any fabric such as a clean handkerchief, a towel, or if necessary an article of clothing is acceptable. In a large wound the dressing or cloth should be placed directly into the wound so that the mesh of the material can encourage blood clotting. By holding the hand over the dressing for two to five minutes the bleeding can be controlled by this local pressure and then, after cessation, may be sustained with a circular bandage if an extremity is involved. Immobilization of the injured part will aid blood control. If an extremity is involved, elevation is advisable.

DIRECT FINGER PRESSURE IN THE WOUND. When a major artery has been severed, direct pressure with the hand (preferably with a freshly ironed towel or handkerchief) against the bleeding artery is often the most effective method of controlling hemorrhage. If no dressing is available, the fingers may be inserted directly into the wound until by trial and error bleeding has been controlled by pressure between the fingers and some bony portion of the body. After the profuse bleeding has stopped, other methods may be sought to maintain this pressure. In certain areas such as the neck or the upper portions of either the arms or the legs tourniquets or pressure dressings may not be efficient, and the person rendering first aid will have to accompany the injured person to a place where more complete medical attention can be obtained, maintaining finger pressure within the wound until proper assistance is available. No matter what the contamination may be, the risk of continual major bleeding outweighs a possible future wound infection.

ARTERIAL PRESSURE POINTS. Certain areas of the body do not lend themselves to the application of a tourniquet or tight pressure dressing. These are regions of the head and neck, shoulder and armpit, and the groin and hip. While direct pressure over the bleeding point as described above is more efficient in control of hemorrhage than pressure over major arteries supplying a bleeding area, there are, nevertheless, instances when a knowledge of arterial control points is beneficial. These are all in locations where the major artery of supply can be compressed between the fingers and a bony prominence (Fig. 1). A prior knowledge of these locations is of course necessary, and the first aid worker should explore such vessels on himself and practice compression. These arterial pressure points are illustrated in Figure 2, and the methods of locating them are described below.

COMMON CAROTID ARTERY (Fig. 2A). Wounds of the neck,

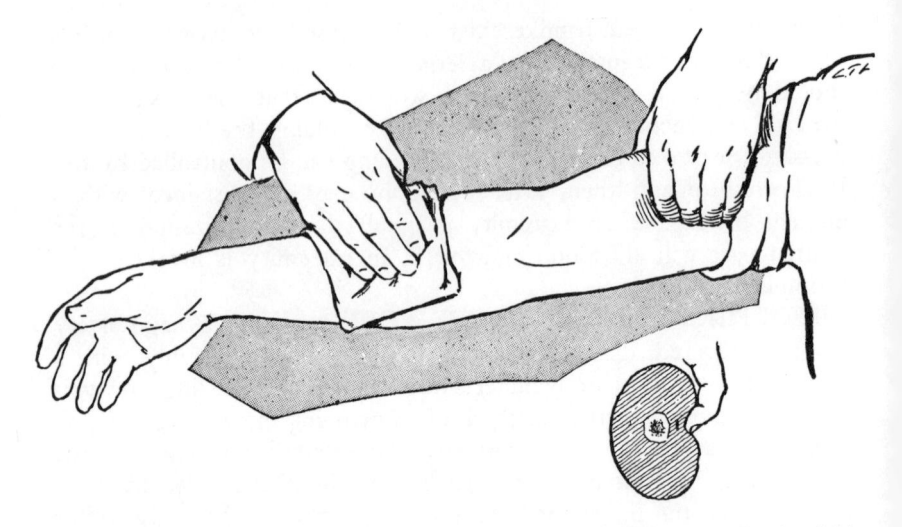

Fig. 1. Bleeding from a wound controlled by pressure on the forearm. The brachial artery may be compressed in the arm as indicated to assist in controlling the bleeding. Insert shows how the artery is compressed against the bone.

mouth, and throat may be controlled by compression of the common carotid artery. To facilitate compression of this vessel a pad of some sort may be placed under the patient's shoulders, throwing the head back and bringing the neck into more prominence. Feel for the trachea (windpipe) and thyroid cartilage (Adam's apple) in the midportion of the neck. Then feel lateral to the firm thyroid cartilage until the tips of the fingers feel a very prominent pulsation. This is usually just at the edge of a very large muscle (sternomastoid). By exerting pressure with the first three fingers of the hand downward toward the back of the neck, the vessel may be compressed without compressing the windpipe.

BRACHIAL ARTERY (Fig. 2D). This vessel is the main artery of the arm. Move the arm to a position at right angles from the body, and rotate it so that the palm of the hand faces upward. In the upper or midportion of the arm from the elbow to the armpit there is a groove created by the large biceps muscle and the bone. In this groove one can compress the brachial artery against the bone (Fig. 1). To check on correct application, if the brachial artery is compressed there will be no pulse at the wrist.

FEMORAL ARTERY (Fig. 2C). The femoral artery is the main vessel of the lower extremity, and it can readily be felt in the mid-portion

Methods of Controlling Hemorrhage / 119

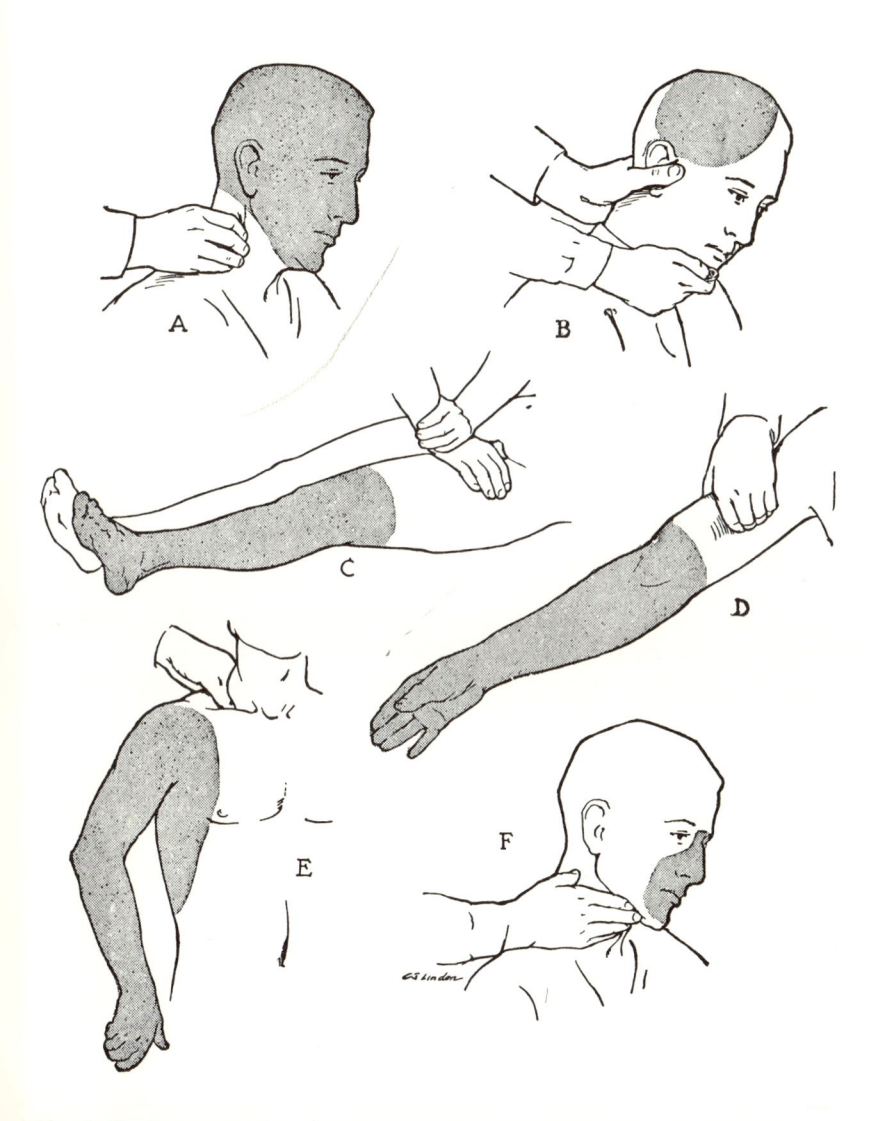

Fig. 2. Illustration revealing the six major pressure points, indicating compression of the artery for control of hemorrhage. Pressure over A, the carotid artery; B, temporal artery; C, femoral artery; D, brachial artery; E, subclavian artery; and F, external maxillary or facial artery. The shaded portions represent the areas where the arterial circulation is impaired by the pressure. As stated previously, pressure directly over the wound with some type of pad is superior to pressure over the artery above the wound for the control of bleeding and with few exceptions should be tried first.

of the crease of the groin. The femoral artery can then be compressed between the hand and the pelvic bone.

OTHER ARTERIES (Fig. 2B, E, F). Three other arterial pressure points are the temporal, subclavian, and facial arteries. The location of these vessels is illustrated but their use is not common. Compression of the temporal and occipital arteries is not effective because of their extensive communications with other vessels; likewise compression of the subclavian artery is not practical because of its location behind the collar-bone (clavicle).

TOURNIQUET. A tourniquet is a device for stopping all blood flow in an extremity by means of an encircling band which can be tightened. Although frequently a lifesaving procedure, an unnecessary or improperly applied tourniquet may be both dangerous and inefficient.

The correct sites of tourniquet application are (1) for the upper extremities, one hand's breadth below the armpit; and (2) for the lower extremities, one hand's breadth below the groin. Ideally a tourniquet should be a flat band at least one inch in width and preferably more. Articles such as a necktie, folded handkerchief, belt, scarf, towel, or torn strips of clothing are usually available. If hospital or first aid equipment is present, a wide rubber band roll (Esmarch bandage) or rubber tubing is excellent material. Before applying a tourniquet, wrap several layers of cloth, such as a folded towel, around the extremity at the level the tourniquet is to be applied (Fig. 3). This prevents the pinching or bruising of the skin and widens the pressure points. A small pad of tightly folded cloth, a stone, or a small block

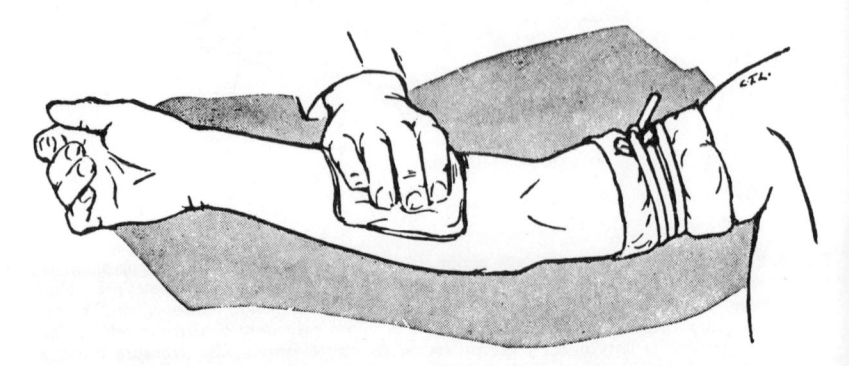

Fig. 3. Application of a rubber tube tourniquet on the arm for control of hemorrhage in the forearm.

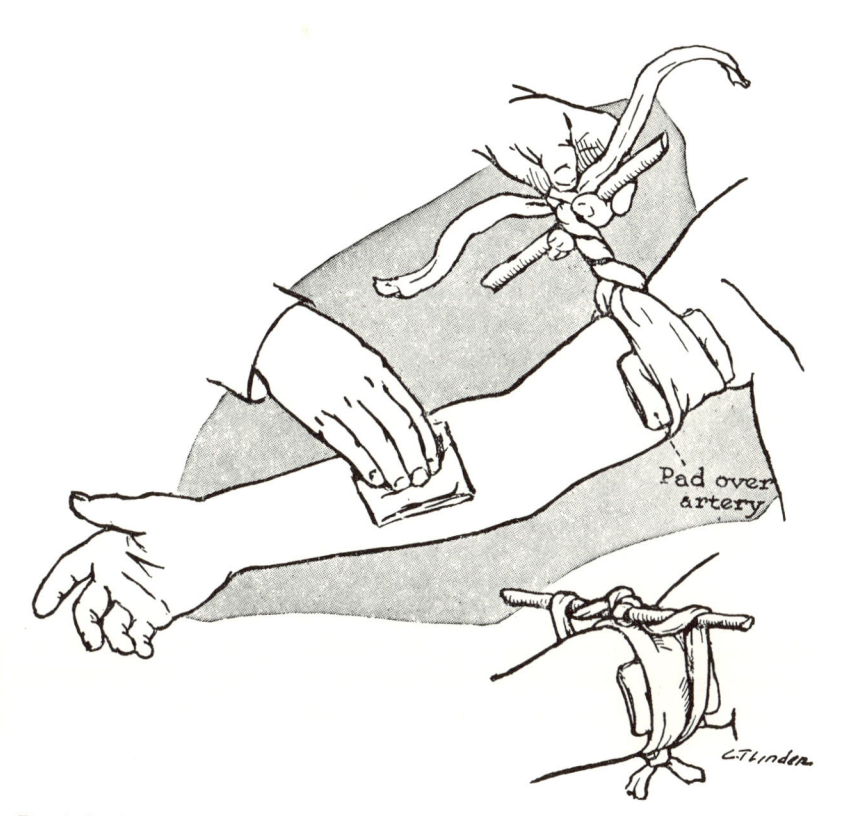

Fig. 4. Application of a handkerchief tourniquet on the arm for control of hemorrhage in the forearm.

of wood may be employed. If this device is cloth, the pad may be applied underneath the encircling material. Locate the arterial pulsation, in these instances the brachial artery for the upper extremity and the femoral artery for the lower extremity, and apply the pressure pad directly over the pulsation (Fig. 4). This small localized pressure device will improve the efficiency of the tourniquet and reduce the amount of constriction necessary to stop arterial bleeding.

If a nonelastic material such as handkerchief, tie, or belt is used, it should be wrapped around the limb and knotted once (Fig. 4). Place a short stick or similar device inside the two ends of the material, tie a square knot over this device, and then elevate the extremity. With the limb elevated, twist the stick rapidly to tighten the tourniquet. Tighten only enough to stop bleeding.

Errors in Tourniquet Application.

Excessive tourniquet application time. The commonest and most dangerous error in the use of a tourniquet is that it is applied for too long a period of time. No tourniquet should be tightened for longer than 30 minutes consecutively. Therefore, the tourniquet should be loosened for approximately 5 minutes every 30 minutes when possible. If arterial bleeding occurs whenever the tourniquet is loosened, the periods of tightness should be short and the periods of release only a few seconds in duration. Excessive tourniquet time may result in the loss of an arm or leg or cause severe nerve damage with permanent pain and/or paralysis of the extremity. If at any time when the tourniquet is loosened arterial bleeding is no longer present, control the remaining ooze by a direct pressure bandage.

Loose tourniquet. If a tourniquet is too loose, an increase in bleeding will result, since there is not enough pressure to compress the arterial inflow, but just enough to interfere with the venous outflow of the extremity. In addition the extremity below the tourniquet will become swollen and bluish in color.

Tight tourniquet. The tourniquet should be adjusted so that it is only tight enough to stop all bleeding from the wound. By tightening the tourniquet excessively the skin may be cut, muscles bruised, and nerves and blood vessels permanently damaged.

Obscured tourniquet. If clothing is placed over the patient after a tourniquet is applied and the patient then passes into other hands, a considerable period of time may elapse before the presence of the tourniquet is known. Where possible write the letters "TK" in a conspicuous place, such as the patient's forehead, and have a portion of the tourniquet showing underneath any covers so that it may be constantly observed.

10 / Thermal Injury: Burns, Chemical Burns, Electric Injuries, Heatstroke, Heat Exhaustion, Cold Injury

CURTIS P. ARTZ

Burns

Burns are rather common injuries. They may vary from minor sunburns to catastrophic injuries. Data from the National Health Survey for the years 1957-1961 show that the average number of burn injuries annually is 1,973,000. Of these, 937,000 are activity-restricting injuries and 268,000 are classified as bed-disabling injuries. Each year in the United States about 7.5 persons per 1,000 population are injured by coming into contact with hot objects or open flames. In children under 15 years of age (31 percent of the population) 29 percent of deaths are from fire and explosion. In persons over 65 (9 percent of the population) 28 percent of deaths occur from fire and explosion. Accidents in the home are responsible for more than three fourths of all deaths from fire. Burn injury is a major entity in the United States. Although the number of deaths is small in comparison to the number caused by the great killers, heart disease, stroke, and cancer, the number of working years lost is appreciable because of the younger age group in which burns take their toll.

CAUSES OF BURNS. In a study of 231 burned patients hospitalized in the University Hospital, Oklahoma City, it was found that the burns were caused by stoves in 69 cases; flammable liquids in 43; open fires in 49; scalding liquids in 43; miscellaneous causes in 29; and causes unknown in 19. Gas heaters and stoves accounted for 40 of the 69 stove burns. Of the 231 patients burned, 66 percent involved ignition of clothing.

In general, it may be stated that for children under three years of age, the most common cause of burns is scalding. From 3 to 14 years, flame burns due to ignited clothing predominate. From 15 to 60 years, industrial accidents account for a large number of burns; for those over 60 years of age, accidents associated with momentary blackouts, smoking in bed or house fires are the most common causes. About 80 percent of burn accidents occur in the home. In young children, scalds are probably more common in boys because boys are more curious. Clothing burns are more common in girls because their clothing is more flammable.

The leading cause of accidental death in homes is burns. It is an injury which is highly feared by most individuals because of the amount of disability and scarring that frequently follow a severe burn injury. The psychologic effects of the burn are usually far reaching especially when convalescence is long and distressing physical defects occur.

PREVENTION OF BURNS. Burns are usually the result of carelessness. There are two major factors worthy of consideration for improving prevention, namely, the type of heating appliance used in the home and the type of clothing. Greater emphasis should be placed upon the adequate guarding of household heating units. Such units should be designed with the safety of a child in mind as well as the safety of the house. Fire extinguishers should be available in danger spots. Sometimes a garden hose placed near a faucet for use in case of fire is advantageous. There should be guards for fireplaces and insulation wherever a dangerous heating surface is near a wall or flammable material. One should watch that the curtains are placed so that they cannot blow into or near flames. If one is buying an older home, a competent electrician should check the wiring. Electric circuits should not be overloaded.

Greater emphasis must be placed upon the development and sale of safer clothing for children. Mothers must be made aware of the flammability of various fabrics and taught to demand flame resistant garments for their children. The most critical garments are the night clothes of children and girls' and women's dresses. Certain fabrics are highly combustible. It is now practical to treat various flammable fabrics with chemicals which make them sufficiently flame resistant. It is expected that the adoption of nonflammable fabrics for clothing would considerably reduce the number of deaths from burns.

Mothers should be careful not to allow trash to accumulate anywhere in the house. Small children should be kept away from the stove during cooking; handles of pots should be turned away from the edge of the stove. Matches and cigarette lighters must be kept out of a child's reach. Curious little boys can rapidly turn an innocent box of matches into a severe burn. One should not use flammable cleaning fluids near an open flame or while smoking. Smoking in bed should be discouraged since many serious burn accidents follow this procedure, especially in older individuals. Flammable liquids should not be used to start a coal or a charcoal fire. The children should have special educational sessions to teach them fire prevention and what to do in case of fire. Every family should have a plan for escape in case of a home fire.

Sunburns are caused by errors in judgment by the individual involved. Most sunburns can be prevented by simply increasing gradually one's daily exposure to the sun's rays. There are many good protective ointments commercially available to prevent sunburn of sensitive skin.

RESCUE FROM FIRE. Rapid and clear thinking are important in removing a person from a fire. The air near the floor is best. Do not hesitate to crawl on the floor if the room is filled with smoke. Tying a wet handkerchief over the mouth will keep out some of the smoke and at the same time minimize the risk of inhaling flames or superheated air. When the fire begins make sure that there is no delay in notifying the Fire Department. Firemen are very adept at rescue.

When the clothing catches on fire, the person should not stand. He should lie down and try to smother the flames with a rug, coat, or blanket. He should cover his head first, thereby minimizing damage to the face and preventing any inhalation of flames and smoke. Injury to the respiratory tract is a prime killer in burned patients and therefore every effort should be made to lessen the inhalation of smoke and other noxious gases from the fire.

It is important to be sure that the fire is completely out with no smoldering clothing left on the patient. Too often a fire is partially put out and a smoldering garment continues to injure the patient. One should always be aware that when there is a smoldering fire there is probably carbon monoxide also. The fire victim who has inhaled an appreciable amount of carbon monoxide may not act rationally in his attempt to escape from a burning building. It is not uncommon that such individuals attempt to return to the building for some minor purpose which in their right minds they would never think of doing.

CLASSIFICATION AND DESCRIPTION OF BURNS. The skin is composed primarily of a superficial layer, the epidermis with its appendages (sweat glands, hair follicles, and sebaceous glands) and the corium, more commonly known as the dermis. The skin is composed of these two layers and its thickness varies from 0.5 mm over the eyelids to about 6 mm on the soles of the feet and the palms of the hands. Although different classifications have been used to differentiate various depths of burns, it has been common practice to divide burns into three categories according to depth namely, first degree, second degree, and third degree (Fig. 1).

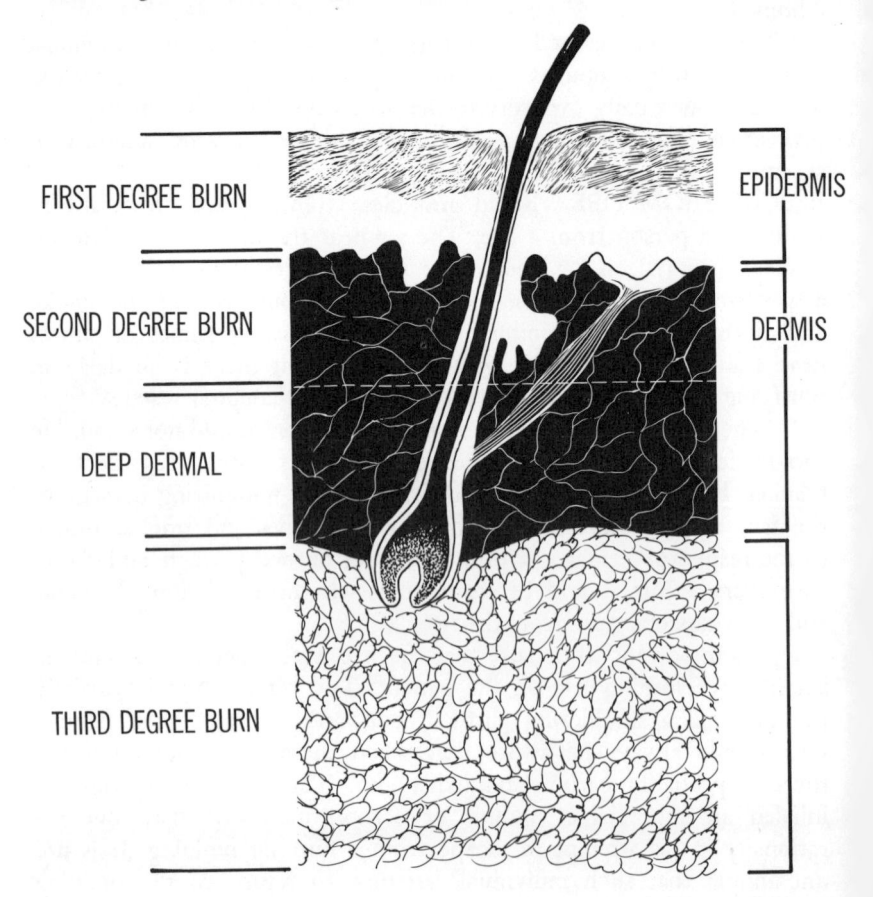

Fig. 1. Schematic cross section of skin. The depth to which burns extend determines the degree.

A *first-degree burn* involves only the epidermis. It is characterized by redness that appears after a variable period of time. A first-degree burn usually follows prolonged exposure to bright sunlight or instantaneous exposure to a more intense heat. Destruction is superficial and therefore the patient is usually not very ill. A slight amount of swelling and some pain are the chief problems. There may be an uncomfortable burning sensation along with slight pain but this usually subsides after 48 hours unless the first-degree burn is extensive. Healing usually takes place uneventfully in about five days. At this time the outer layer peels off in small scales and some redness remains for a few days but there is no permanent scarring.

A *second-degree burn* is a deeper injury and involves all of the epidermis and much of the corium. Blisters characterize second-degree burns and there is usually a moderate amount of swelling. The rate of healing is dependent upon the depth of skin destruction and on whether or not infection occurs. Most second-degree burns heal in 10 to 14 days irrespective of the method of treatment as long as there is no infection. Some very deep second-degree burns are known as deep dermal burns. These deep second-degree burns may be converted with very little infection into a third-degree burn and require grafting. Most deep second-degree burns require 25 to 35 days to heal.

Third-degree burns are a very severe form of injury. The entire skin, the epidermis and dermis down to the subcutaneous fat, is destroyed by heat. Thrombosis occurs in the small vessels of the underlying subcutaneous tissues. There is increased permeability of the capillaries and therefore significant loss of fluid into the subcutaneous tissue. This makes for considerable swelling in and around the burned areas. In two to three weeks the dead skin liquefies and slowly comes off. Usually there is a certain amount of infection associated with this process. Underneath this dead burn eschar is a granulating surface which is composed primarily of buds of capillaries

TABLE 1. *Characteristics of Various Depths of Burn Injury.*

Depth of Burn	Cause	Surface	Color	Pain Sensation
First degree	Sun or minor flash	Dry, no blisters	Erythematous	Painful
Second degree	Flash or hot liquids	Blisters, moist	Mottled red	Painful
Third degree	Flame	Dry	Pearly white or charred	Little pain, anesthetic

From Artz, C. P. and Moncrief, J. A. *The Treatment of Burns,* 2nd. ed. Philadelphia, W. B. Saunders Company, 1969.

128 / Ch. 10: Thermal Injury

and some fibrous tissue. This is usually covered by a skin graft. The characteristics of various depths of burn injury are summarized in Table 1.

THE SERIOUSNESS OF THE INJURY. The extent of burn is usually expressed as a percentage of the body surface that is injured. There are charts for rather accurate assessment of percentage of body surface burn but the simplified method usually used is the Rule of Nines (Fig. 2). According to this rule the body surface is divided into

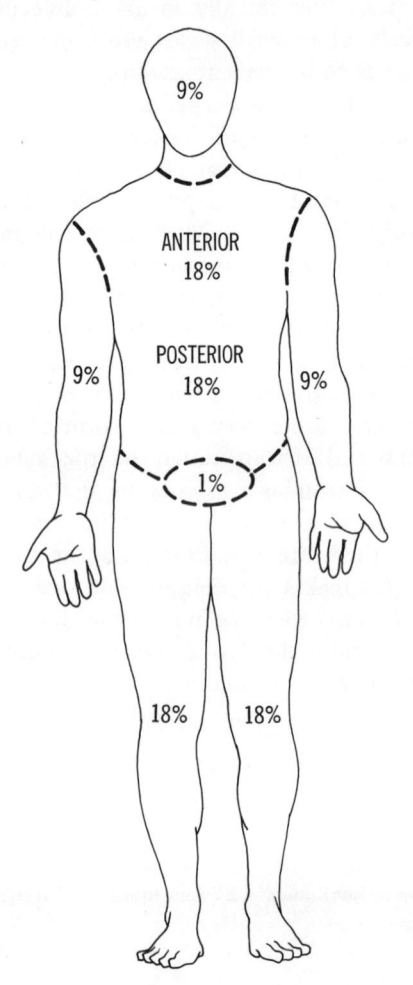

Fig. 2. Rule of Nines which provides a rapid means of estimating percentage of body surface burned.

areas representing 9 percent or multiples of 9 percent: the head and neck–9 percent; anterior trunk–double 9 or 18 percent; posterior trunk–18 percent; each lower extremity–9 percent; and the perineum –1 percent. The Rule of Nines has been widely accepted as a very useful guide in estimating percentage of body surface burned. It is usually believed that an area equivalent to one side of the hand is about 1 percent of the body surface.

Obviously a third-degree burn is much more serious than second- and first-degree injury. The age of the patient is important in estimating seriousness of the injury. A 20 percent third-degree burn in a 60-year-old individual usually results in death while in a younger person with the same size injury, recovery most often occurs unless there is some unusual complication. In burns involving up to 30 percent of the body surface, in patients under the age of 50, the mortality is quite low. As the extent of body surface involvement goes above 30 percent, the mortality rises in all age groups but as the age increases beyond 50, the mortality rises even in burns of less than 30 percent.

In some parts of the body burns of small extent may result in such crippling deformities that they must be regarded as serious. The critical anatomic areas are the face, hands, feet, external genitalia, neck, and joint surfaces. Respiratory tract injury which occurs when the patient inhales noxious fumes or gases may be fatal regardless of the amount of surface area burned. Patients who have preexisting renal, cardiovascular, or pulmonary disease cannot tolerate burns of even moderate extent. In patients with occlusive vascular disease burns of the lower extremities, especially the feet, are particularly serious. Gangrene, requiring amputation, is not uncommon after a burn of the feet and lower legs in a patient with peripheral arteriosclerosis of the lower extremities.

TRANSPORTATION OF BURNED PATIENTS. The transportation of a burned patient from the scene of the accident to a physician's office or hospital should be conducted in a comfortable and orderly manner. If the hands are burned, rings should be removed. Burned shoes or constricting clothing should be taken off. If the clothing is still smoldering, it should be removed. The area of the injury should be covered with a clean sheet or bandage (Fig. 3). It is usually unnecessary to rush the patient to the hospital. Speeding is frowned upon because frequently it can result in a greater accident or injury than the initial burn.

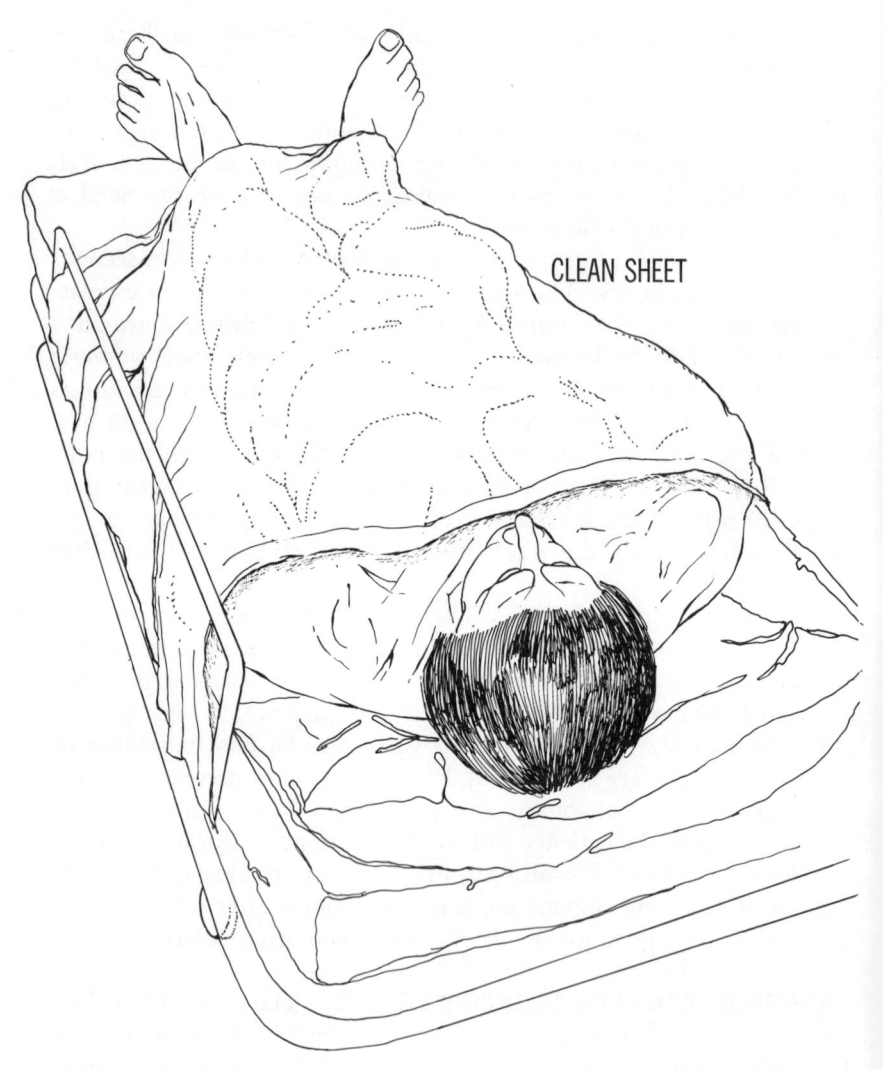

Fig. 3. For transportation of patient from scene of accident to physician or hospital, remove burned shoes or constricting clothing and cover wound with a clean sheet.

Most burned victims are able to perform a moderate amount of activity for the first hour or so after the accident. In fact, it is not unusual for an individual with 30 percent of his body surface burned to drive a car 20 miles for help. Since the burned victim remains in relatively good condition for some time after the accident, the problem of transportation from the scene of the injury to a hospital is not difficult. If this is a short distance it can usually be accomplished in an automobile. No stimulants or liquids should be given by mouth. It is important to make sure that the patient does not have other complicating injuries. If the burn is rather large, it is wise to make a telephone call to the emergency department of the hospital to notify the personnel that a burned patient is on the way.

EARLY CARE OR FIRST AID. The primary aims in first aid are to relieve pain and to prevent infection. In burns of more than 4 square inches of the body surface, the patient should be taken to a physician. In smaller burns the best immediate treatment is to put the injured part in cold, clean water. This neutralizes the heat, provides comfort, and prevents damage to deeper tissues. All burns and scalds should be cooled as quickly as possible after injury. The best way is to place the affected part, if convenient, under cold water. Application of towels soaked in ice water brings almost immediate pain relief (Fig. 4). Cooling should be continued for about 10 minutes.

The wound should be covered as soon as is reasonable. This minimizes contamination and inhibits pain by preventing air from coming in contact with the injured surface. Medicaments or home remedies should not be applied. Stimulants must not be used. Burned patients are usually frightened and need to be reassured. They have mental pictures of disastrous end results—scarring of the face and inability to move the hands. If there is minimal injury to the face, it is always nice to reassure the patient that there is very little injury there and that scarring will not occur. It is wise to remember that a burn always looks worse several hours after it has occurred than immediately after injury. It may be one or two hours before blisters develop; edema forms slowly; and with swelling the patient always appears much worse. Any person who has been burned as a result of an explosion or a blast of superheated air must be assumed to have sustained inhalation of noxious agents and gases. Such victims must be carefully observed since symptoms do not always appear immediately. In some instances inhalation of smoke may cause considerable respiratory tract difficulty.

Chemical burns, caused by acid or alkali, should be washed immediately with large quantities of water to remove the injurious agent. One should not waste time looking for a specific antidote. All clothing should be removed. If a large quantity of a chemical burning agent has come in contact with the skin, the patient should get into a

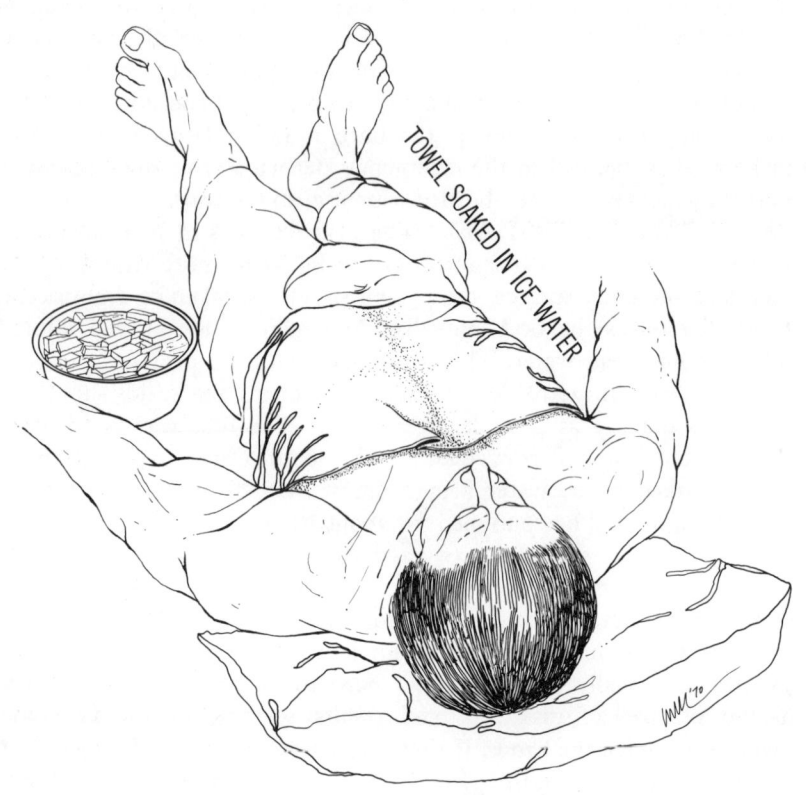

Fig. 4. The application of towels soaked in ice water helps to relieve pain and may reduce further injury.

bathtub or under a shower immediately. If the wound is minor, it should be cleansed with soap and water and bandaged with some type of greased gauze or anesthetic ointment. Patients with larger burns or burns around critical areas, such as the face and hands, should be taken to a physician's office or a hospital emergency room.

Sunburns should be treated by gentle washing with soap and tepid water and the application of a water-soluble anesthetic ointment. Large quantities of water should be given by mouth. Aspirin may be of value in relieving the general discomfort.

INITIAL MANAGEMENT OF MINOR BURNS. Minor burns—those of less than 2 percent of the body surface, unless critical areas are involved—are usually treated in a physician's office, in an industrial or military dispensary, in a first aid facility, or in an emergency room.

One of the very distressing problems in small superficial burns is pain. Sometimes pain can be controlled by the application of cold, wet towels. Such treatment is particularly effective in second-degree burns of the face. Even with minor burns there may be a great deal of apprehension. Morphine given intravenously is advantageous. Most of the pain disappears when the wound is covered by a comfortable dressing. If the patient needs something for pain after the wound is dressed, aspirin is usually sufficient.

All burn wounds should be thoroughly cleansed. This is best accomplished by warm water and a bland soap. There is no place for the use of an antiseptic in the cleansing of burned areas. The washing should be done gently so that it will not damage any remaining viable epithelium. Every attempt should be made to remove all foreign substances and dirt. In general it is best to pull off or cut away any blisters. Minor burns of the hand that involve very thick blisters, particularly on the palm, do best when the blisters are left unruptured.

After the area has been thoroughly cleansed, a dressing should be applied. Some superficial burns on small infants and burns of the face probably do better when exposed. A dressing should cover the entire wound, splint the area, be easily removable and comfortable. It should also be absorptive because superficial wounds weep serum and the aim of the dressing is to absorb this fluid so that the wound surface will be kept as dry as possible. Some type of water-soluble ointment or ointment gauze placed next to the wound will usually keep the dressing from sticking. Many preparations are commercially available. Over the initial layer of gauze, should be placed an appropriate amount of absorptive material and then the entire dressing held in place with an elastic-type bandage. The dressing should be made to look as neat as possible but, above all, it should be put on in such a way that it will not come off. By leaving the tips of the fingers or toes out of a dressing, the circulation can be easily observed. Unless there is third-degree injury or an associated injury, no tetanus prophylaxis is necessary.

Dressings are usually changed about every five days. If the dressing is thin, or if there has been a particularly large amount of serum oozing from the surface, it may be necessary to change the dressing every two or three days. Gentle removal of a dressing prevents pain and protects any thin, viable epithelium. Usually it is wise to soak off the inner layer of gauze rather than manually pull it away.

Burns of the eyes should receive special consideration. They appear to be a minor burn but in most instances they should be seen by a competent physician. If the injury occurred as the result of a chemical, the eye should be irrigated with clean, warm water. If there appears to be damage to the eye, a clean cloth or bandage should be placed over it and medical aid sought immediately.

Chemical Burns

When strong acids or strong alkalies come in contact with the skin, changes are produced similar to those resulting from heat. Although it would seem reasonable to attempt to neutralize an acid or an alkali as initial therapy, it is probably best to wash the area thoroughly with large quantities of water. Damage is frequently produced by a neutralizing agent so it is safer to use large quantities of water. When a major portion of the body has come in contact with a chemical the patient should be put under a shower after the soiled clothing has been removed. It is imperative that the clothing contaminated with the chemical be removed as quickly as possible.

Extensive burns due to chemicals occur primarily in industrial accidents or during military conflict. Certain laboratory and domestic mishaps do lead to chemical burning accidents. Burns from acids are

TABLE 2. *Initial Procedures for Chemical Burns.*

Agent	Cleansing	Neutralization
Acid Burns		
Sulfuric	Water	Sodium bicarbonate solution
Nitric		
Hydrochloric		
Trichloroacetic		
Phenol	Ethyl alcohol	Sodium bicarbonate solution
Hydrofluoric	Water	Same as other acids plus magnesium oxide, glycerin paste, local injection, calcium gluconate
Alkali Burns		
Potassium hydroxide		
Sodium hydroxide	Water	0.5-5.0% acetic acid or 5.0% ammonium chloride
Lime	Brush off powder	0.5-5.0% acetic acid or 5.0% ammonium chloride
Phosphorus	Water	Copper sulfate soaks
Mustard gas	Water	M-5 ointment
Tear gas	Water	Sodium bicarbonate solution

extremely painful and the pain often persists for long periods because of the continued chemical reaction. The appearance of a chemical burn is somewhat different from that of a thermal burn. The more superficial injuries have a redness but this turns to a yellowish-brown or black if the injury is deeper and more severe. In industrial accidents one should watch for the signs of inhalation of acid fumes which will give the patient a chemical tracheobronchitis. Unless the injury is very small, it is usually wise to wash the chemically injured areas with large quantities of water, apply some type of clean dressing or covering, and take the patient to a physician. The initial procedures for the care of chemical burns are listed in Table 2.

Electric Injuries

Electric injuries may vary from a rather mild tingling sensation with a minor injury at the point of contact to a more extensive, destructive injury and even death. Severe damage to the heart or respiratory mechanism may occur at the initial time of injury. Respiratory paralysis and ventricular fibrillation are the principal causes of immediate death. If the patient is not breathing, artificial respiration should be started immediately. Mouth-to-mouth resuscitation has saved many lives. If the heart is not beating, there is probably ventricular fibrillation and cardiac massage should be instituted until the patient can be taken to a hospital where defibrillation is possible.

It is important that the victim of an electric shock be freed from the current as quickly as possible. Care must be taken by the rescuer that the current is off before touching the victim or he will become injured. The current may be switched off, or the wires may be cut with a wooden-handled axe or properly insulated pliers. Above all the rescuer must take every precaution to prevent the electric current from attacking his body.

Electric injury to the skin and underlying tissue is always greater than first anticipated. It is usually wise to take the patient with any significant electric injury to a physician as soon as is reasonable. The local wound may be washed and a dry, clean covering placed over it. Usually electric burns are not painful because they have burned through all the layers of the skin and rendered the nerve endings insensible to pain. Frequently at the time of an electric injury, clothing may catch on fire. In such instances there is a combination of electric injuries and flame burn. The initial management of such a patient should be the same as that for a thermal burn.

Heatstroke

Heatstroke or sunstroke usually follows a long exposure to heat either in the hot sun or in particularly hot areas, such as certain factories. It occurs more often in males than in females and is more frequent in elderly individuals. Physical exertion may be a contributing factor and it is more common to occur in high humidity rather than in low humidity. The symptoms in heatstroke are: headache, dry skin, rapid pulse, dizziness, and sometimes nausea. There is usually a rapid rise in body temperature. Sweating ceases and the high fever that follows may cause permanent damage to various organs. Sometimes the patient will collapse. Usually his skin appears to be flushed, dry, and hot. His fever may rise to 106° F or above. Heatstroke is a very serious condition especially when it occurs in elderly individuals. Treatment must be started immediately. Every effort must be made to diminish the patient's general body temperature. He should be placed in a tub of cold water with ice added. Sometimes this is not possible and one should sponge the body freely with water or with alcohol in an attempt to reduce the body temperature. Ice bags to axillas and groins may be helpful. Occasionally ice water enemas will diminish the fever. The principles for the treatment of heatstroke are: diminution of body temperature as quickly as possible by any means available and the movement of the patient to a hospital as soon as is reasonable.

Heat Exhaustion

Heat exhaustion is not as serious as heatstroke. Exhaustion occurs most often in people who are not used to hot weather and more often in women than in men. The patient usually feels tired, nauseated, and somewhat faint; he may have a headache. There is usually a clammy perspiration with whiteness of the skin and a weak, thready pulse. Usually the patient has a very prostrate appearance. His body temperature is not elevated.

Have the patient lie down in some comfortable place with his head down and his feet elevated. His clothing should be removed. As soon as he improves, he should be permitted to rest and then given some fluids along with salt. The condition is usually associated with a depletion of the body's salt, therefore, a one-half teaspoon of salt in a glass of water may be very beneficial. If the patient's condition does not quickly return to normal, he should be taken to a physician. Heat exhaustion can usually be prevented by those people working in particularly hot areas if they take two or three 5-grain salt tablets a day along with ample quantities of water.

Cold Injury

Freezing may produce frostbite of various parts of the body; the nose, ears, cheeks, fingers, and toes are affected most often. Elderly

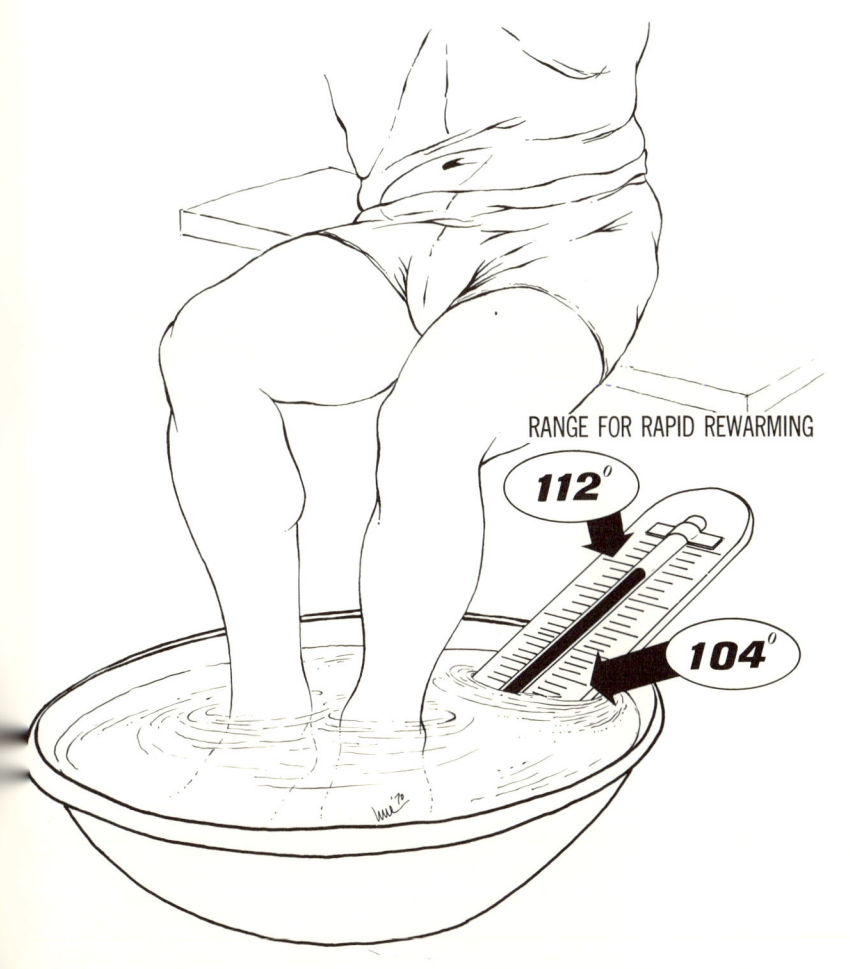

Fig. 5. For cold injury, or frostbite, rapid rewarming is advocated. The temperature of the water should be between 104° and 112° F.

individuals with poor circulation to the extremities are easily affected. Intoxicated persons often suffer extensive injury, particularly to the toes and fingers. When tissue begins to freeze, there is a tingling sensation; then it becomes numb and finally totally anesthetic. Frozen tissue usually has a dead white color.

Every effort should be made to prevent undue exposure to cold. One should beware of cold climates with high winds. Alcohol should be avoided. One should make every effort to provide adequate clothing, especially socks, shoes, and mittens. It is wise to keep up some physical activity of parts of the extremities, especially the fingers and toes, when one is in a very cold environment.

If it appears that any part of the body is frozen, the patient should be removed from the freezing temperature as soon as possible. Every effort must be made to protect the frozen area from further injury. Rubbing in an attempt to restore the circulation is not of any value and frequently increases the damage to the local area.

If there is damage to the feet, the patient should not be allowed to walk. Rapid rewarming of the tissue is advocated (Fig. 5). This should be done in warm water at a temperature between 104° and 112° F. As soon as the frozen tissues are thawed, a little more heat is applied. The area should be kept scrupulously clean to prevent any infection. After cleansing the best treatment is to allow the area to remain exposed so that it will stay dry. It may take a few days before one knows exactly the extent of the damage process. If it has been severe, blisters will form and later there may be gangrene. As soon as rapid rewarming has been accomplished, the patient with suspected frostbite should be taken to a hospital.

11 / Transportation of the Injured

JOSEPH D. FARRINGTON

The term "Transportation of the Injured" has become synonomous with emergency care both for the injured and critically ill at the scene and during transport to medical facilities. Such care is provided by an ambulance service, an essential part of the Emergency Medical Services system of any community.

Few ideal Emergency Medical Services systems exist today. Evaluation of the existing services of a community is necessary and should be carried out by a Council on Emergency Medical Services. Such a council should be active in every community or in a group of closely related communities as an advisory, but not regulatory group. Effective organization of such a council depends upon a concerned citizen, a missionary, and hopefully a physician who will give time and effort as part of his civic duty.

Many essentials are required of an effective ambulance service in its role as an important part of the Emergency Medical Services system. These include

1, proper organization; 2, suitable vehicles; 3, adequate equipment; 4, approved training of technicians; 5, effective communications; and 6, close relationship with medical facilities.

Proper Organization

The scope of an ambulance service will depend upon the day to day experience of such a service. In large cities one or more services will be required, while in rural or less populated areas a service will, of necessity, provide for the needs of a number of closely related communities. Evaluation of the ambulance service should result in any necessary improvement or, in the choosing of the proper type of service for the area if none exists. No one type of service will satisfy the needs of the entire country. The types of service in existence today are:

1. Mortician service. Until recently 50 percent of the services of this country were this type. While many provide effective service a great number, hampered by inadequate vehicles, poor equipment, and high turnover of untrained personnel, are discontinuing their operation.
2. Commercial service. For this type of service to survive without a subsidy, a monopolistic operation serving a population of not less than 60,000 is necessary.
3. Municipal service. Police department, fire department, separate service. While a municipal service may be part of an existing organization to be of maximal effectiveness, it must function separately, neither the vehicles nor the manpower serving in a dual capacity.
4. Voluntary service. Such organizations have been in operation for years and as a rule provide very adequate service. Many are resistant to outside regulation but it should be evident that state standards and regulations must be established for all ambulance services, just as exist for all fire departments, voluntary or not.
5. Hospital-based service. Regardless of the type of service the ambulance may be hospital-based though the organization of such service is not necessarily hospital-oriented. The technicians serve in a dual capacity by working in hospital areas when not involved in ambulance service. Such an organization is particularly effective in the less populated and rural areas where so frequently the day to day experience is low. The technicians by serving in two areas keep occupied, gain stature and a better pay scale since they are working with and around patients and their remuneration comes from two sources. As a result, a higher caliber, career-minded individual is attracted to ambulance service in these areas.
6. Air ambulance service. Fixed wing air ambulances have been in service for years, being used for the most part in the transfer of patients from small outlying hospitals to medical centers. The use of helicopters in recent wars as ambulances has appealed to the uninformed to the point of recommendations that they replace all surface vehicles. A number of factors such as high initial and operating cost, inability to operate in minimal inclement weather, obstructions to landing in urban areas, and difficulties as to emergency

care in the aircraft, prove this concept to be a poor recommendation and of questionable value in civilian practice.

Helicopter ambulance services may be effective in emergency care for patients on crowded expressways and highways through vast nonpopulated areas if part of a multi-purpose service, including search and rescue, highway surveillance, and fire-fighting to name a few.

7. Intensive care service. Specialized care units have not been in existance long enough for fair evaluation of their feasibility. At first glance it would seem that such a specialized service does nothing but dilute the efforts to increase the effectiveness of all emergency care. Our goal should be to equip every ambulance and train every technician sufficiently to care for any problem.

Suitable Vehicles

To be termed an ambulance, the vehicle must carry the personnel and equipment necessary to provide both emergency care and transportation of the critically ill and injured. Vehicles which merely provide transportation to and from medical facilities should be recognized by another name, i.e., invalid coach, clinic bus, or hospital van.

A nationally uniform color for the exterior surface of white in combination with a cross of reflectorized Omaha orange and the word "Ambulance" in black lettering on each side of the vehicle, has been recommended.

The vehicle need not be the expensive, high-powered, status symbol type so prevalent today. Power should be such that the vehicle may safely proceed in the flow of traffic and pass as necessary. The popular commercial van type vehicle is relatively inexpensive and of sufficient power to meet these requirements.

The outstanding fault in the majority of vehicles in use as ambulances today, is the patient compartment size. This compartment should be of sufficient size to carry two litter patients and provide room for two Emergency Medical Technicians, space for administering life-saving care, and storage of necessary equipment. There must be a minimum of 54 inches floor to ceiling height (60 inches being preferable); there must be 25 inches of space at the head end and 15 inches of space at the foot end of an average length litter (76 inches), and there must be 25 inches of available space along side the litter at the patient chest level so that a technician may kneel at right angles for the performance of cardiopulmonary resuscitation.

There must be sufficient storage compartments for the equipment listed below and provision for the more sophisticated items of the future.

There should be windows in the rear doors of the patient compartment, but side windows are considered not only unnecessary in that they take up space needed for storage of equipment, but are dangerous sources of added injury in case of an accident.

There must be adequate environmental control and lighting in the patient compartment.

The tires of the vehicle should be puncture proof as immobilization of ambulances is frequent due to deflated tires caused by the debris of natural disasters.

In addition to an adequate standard electric power supply, there should be a 110 volt, 60 cycle, at least 3,000 watt power supply for installed and portable equipment, such as flood lights and electric access equipment. Such a power supply is easily obtained by replacing the standard alternator-generator with a specialized unit, many types of which are available and require no additional space in the engine compartment.

Types of Equipment

BASIC. All ambulances should carry one wheeled stretcher, a folding litter, and an adjustable device for moving patients in narrow and confined areas where a rigid stretcher cannot be used. The folding litter and adjustable device may be combined as one item.

The head of the wheeled stretcher must be capable of being tilted upward to a 60° semisitting position and the entire litter should be capable of being tilted to head down position of at least 10°. The frames or handles should be designed for fasteners to secure it firmly to the floor or side of the vehicle. Restraining devices must be provided to prevent dislodgement of the patient during transport.

There must be a fixed suction unit, powered preferably by the automobile engine manifold, powerful enough to provide an airflow of over 30 liters per minute at the end of the delivery tube and a vacuum of over 300 mm of mercury, to be reached within four seconds when a tube is clamped.

Necessary accessories should be stored in space near the head end of the litters.

There must be fixed oxygen supply with the necessary equipment for administration.

Other basic equipment consists of: pillows, pillowcases, sheets, blankets, towels, emesis bags, tissue, bedpan, urinal, and paper cups. It is best that the blankets be fire-resistant and that a body bag be stored.

SAFETY EQUIPMENT. A limited amount of safety equipment must be carried by every ambulance so that the technicians may secure the area and protect the patients and themselves from additional injury until authorities or specialized help to provide such service arrives. Flares with life of 30 minutes, flood lights and flashlights, fire extinguisher BC dry powder type, and insulated gauntlets are essential.

ACCESS EQUIPMENT. Unless a rescue vehicle accompanies an ambulance on every emergency call, certain access and extrication equipment should be carried since the time element in life-threatening problems is so critical that if the technicians must await the arrival of such equipment, lives that might be saved will be lost.

Lifting, prying, battering, cutting, and pulling tools should be carried in a compartment accessible from outside the ambulance. Specifically these items are:

One wrench 12″ adjustable open end
One screw driver 12″ regular blade
One screw driver 12″ Phillips type
One hacksaw with 12 wire (carbide) blades
One pliers 10″ vice-grip
One hammer 5# 15″ handle, one fire axe butt 24″ handle, one wrecking bar 24″; separate or as one combination tool.
One crowbar 51″ pinch point
One bolt cutter 39″ jaw opening 1¼″
One portable power jack and spreader tool
One shovel 49″ pointed blade
One double action tin snip minimum 8″
Two ropes, manila, 50′ × ¾″ diameter

An optional power winch, front mounted, minimum two ton capacity is recommended particularly in areas where such a unit is not readily available. In addition to the rated wire cable, there should be a 15-foot chain with one grab hook and one running hook.

EMERGENCY CARE EQUIPMENT. There are various categories of emergency care equipment essential in all ambulances.

Resuscitation. Portable suction units of sufficient power for adequate pharyngeal suction, with wide bore tubing and pharyngeal suction tips.

Portable oxygen units with transparent, semiopen, valveless masks in infant, child, and adult sizes.

Bag-valve-mask, hand operated, artificial ventilation unit with infant, child, and adult masks and attachments for connection to an oxygen supply.

Airways, both oropharyngeal and two-way.

Mouth gags, either commercial or made of tongue blades, taped together and padded.

15 mm male tracheostomy adaptors.

Short spine board used to provide firm surface for cardiac compression.

Intravenous fluids with necessary administration units. (Type and use of fluids to be determined by local physicians, preferably by radio control).

Blood pressure manometer, cuff, and stethoscope.

Immobilization of Fractures. Half-ring lower extremity traction splint with commercial support slings, ankle hitch, and traction strap.

Long and short padded board, card-board, wire ladder splints.

Uncomplicated inflatable splints, arm and leg size.

Triangular bandages.

Long and short spine boards with accessories.

Wound Dressings.

Gauze pads 4" × 4".

Universal dressings 10" × 36", packaged folded to compact size.

Roll of aluminum foil (nonadherent occlusive dressing).

Soft roller, self-adhering bandages 6" × 5 yards.

Adhesive tape in 3" rolls.

Safety pins.

Bandage shears.

Burn sheets, packaged folded and sterile.

Emergency Childbirth. Sterile gloves, scissors, umbilical clamps or tape, sterile dressings, and towels.

Aluminum foil provides excellent incubator for newborn infants, especially premature infants when wrapped about the entire body leaving the face free.

POISONING TREATMENT SUPPLIES. Syrup of Ipecac and activated charcoal in prepackaged doses.

Snake bite kits, where applicable.

Drinking water.

SPECIAL EQUIPMENT. In anticipation of more advanced training of a greater number of technicians in the use of specialized equipment and the occasional presence of physicians at the scene of the emergencies, the following items may be carried in a sealed container to prevent use by the unauthorized: tracheal intubation kit, pleural decompression set, drug injection kit, venous cut-down kit, tracheostomy or cricothyrotome set, minor surgical kit, urinary catheters, and portable cardioscope and defibrillator.

Improved Training of Technicians

Improvement in emergency care with the resultant saving of lives is dependent upon better training of the Emergency Medical Technician. For too long the medical profession has not involved itself directly in such training. The American Red Cross and other similar "first-aid" organizations have done an excellent job in the past but such training is not sufficient if lives are to be saved. The status of care at the emergency scene and during transport is the direct responsibility of the physicians of this country and until actual teaching of the technicians on a community basis by physicians becomes an integral part of the Emergency Medical Services system, the marked improvement possible will not materialize. Only a few hours each week is involved and this is a small price to pay for the saving of an estimated 10,000 lives each year.

To outline and develop any training program, the capabilities of the technician from a medical standpoint must be defined. Regardless of the duration of a planned program, the curriculum should remain the same, but expanded as the scope of the course increases. The capabilities which Emergency Medical Technicians may be expected to achieve can be divided into three main categories:

1. Capabilities in the care of life-threatening conditions
    a. Establish and maintain a patent airway
    b. Provide correct oxygen inhalation

c. Provide intermittent positive pressure ventilation
   d. Perform cardiopulmonary resuscitation
   e. Control accessible bleeding
   f. Treat shock with intravenous fluids
   g. Provide care for patients with poisoning
2. Capabilities in the care of nonlife-threatening conditions
   a. Dress and bandage wounds
   b. Immobilize fractures properly
   c. Care of emergency obstetrical problems, the newborn and premature infants
   d. Management of the unruly patient
3. Capabilities in areas of a nonmedical nature:
   a. Rescue and extrication
   b. Care of equipment
   c. Use and maintenance of supplies
   d. Knowledge in appropriate medicolegal problems
   e. Emergency and defensive driving
   f. Communications, verbal and written

Evaluation of the training requirements and regulations for other types of personnel providing services to the public are very enlightening. When one realizes that in some states a bartender is required to have 40 hours of training, and a barber required to have 1,248 hours of training, completed in not less than 9 months, it certainly is not too much to ask that the training of emergency-care personnel goes beyond the 26 hours required in the Advanced American Red Cross first aid course or its equivalent. A new profession must be created, and the Emergency Medical Technician eventually must be trained to the level of the diploma registered nurse. To do this, training will progress through the basic and advanced stage to a two-year program. After some years of study, a satisfactory basic training program has been developed and field tested in many areas. The program is on-going in nature, lasts many weeks, and is easily presented at the community level. The curriculum consists of 70 hours of lectures, demonstration, and practice sessions, presented in periods three hours long over 12 to 24 weeks. In addition, there are 10 hours of in-hospital training. The American Red Cross Advanced First Aid Certificate, or its equivalent, is a prerequisite to this training. An additional 100 hours of actual patient care, 20 hours of which would be in-hospital, should be required before the technician may stand for examination and subsequent certification. Such training is only the beginning. If the estimated 10,000 savable patients dying each year as the result of accidents are to be saved, there must be advanced training to instruct the more capable technicians in the techniques of intubation, infusions, advanced cardiopulmonary resuscitation, consisting of the administration of drugs for cardiac irregularities and defibrillation under physicians' orders by radio.

Communications

Direct voice communication between the authorities, ambulances, and hospital emergency departments is essential for improved ambulance service. Voice communication with a man on the moon has been possible, yet too few technicians in this country are able to speak directly to the emergency departments of hospitals from the emergency scene or during transport to such hospitals. Availability of such communication allows physician direction of more complicated life-saving care, proper distribution of patients, treatment of complications during transport, and more effective activity in natural disasters.

In addition to such communication, which should be state-wide, technicians separated by circumstances at the emergency scene should be equipped with short range walkie-talkies to allow more efficient action.

Close Relationship with Medical Facilities

Close relationship between the Emergency Medical Technician and the medical staff of the emergency departments of hospitals is essential and involves three areas: reports, exchange system, and critiques.

On delivery of the patient to the emergency department, the technician should report verbally as to important events and actions at the emergency scene and during transport. Such reports should cover life-threatening problems and complications. On completion of required activity in the emergency department, the technician should have available an area where he may, in writing or by dictation, complete in detail the report for the patient's record, for his organization, for his protection, and for interested authorities.

An exchange system is of particular importance and easily established at hospital emergency departments. The technicians should be supplied with duplicates of any equipment used and in place on the patient. This precludes premature and dangerous removal of equipment from patients and prevents loss of time on the part of the technicians, as they do not have to wait for or return at some later date for such equipment.

Improved rapport between emergency medical technicians, emergency department personnel, and physicians will result from regular critiques, the frequency of which will depend upon the day to day experience of an area. Evaluation of action at the scene and during transport, commending proper care, pointing out errors of commission and omission, and the discussion of the results of definitive care will lead to better understanding and improvement in the emergency care of the critically ill and injured.

12 / Special Weapons Effects

GERRIT L. HEKHUIS

This discussion of special weapons effects includes three categories: nuclear weapons, chemical, and biologic agents.

Nuclear Weapons Effects

The effects of nuclear weapons which produce casualties are those of blast, thermal, and ionizing radiations. The first two, blast and thermal, are concerned with phenomena similar to those observed in high explosive and incendiary-type weapons. The third category deals specifically with the effects of ionizing radiation. While this arbitrary categoric separation facilitates the discussion of the problems, it must be remembered that the effects are practically simultaneous, and any casualty could be the victim of multiple injury causes.

Since the early nuclear (fission) weapons, there have been developed thermonuclear (fission + fusion) weapons, and the TNT equivalents have increased from that of the "nominal atomic bomb" (20 kilotons) to multimegatons (millions of tons of TNT). The expected medical problems from these later, larger weapons must be scaled upward appropriately in size, type, and duration from the effects described below as produced by "nominal" nuclear detonations.

BLAST EFFECTS. Blast effects following the World War II experience were often characterized by relatively severe internal damage with minimal external damage visible. At autopsy, frequent findings included multiple internal hemorrhages involving many organ systems, with fairly consistent involvement of the lungs, brain, and adrenal glands.

After a nuclear explosion very high pressures and resulting winds of very high velocity are recorded near the epicenter of the explosion.

The rapidly expanding pressure wave acts like a moving wall, exerting extreme stresses on structures and personnel in its path. The positive pressure impact wave is followed by a relatively long (compared to TNT explosions) phase of positive pressure engulfment before the development of a negative pressure, or "suction" phase.

(Blast effects are divided into the primary or direct blast effect and the secondary or indirect effect due to flying debris, flying glass, and structural collapse.)

Peak overpressures of one and one half to three pounds per square inch (psi) will fairly completely destroy residential structures, whereas primary pressures of over 100 psi are required to produce significant internal damage to the human body.

The amount and distribution of the secondary, or flying missile effects are dependent on the distance from the explosion; and the clinical results are the expected multiple contusions, lacerations, and fractures. The contusions and fractures present no unique problems of importance except in their combination with other simultaneous injuries. There is a high incidence of lacerations due to flying glass, and these are often extremely small and numerous.

Treatment of these casualties presents no new problems, and first aid treatment may not be significantly important in affecting mortality rate. Alertness should be maintained for secondary effects such as shock. Intensive definitive treatment is advisable for the alleviation of pain, preparation of the patient for surgery, and promotion of rapid healing to minimize possible complications of radiation sickness. However, the vast number of casualties is a problem seen only in disaster medicine, and adequate surveillance may well be a task far outshadowing the adequacy of even minimal care.

THERMAL EFFECTS. Thermal radiation effects are divided according to the method of production into primary (flash) burns and secondary (flame) burns. It is emphasized that these burns in no way differ from burns caused by conventional weapons.

Primary thermal radiation effects are due to absorption of energy with large components of infrared and visible wave lengths (with a very small component of ultraviolet) applied during a brief exposure, and result in flash-type or profile burns since they occur only on the surface facing the detonation. The thermal effects are related to the distance from the center of the explosion and atmospheric conditions. In Japan, the most severe burns were noted within a one-half-mile radius, with diminishing to negligible effects at a two and one-half-mile radius. Burns were modified by shielding, shading of structures, and angle of incidence. At distances greater than three-quarters of a mile, in many cases clothing served as adequate protection. A greater degree of protection was afforded by loose fitting, light colored materials. Dark colored clothing absorbed heat, thereby transmitting it to the body or bursting into flame. Burns varied from mild erythema without vesication occuring usually beyond two and one half miles, to severe second- and third-degree burns closer to the center. The second-degree burns usually showed an intense erythema within a few days, then showed increased pigmentation and darkening which persisted for varying periods of time. Second-degree burns frequently involved large areas of body surface and were similar to "moderate-temperature" burns except that the associated mortality was not as high as might have been expected. Vesication often appeared within a few minutes after exposure. Beyond two and one-half miles from ground zero, burns were insignificant and beyond one and three-quarters miles, very few burns required treatment. Improper healing of these burns was influenced by lack of treatment. Common sequelae were contractures and keloid formation. One half of the Japanese deaths attributed to burns occurred within the first week and three quarters occurred within two weeks. It can be stated that it requires 3 cal per cm^2 delivered in a three-second period of time to produce a partial thickness (second-degree) burn of human skin. It is to be noted that 9 cal per cm^2 is required to ignite cotton and 14 cal per cm^2 is required to ignite wool.

Secondary (flame) burns occurred in Japan, associated with secondary fires which developed in the city buildings, as well as flame burn due to actual burning of clothing. These secondary burns were responsible for many fatalities, especially in persons who were so injured by secondary blast effects that they could not escape.

The treatment of burns may represent the biggest problem. Under field conditions unshielded personnel will sustain large numbers of burns involving exposed body surfaces, i.e., face and hands. Under these conditions, the initial treatment should consist of an occlusive dressing and sedation as required. The important consideration is evacuation to medical facilities where surgical technique and extensive supportive treatment are available. If the burned area involves over 20 percent of the body surface or if there are medical indications, fluid replacement should be started before evacuation.

It must be emphasized that mechanical and thermal injuries con-

stitute the great majority of casualties, and thus the care of these casualties will require the majority of emergency care in the event of an atomic bomb detonation.

First-degree burns may involve mainly the normally exposed skin surfaces—the face, neck, and hands. They usually are quite painful. Prompt dressing of the burn will do much to alleviate the pain, followed by administration of analgesics or sedatives.

Second- and third-degree burns, usually the result of secondary flame injury, are more severe in injury produced area involved, and are often infected. Care to aseptic technique in dressing, prevention and treatment of shock, restoration of fluid and electrolyte balance, sedation, and use of fluids, blood, plasma as indicated, are part of the treatment problem, as well as the provision, if possible, of skilled nursing care. In a nuclear-weapon-produced disaster, these specialized care facilities will likely not be immediately available, and the application of an adequate sterile dressing using aseptic technique and following the closed dressing principle is probably the best initial care that can be advised.

RADIATION EFFECTS. The effects of ionizing nuclear radiation can be divided into "immediate" and "residual." The immediate radiation is that produced by the bomb detonation, and coincides in time with the release of the blast and thermal energies, thus the production of simultaneous injuries. The residual or delayed radiation results from the particulate matter which falls out from the atomic cloud, or from radioactive elements produced when the explosion is near enough to the earth surface to induce such radioactivity.

Aside from evacuation, shielding or adequate shelter are the only practical methods of protection from ionizing radiation.

The effects on the body of nuclear explosion ionizing radiation are similar to those produced by deep x-rays, except that in the case of the explosion, whole body exposure is produced as contrasted to very small volume, single organ exposure—the aim in deep x-ray therapy. Ionizing radiation affects different tissues and organs of the body with different degrees and results, and the composite picture of a total body exposure becomes a most complex one.

The effects of radiation on the body depend on the amount of radiation absorbed, the rate of this absorption, the duration (length) of the exposure, the volume and location of the exposed tissues, and the previous condition of the individual. Deep organ effects are produced mainly by gamma rays and neutrons from the immediate phase of the radiation; and both surface and deep exposures can result from the beta-particles and gamma rays from the residual exposures.

The changes produced are fundamentally biochemical as the radiations alter the proteins, nucleic acids, enzyme systems, cell development and maturation, and other important biologic and biochemical processes.

The clinical and laboratory findings resulting from exposure to radiation are functions of the amount of radiation, the rate of exposure, and the dosage absorbed in various parts of the body. Both acute and chronic effects may result from either internal or external sources of radiation. While the overall effects of radiation can be described fairly accurately, it must be recalled that these changes in the body are a physiologic response to damage from absorbed energy and are not pathognomonic of radiation exposure. The type and penetration of the radiation will determine the location of effect.

The symptomatology in man after exposure to radiation can be summarized as follows. A few hours following exposure to ionizing radiation, anorexia, nausea, and vomiting appear, which last from 1 to 48 hours and then subside for a variable latent period of days. The shorter the latent period the more severe are the symptoms of recurrent anorexia, nausea, vomiting, and diarrhea. Later, mucous or bloody discharges from the body orifices and secondary hemorrhages occur resulting in death. In general, the rapidity of onset of symptoms and the rapidity of progression of the illness are in direct proportion to the amount of radiation received. The duration of the latent period is inversely proportional to the degree of radiation exposure. With large doses the latent period may become very short or even disappear and death can occur within 24 hours. It is important to remember that with short latent periods, death may occur before the full radiation syndrome develops. The latent period is also modified by species and individual characteristics.

The hematologic responses to intense penetrating radiations are quite uniform, but exposure to less penetrating (low energy) radiations may result in blood changes which may be of short duration, slight or undetectable, even in the presence of severe superficial body damage. Beginning shortly after exposure to radiation, there is a prompt decrease in the total white-cell count, with its maximum effect within 24 to 72 hours, depending partially on the amount of radiation received. Not so regularly seen are reduction in the platelet count, morphologic changes in the white cells and reduction in red-cell count. A strict schedule of changes following acute or chronic radiation cannot be compiled because of the marked "normal" variations in blood constituents in addition to the multiple variable factors associated with the radiation itself.

The description of the clinical symptomatology or radiation syndrome is facilitated by dividing into three categories patients observed who have suffered from radiation overexposure. These divisions are inexact in their differentiation, but may present a guide to the clinical picture.

Patients who died within the first two weeks showed histologic evidence of radiation effects on the skin, gastrointestinal tract, lymphoid tissue, bone marrow, or gonads, but these changes were not observed grossly or clinically. Nausea and vomiting were noted on the first day of exposure, followed by anorexia, malaise, severe diarrhea, thirst, and the development of fever. There was no epilation or purpura. Fever continued to rise and death occurred with the patient in delirium. The earlier the fever, the more severe the symptoms and the poorer the prognosis.

Patients who died during the third to sixth weeks, or who survived the severe symptoms, showed the maximum changes in the anatomic and clinical results of radiation. Most prominent were epilation and the depressive effect on the bone marrow. The hemorrhagic and necrotizing lesions were comparable to those seen in aplastic anemia and agranulocytosis, and occurred in the gums, respiratory and gastrointestinal tracts. The nausea and vomiting occurred on the day of exposure followed by marked malaise. The patient then experienced a period of improvement which continued until about the second week, when epilation marked the beginning of the relapse phase. Malaise again appeared followed by fever which increased in step-like fashion, onset of pharyngeal pain and often a bloody diarrhea. There was a profound anemia with low levels of leukocytes and platelets and a general debilitated condition which lasted, in some cases, for a long period of time.

In a few individuals in whom the bone marrow failed to recover, the debilitated condition and profound anemia, leukopenia, and malaise continued and progressed; and the patients died after a chronic illness of extreme emaciation. In other words, associated with the apparent recovery of the bone marrow, the marked anemic picture disappeared but the patients later succumbed to intercurrent infections or complications such as tuberculosis, lung abscess, or pneu-

TABLE 1. *Clinical Radiation Illness.*

Days after exposure	Lethal exposure (Over 600 r)	Mid-lethal exposure (450 r) 50% deaths	Nonlethal exposure
0	Nausea and vomiting with 1-3 hours	Nausea and vomiting after 2-4 hours	Variable depending on individual
1	Generalized malaise	No definite symptoms	do.
2	Malaise and anorexia	do.	do.
3	Anorexia and nausea	do.	do.
4	Nausea and vomiting	do.	do.
5	Vomiting and diarrhea	do.	do.
6	Inflammation of mouth and throat	do.	do.
7	Fever	do.	do.
8	Rapid emaciation	do.	do.
9	Death	Beginning epilation	do.
10	Mortality probably 100%		do.
11			do.
12			do.
13			do.
14			do.
15			do.
16			do.
17		Anorexia and malaise	do.
18			Beginning epilation
19		Fever	Anorexia and malaise
20		Mucosal inflammation	
21			Sore mouth
22			Pallor
23		Pallor	Petechiae
24			Diarrhea
25		Petechiae	Moderate emaciation
26		Mucosal hemorrhage	
27		Diarrhea	(Recovery unless complicated by previous poor health or superimposed injuries or infections)
28			
29			
30		Rapid emaciation Death, mortality probably 50%	

Note. *These signs and symptoms suppose no medical intervention and ignore individual biologic variations.*

monia. Table 1 is a summary of the clinical signs and symptoms which can be expected as a result of whole body gamma radiation delivered within one hour.

Chemical Agents

This category includes solids, liquids, and gases, which through their chemical properties, produce damaging or lethal effects on man. These effects include irritating, blinding, blistering, or toxic characteristics.

Chemical agents are classified in various ways, but their physiologic effect is pertinent to this discussion. In order of decreasing severity, the physiologic effects would be:

NERVE AGENTS. These agents, when absorbed into the body by inhalation, ingestion, or through the skin, affect bodily functions by an irreversible reaction involving tissue fluids, producing interference with passage of nerve impulses, thus disturbing essential body functions such as breathing, vision, and muscular control.

BLISTER AGENTS. These are readily absorbed by both exterior and interior surfaces of the body and cause inflamation, blisters, and general destruction of tissues. The vapors, besides affecting the skin, attack the respiratory tract, most severely in the upper tract. Eyes are also very susceptible to blister agents.

CHOKING AGENTS. These cause irritation and inflammation of the bronchial passages and the lungs. Their primary effect is limited to the respiratory tract with injury extending to the deepest parts of the lungs.

BLOOD AGENTS. When these are absorbed into the body, primarily by breathing, they affect bodily functions through action on the oxygen-carrying properties of the blood and interfere with the normal transfer of oxygen from the lungs via the blood to body tissues.

VOMITING AGENTS. These agents primarily cause vomiting but may also cause coughing, sneezing, pain in the nose and throat, nasal discharge, tears, and usually a severe headache.

TEAR AGENTS. Contact with these agents results in a copious flow of tears and intense, although temporary, eye pain. In high concentrations, these agents are also irritating to the skin and cause a temporary burning and itching sensation. High contact concentrations can also produce chemical type burns.

Important factors in determining the degree of exposure and

absorption of these agents include their physical properties, especially volatility, their persistence and resistance to dispersion or deterioration, the weather conditions at time of dispersal, the method of dissemination, and the conditions of the terrain or the target area.

Protection against chemical agents is based on prevention of exposure, and usually involves use of gas masks, and completely-covering, protective clothing. Special comments for each group are:

NERVE AGENTS. Protective mask and protective clothing. Ordinary clothing gives off nerve agent vapors for about 30 minutes, and their evaporation rate is similar to that of water. This should be considered before unmasking.

BLISTER AGENTS. Protective mask and permeable protective clothing for vapors, impermeable clothing for liquids.

CHOKING AGENTS. Protective mask.

BLOOD AGENTS. Protective mask.

VOMITING AGENTS. Protective mask.

TEAR AGENTS. Protective mask.

Physiologic symptoms of the characteristic agents are:

NERVE AGENTS. Individuals exposed to nerve agents will generally show the same sequence of symptoms regardless of the route by which the agent enters the body. These symptoms in normal order of appearance are running nose, tightness of chest, dimness of vision and pinpointing of eye pupils, difficulty in breathing, drooling and excessive sweating, nausea, vomiting, cramps, and involuntary defecation and urination, twitching, jerking and staggering, headache, confusion, drowsiness, coma and convulsion. These symptoms are followed by cessation of breathing and death.

Symptoms appear much more slowly from skin dosage than from respiratory dosage. Although skin dosage absorption great enough to cause death may occur in one to two minutes, death may be delayed for one to three hours. Respiratory lethal dosages kill in 1-10 minutes, and liquid in the eye kills nearly as rapidly. The number and severity of symptoms which appear are dependent upon the quantity and the rate of entry of the nerve agent into the body.

BLISTER AGENTS. Most blister agents are insidious in action; there is usually little or no pain at the time of exposure, and the development of casualties is usually somewhat delayed.

DISTILLED MUSTARDS. First symptoms in four to six hours; the higher the concentration the shorter the interval. The local reaction results in inflammation or conjunctivitis of the eyes, redness of the skin which may be followed by blistering or ulceration; and inflammation of the nose, throat, trachea, and so on.

NITROGEN MUSTARDS. Irritates the eyes in dosages which do not significantly damage the skin or respiratory tract. After mild exposure, there may be no skin lesions. With higher doses, there may be redness, irritation, and itching, with blister formation following. Effects on the respiratory tract include irritation of nose and throat, hoarseness, persistent cough. Pneumonia may develop. After systemic absorption, there may be injury to the blood-forming mechanisms, and there may be diarrhea, often hemorrhagic.

PHOSGENE. A powerful irritant which produces *immediate* pain, varying from a mild sensation to a feeling resembling a severe bee sting. It causes violent irritation to the surfaces of the nose and eyes. On the skin it produces a blanched, then reddened area in about a week.

LEWISITE. Effects similar to distilled mustard, but is additionally a systemic poison, causing lung edema, diarrhea, restlessness, weakness, subnormal temperature, and low blood pressure. In order of severity and appearance of symptoms it is a blister agent, a toxic lung irritant, and when absorbed, a systemic poison.

CHOKING AGENTS. They exert their effect solely on the lungs, and result in damage to the capillaries. The air sacs become so flooded that air is excluded and the victim dies of oxygen deficiency. Severity of poisoning cannot be determined from the initial symptoms since the full effect is not usually apparent until three to four hours after exposure. Most deaths occur within 24 hours.

BLOOD AGENTS. The cyanide-type agents interfere with the utilization of oxygen by the body tissues by inhibition of enzyme systems and produce a marked stimulation of the breathing rate. Arsine interferes with the functioning of the blood and damages the liver and kidneys. Increasing exposure causes headache and uneasiness to chills, nausea and vomiting, and blood damage and anemia.

VOMITING AGENTS. Symptoms, in progressive order, are irritation of the eyes and mucous membranes, viscous discharge from the nose, sneezing, coughing, severe headache, acute pain and tightness in the chest, nausea and vomiting.

TEAR AGENTS. Cause irritation and profuse tear formation. Headache, coughing, dizziness, and sometimes nausea and vomiting may occur.

The treatment of injuries caused by chemical agents is as follows:
NERVE AGENTS. Atropine, intravenously or intramuscularly, in 2 mg dosage, given immediately and repeated at 10 minute intervals in moderate to severe exposure, and at 20 minute intervals in mild exposure, if symptoms are not relieved or symptoms of atropine action (dry mouth and skin) do not appear. Not more than 3 doses (6 mg) should be given without advice of a physician.
BLISTER AGENTS. Separation from other casualties; contaminated clothing carefully cut away; and the skin washed abundantly with water. Protective ointments specific for these agents, when available, should be applied (BAL ointments).
CHOKING AGENTS. Removal of casualty from contaminated areas, close observation, rest, supportive treatment as indicated. Oxygen, sedation, and fluid balance maintenance should be considered.
BLOOD AGENTS. Amyl nitrate for inhalation is the first step in emergency treatment, repeated as necessary. Artificial respiration may become indicated.
VOMITING AGENTS. Remove casualties from contaminated area and provide adequate fresh air.
TEAR AGENTS. Removal of patient from hazardous area, provide plenty of fresh air.

Biologic Agents

Biologic agents are living organisms which cause disease in man, animals, or plants; or they cause deterioration of material. A number of these biologic agents have been mentioned as possible enemy threats. The agents mentioned fall into the categories of bacteria, rickettsia, fungi, viruses, toxins, and other biologic products.

Biologic and chemical agents are similar in that they are directed mainly against living things, they can be disseminated in the air and are capable of contaminating terrain, clothing, equipment, food, and water. Man, animals, and plants vary in their susceptibility.

Biologic agents differ from chemical agents in that they require the ability to multiply after entry into the target host; they have a delayed action of hours or days; and their response in the target material is similar in appearance to many naturally-occurring diseases.

Detection and recognition become most important factors in the prevention and control of the use of these agents. On-site identification of biologic agents is difficult, if not impossible at the present time; and even when facilities are available, the process is detailed and time consuming.

Principles of preventive medicine and public health will be most effective as means of protection in a general approach, and early diagnosis of the situation will be necessary to provide protection and treatment in connection with the specific condition encountered.

13 / Fractures, Dislocations, and Sprains

OSCAR P. HAMPTON, JR.

Fractures

DEFINITIONS. A fracture is a broken bone. Each bone of the skeleton may be the site of a fracture. A fracture is either complete or incomplete. In a complete fracture the bone is broken into two pieces, although they may not be separated or displaced. In an incomplete fracture, the line of fracture does not extend completely across the bone.

Every fracture is either *closed* (formerly called simple) or *open* (formerly called compound). In an open fracture, a wound extends through the skin and deeper structures into the fracture site. In a closed fracture, such a wound is absent. A closed fracture may have an associated overlying wound through the skin, but if this wound does not extend into the fracture site, an open fracture is not present.

Fractures are further classified according to the direction of the line of fracture into *transverse, oblique,* or *spiral* (Fig. 1A,B,D). Other definitions concerning fractures are as follows:

A *comminuted fracture* (Fig. 1C) is present when there are two or more communicating lines of fracture which means, of course, that the bone is broken into more than two fragments. Comminuted fractures are quite common.

A *double* or *triple (segmental) fracture* is present when there are two or three separate lines of fracture, none of which communicates with another.

An *impacted fracture* (Fig. 1E) is present when the fragments are driven into each other so that the bone retains a certain degree of stability. The upper end of the humerus (near the shoulder) is a frequent site of an impacted fracture.

162 / Ch. 13: Fractures, Dislocations, and Sprains

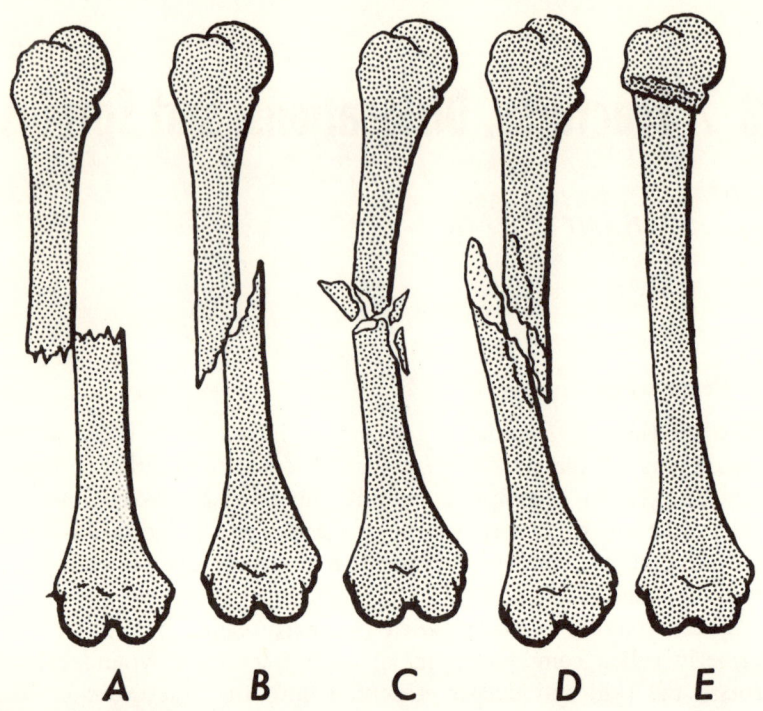

A B C D E

Fig. 1. Classification of fractures according to the direction of the line(s) of fracture. Right humerus in the anterior posterior projection. A, transverse fracture of the middle of the shaft with medial displacement of the distal fragment (the fragments are in poor apposition but are in good alignment). B, an oblique fracture with some overriding or shortening (the fragments are in partial apposition and good alignment). C, comminuted fracture with lateral angulation (the apposition is satisfactory). D, spiral fracture with lateral angulation (both apposition and alignment are poor). E, impacted fracture of the proximal portion of the bone (both apposition and alignment are excellent). (From Rhoads et al. ed. **Surgery, Principles and Practice,** 3rd edition, 1965. Courtesy of J. B. Lippincott Company.)

A *compression fracture* is present when a bone is crushed so that its normal contour is lost. Vertebrae are the most common sites of compression fractures.

A *greenstick fracture* (Fig. 2A) is an incomplete fracture occurring in a long bone in children. The bone is broken through on one side but remains intact on the other. It gets its name because of the way a green twig of a tree may break.

An *avulsion fracture* is present when a small piece of bone is pulled away by a strong ligament. An avulsion fracture is often described as a sprain fracture.

Fractures / 163

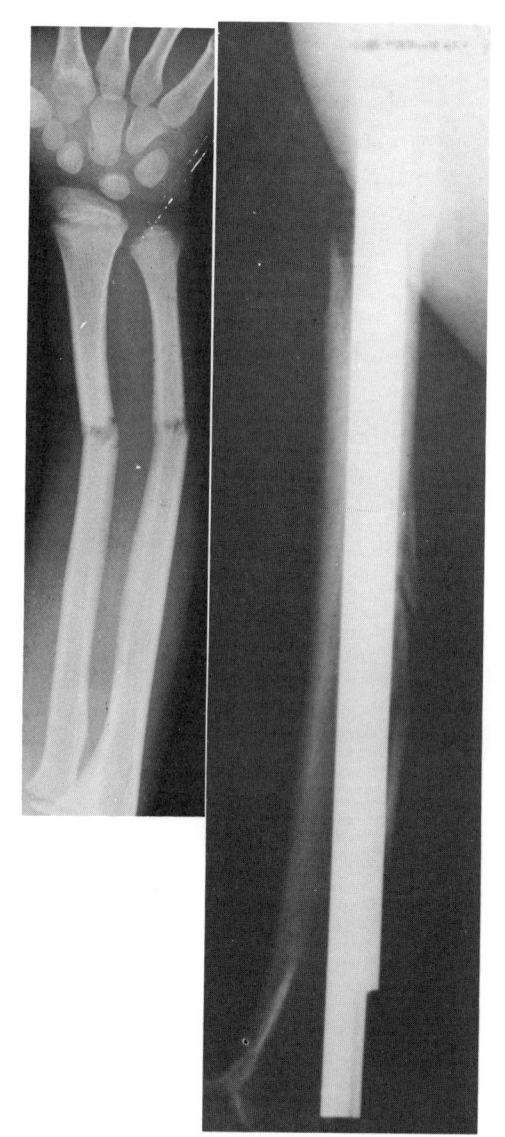

Fig. 2. Other types of fractures. Left, greenstick fracture of both bones of the forearm. (From Hampton and Fitts. **In** Rhoads et al. ed. **Surgery, Principles and Practice,** 3rd edition, 1965. Courtesy of J. B. Lippincott Company.) Right, pathologic fracture of femur at the site of a metastasis from a carcinoma (cancer) elsewhere in the body. (From Hampton and Fitts. **Open Reduction of Common Fractures,** 1959. Courtesy of Grune & Stratton, Inc.)

A *depressed fracture* is present when a portion of a bone is "pushed in." The skull and bones of the face are sites of depressed fractures.

A *pathologic fracture* (Fig. 2B) is present when an area of diseased bone, such as a bone cyst or bone tumor, becomes the site of the fracture. Pathologic fractures may occur in any bone usually with minimal force.

MECHANISMS FOR PRODUCTION OF FRACTURES. A force sufficient to produce a fracture may be applied to a bone in several ways.

DIRECT FORCE. A strong blow is received by an area overlying a bone causing the bone beneath to break. Examples are a blow of an automobile bumper on a leg causing its bones to be broken, or a baseball striking the forearm usually just above the wrist causing the small bone (ulna) to break.

INDIRECT FORCE. A force is received at some distance away from the point where a bone breaks. An individual may step in a hole fixing the foot and ankle while the body continues to move producing a twisting force on the leg so that the bones of the leg break well above the ankle. A child may fall on the outstretched hand, the force of the blow causing the bones of the forearms to break in the middle or upper portion.

DIRECT VIOLENCE TO THE BONE. A force is applied directly to a bone. The blow of an axe cutting through soft tissue may also cut through the underlying bone. A fracture produced by a bullet striking the bone is another example.

THE FORCE OF A POWERFUL MUSCLE CONTRACTION. A piece of bone may be avulsed (avulsion fracture) by the strong pull of a powerful muscle. An example is an avulsion fracture of a prominence of the pelvis caused by strong contracture of thigh muscles which are attached to various prominences of the pelvis.

DIAGNOSIS OF A FRACTURE. Diagnosis, or even a suspicion of a fracture, is based upon certain *symptoms* of which the patient complains and on certain *signs* which are determined by examination of the patient. Of course, the presence of a fracture is definitely ruled in or out on the basis of x-ray examination, although certain signs are often enough to permit the first aid worker or physician in the hospital emergency department to be positive of the diagnosis.

SYMPTOMS. A predominant symptom is pain in the region of the suspected fracture. A second important symptom, especially in an injury to an extremity, is the loss of its use by the patient. If, however, the fracture is incomplete or impacted, use of the extremity may be only partially impaired. Immediately after the injury is sustained, the patient may complain of numbness about the site of the injury.

SIGNS. The following findings on examination of the patient, based upon observation and gentle feeling (palpation) of the area of the injury, are listed somewhat in the order of their importance. (1) Deformity, such as angulation of an extremity at a point away from a joint. (2) False motion—obvious movement at a point away from a joint. (3) Crepitation—audible or palpable grating of bony fragments as the extremity is handled. (4) Localized swelling in the suspected area. (5) Localized extreme tenderness at the site of the suspected fracture. (6) Marked spasm of the muscles about the site of the injury. (7) Bluish discoloration beneath or within the skin.

Angulation and false motion at a point in an extremity well away from a joint and crepitation resulting from bony fragments grating against each other constitute the most convincing signs that a fracture is present. False motion and crepitation should be found incidentally as the extremity is gently handled as part of the examination. Forceful testing should not be made in an effort to find them because of the danger that the bone ends will further damage the tissue about them.

IMMEDIATE COMPLICATIONS OF A FRACTURE. Immediate complications of a fracture include: 1, injury to major arteries; 2, injury to major nerve trunks; 3, injury to organs in the abdomen; 4, injury to the lungs and large blood vessels in the chest; 5, massive hemorrhage and shock; and 6, injuries to the spinal cord associated with fractures of the spine.

INJURIES TO MAJOR ARTERIES OR NERVES. Whenever a fracture occurs, a major artery or nerve in the same area of the extremity may be injured (Fig. 3). Routinely, therefore, anyone giving first aid to a patient with a fracture of an extremity, should always feel for arterial pulsations at the lower end of the extremity and ask the patient to move the fingers or toes. The absence of a pulse at the wrist or ankle (on the front of the wrist on the thumb side; behind the bony prominence on the inner side of the ankle) indicates complete or partial interruption of the major artery to the involved extremity. Loss of the ability to move the fingers and thumb or the toes in all directions indicates injury to a major nerve trunk. Such injuries may be of much more consequence than the fracture itself. They indicate precise handling including appropriate splinting of the extremity and prompt care of a physician.

INJURY TO ORGANS IN THE ABDOMEN. Fractures of the pelvis or the lower ribs may be complicated by injuries to either the solid or

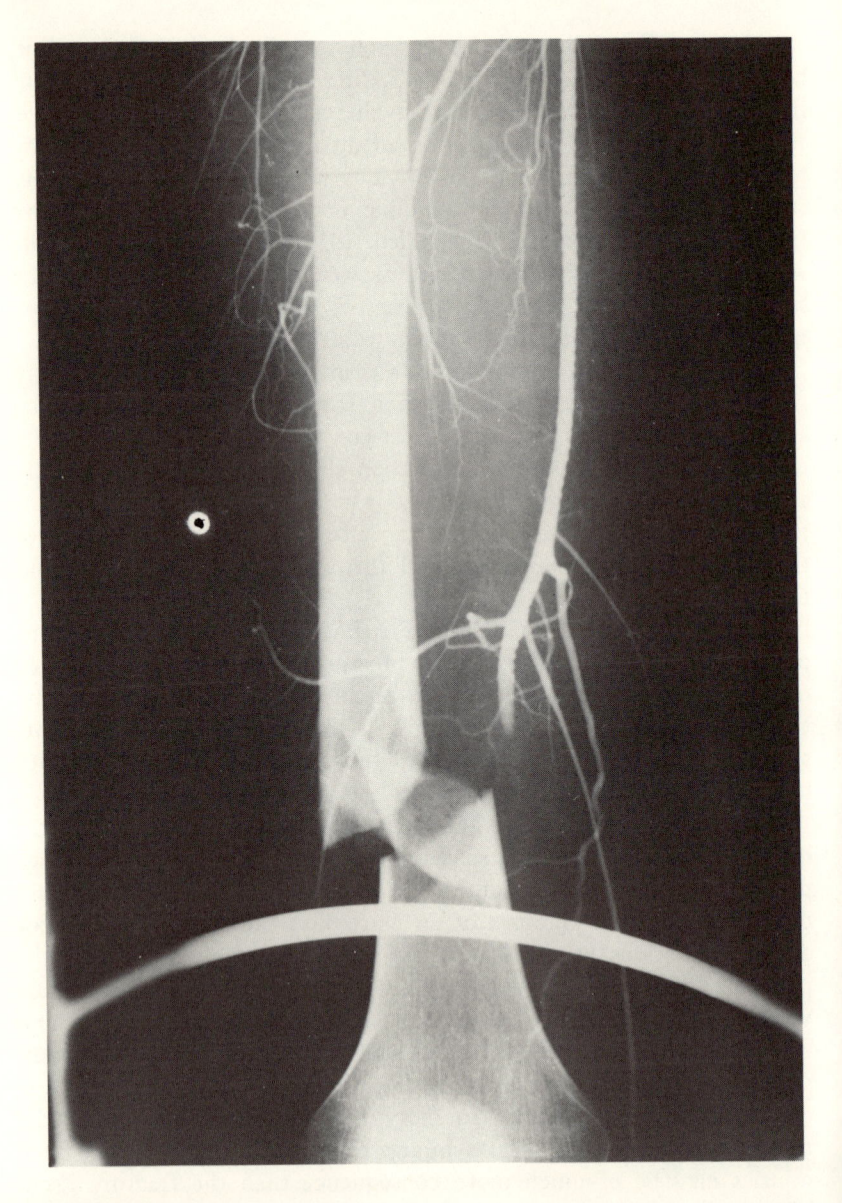

Fig. 3. Fracture of shaft of femur in lower third complicated by a laceration of the femoral artery as demonstrated by an arteriogram (x-ray film) made in a hospital (Dr. James Stokes). (From Artz and Hardy. **Complications in Surgery and their Management,** 1960. Courtesy of W. B. Saunders Company.)

hollow organs within the abdomen, which are of much greater significance than the fracture because of the danger to life. A first aid worker may not be able to recognize such complications, but he may suspect them from the amount of abdominal pain which a patient is having and indications that the patient may be in shock (see below).

HEMORRHAGE AND SHOCK. Loss of blood in large amounts through an open wound, into the abdominal or chest cavities or even into the tissues from a closed fracture of a large bone produces shock (see Chap. 8). Shock due to hemorrhage is often present in injuries of the liver or spleen in the abdomen or of the lung or large blood vessels in the chest. The bleeding from a fracture occurs from the ends of the broken bones and from torn muscle tissue or perhaps a damaged blood vessel about the fracture site. Fractures of the pelvis or spine may be complicated by shock due to hemorrhage. Hemorrhage and shock are life-endangering and demand prompt medical treatment.

INJURIES TO THE SPINAL CORD. An injury to the spinal cord may occur with either a fracture or dislocation of a vertebra. This complication is found most often with injuries to the cervical spine (neck), the thoracic spine behind the upper part of the chest and that area of the spine (low thoracic or lumbar) a few inches above the level of the beltline. An injury to the spinal cord far outweighs a fracture of a vertebra in importance. Such an injury may be suspected when the patient cannot move the toes and foot normally and, in injuries to the neck, also when impaired use of the fingers and thumb is present. Patients with suspected injuries to a vertebra, particularly those with signs suggesting injuries to the spinal cord, must be handled and transported in such a way as to avoid or prevent further damage to the spinal cord (see Chap. 17).

FIRST AID FOR PATIENTS WITH FRACTURES. Although proper first aid care for fractures is exceedingly important, other life-endangering situations take priority. It is crucial that an open airway and adequate breathing be insured and that significant hemorrhage be controlled. An obstructed airway is the greatest cause of death following injury and uncontrolled excessive bleeding ranks second. When a first aid worker or a physician first sees a patient with a fracture, he must divert his attention from the fracture to make certain that the airway is open, that the patient is breathing adequately, and that serious hemorrhage is controlled (Fig. 4).

FIRST AID SPLINTING OF FRACTURES. The emergency splinting

168 / Ch. 13: Fractures, Dislocations, and Sprains

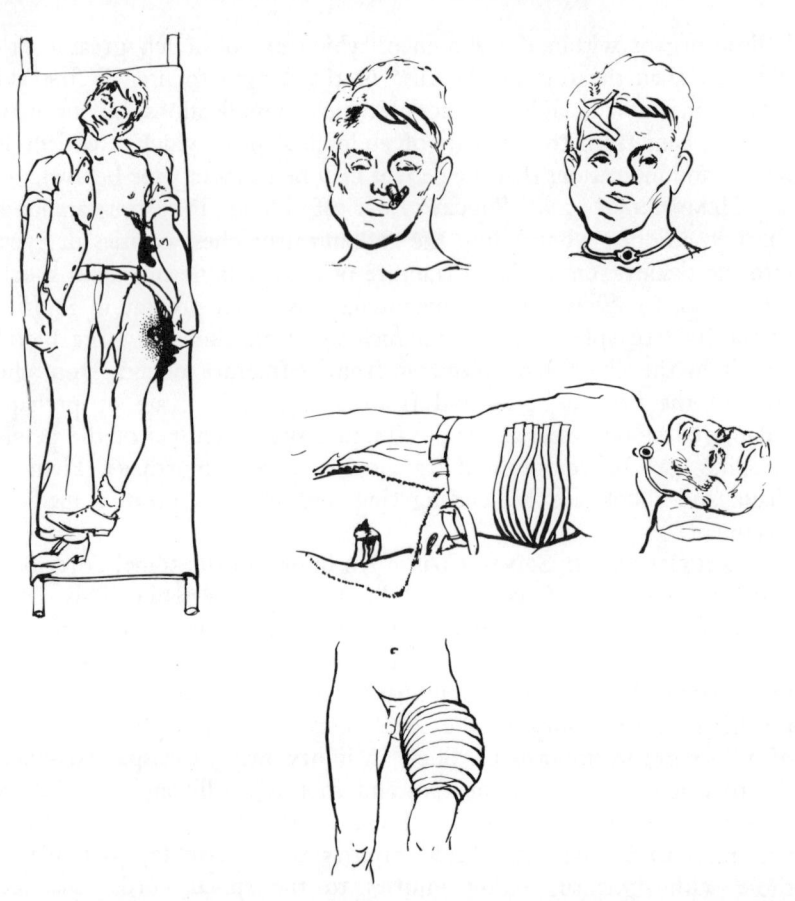

Fig. 4. First aid and emergency medical treatment of multiple injuries (Artist's Drawings). Upper Left, a multiple injured patient with a head (intracranial) injury, fracture of the jaw with displacement, open sucking wound of the chest, and an open fracture of the left femur. 1, procedures to establish an adequate airway may be carried out by a physician in the hospital emergency department. 2, occlusive dressing to close a sucking wound of the chest should be carried out by a first-aid worker or a physician or nurse. 3, compression dressing to arrest hemorrhage should be carried out by a first-aid worker or a physician or nurse.

of a fractured extremity is a highly significant part of first aid treatment. Properly carried out, it tends to minimize or prevent shock and is an important step toward complete rehabilitation of the patient. The guiding principle is "splint 'em where they lie."

The objective of emergency splinting is, of course, not reduction of a fracture, but rather the relief of pain and the prevention of additional damage to muscles and other soft tissues by the fragments

Fractures / 169

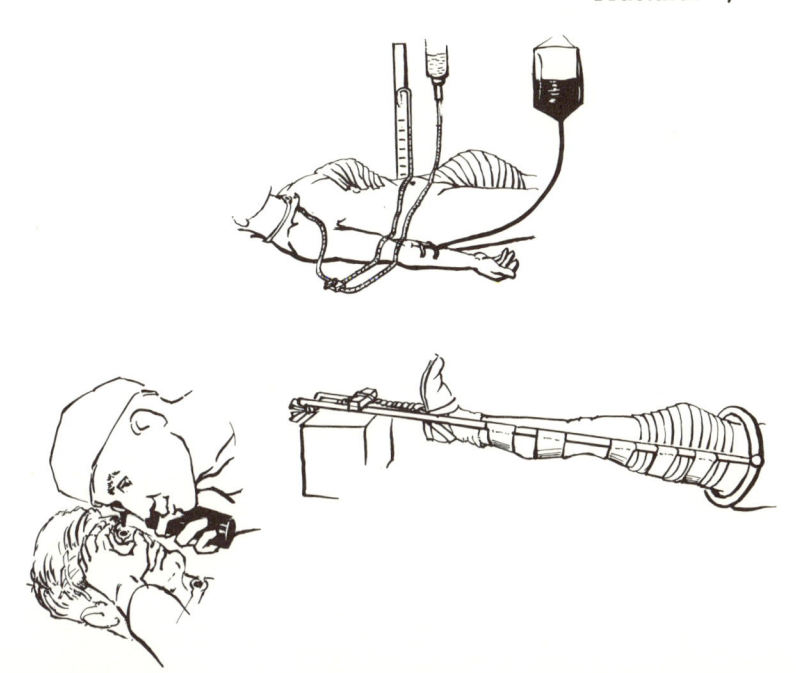

Fig. 4 (cont.) 4, intravenous fluids as administrated by a physician in hospital emergency department and, hopefully, in the near future by well-trained emergency medical technicians (ambulance attendants). 5, fixed traction splinting as should be carried out at the scene of the accident by emergency medical technicians (ambulance attendants) but, if not, by a physician or nurse in the hospital emergency department. 6, examination of the eye grounds by a physician in the hospital emergency department as one means of evaluating status of an intracranial injury. (From Hampton and Fitts. **In** Rhoads et al. ed. **Surgery, Principles and Practice,** 3rd edition, 1965. Courtesy of J. B. Lippincott Company.)

of bone. It may be startling to observe the great relief obtained by a patient with a fracture of an extremity when effective splinting has been provided. Splinting is indicated whenever a fracture of an extremity is suspected, even though the signs may be insufficient to establish the diagnosis definitely.

PRINCIPLES OF SPLINTING. Splinting of an extremity involves the application of some rigid material in such a way as to support the broken bone and, as a matter of fact, the entire extremity. An effective splint, as a rule, must extend beyond both the joint above and the joint below the fracture. Emergency splinting may be classified as 1, coaptation or rigid splinting; and 2, traction splinting.

Coaptation splinting is provided with a properly padded board or a rigid piece of some other material which is bandaged to the extremity in the proper fashion. Actually bandaging of the upper extremity to the chest wall with the forearm supported or unsupported by a sling is a form of coaptation splinting. Inflatable splints may be considered as a form of coaptation or rigid splinting.

Inflatable splints have become available in recent years. These plastic air-tight cylindrical bags with air-intake valves have a definite place among emergency splints for certain fractures of both the upper and lower extremities. Some physicians feel that they are advantageous in open fractures, particularly when bleeding from the wound is brisk. With a dressing over the wound and the air splint applied and inflated, the pressure it provides is said to control the bleeding adequately.

For a fracture of the elbow region, forearm, wrist, or hand in the upper extremity or for a fracture of the knee region, leg, ankle, or foot in the lower extremity, an inflatable splint, properly applied, will provide effective splinting (Fig. 5). It is not applicable, however, for a fracture of an arm (humerus) definitely above the elbow or for a fracture of the thigh (femur) definitely above the knee (Fig. 5B). Efforts to extend its use to such fractures would be hazardous.

Application of an inflatable splint is not difficult but should be carried out by a precise technique. The uninflated splint should be placed so that it lays on the forearm and arm of the first aid worker or physician as he grasps the hand or foot with this hand. Preferably a helper will support the weight of the injured limb and avoid movement at the site of the fracture. While the first aid worker applies gentle traction to the injured extremity with one hand, he slides the air splint on with the other. The splint is then inflated to the desired pressure by blowing into the intake valve. The degree of inflation should be enough so that firm pressure with a thumb on the inflated splint will produce merely a slight indentation. *Never should the splint be inflated with a pump because of the danger of excessive inflation.* The degree of inflation should be checked from time to time to make certain that the pressure is not lost through an unrecognized leak or a defective valve.

Traction splinting involves the use of a special ring splint (Thomas or half-ring) (Fig. 6) by means of which continuous traction (pull) may be applied to a broken lower extremity. Application of a traction splint is a two-man job. A hitch, standard or improvised from a bandage or sling, is placed about the ankle and tied to the distal end of the splint while manual traction is being continued. Some material, perhaps folded slings or towels, are arranged in a

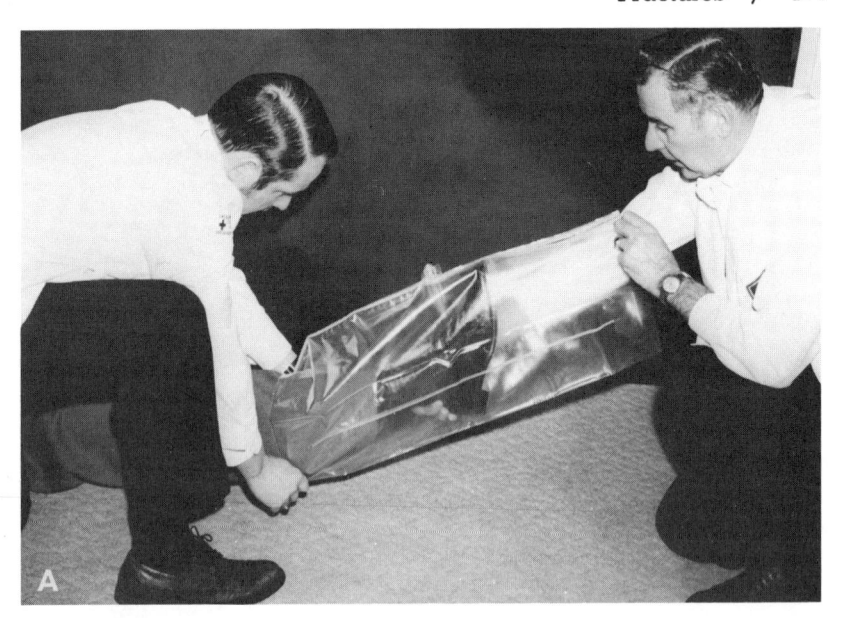

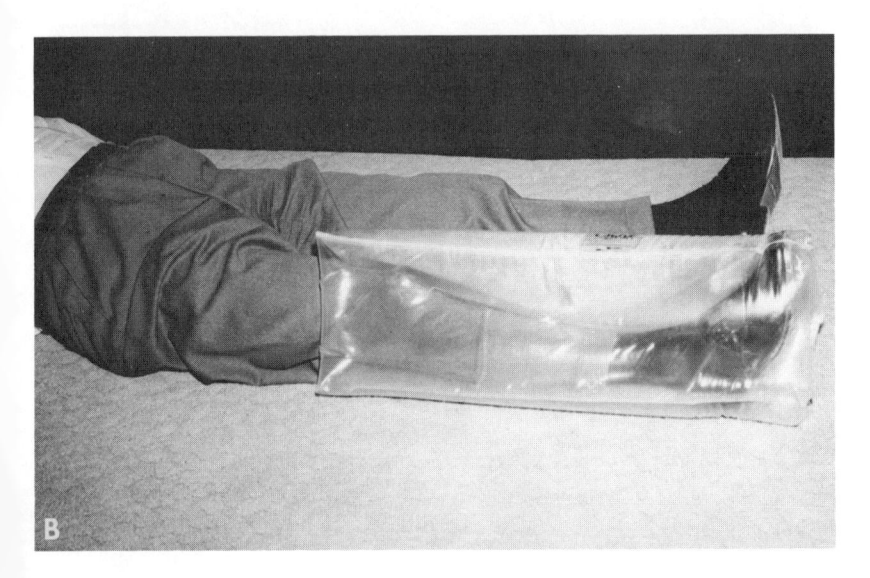

Fig. 5. Inflatable splint for the leg. A, two-man application. Note the uninflated splint is supported on the arm and forearm of one attendant, his hand grasping the foot of the patient. The second attendant then slides the splint over the foot and leg of the patient as far as the length of the splint will permit. B, once in place, the splint is inflated solely by blowing of exhaled air into the intake valve until the splint will provide adequate immobilization.

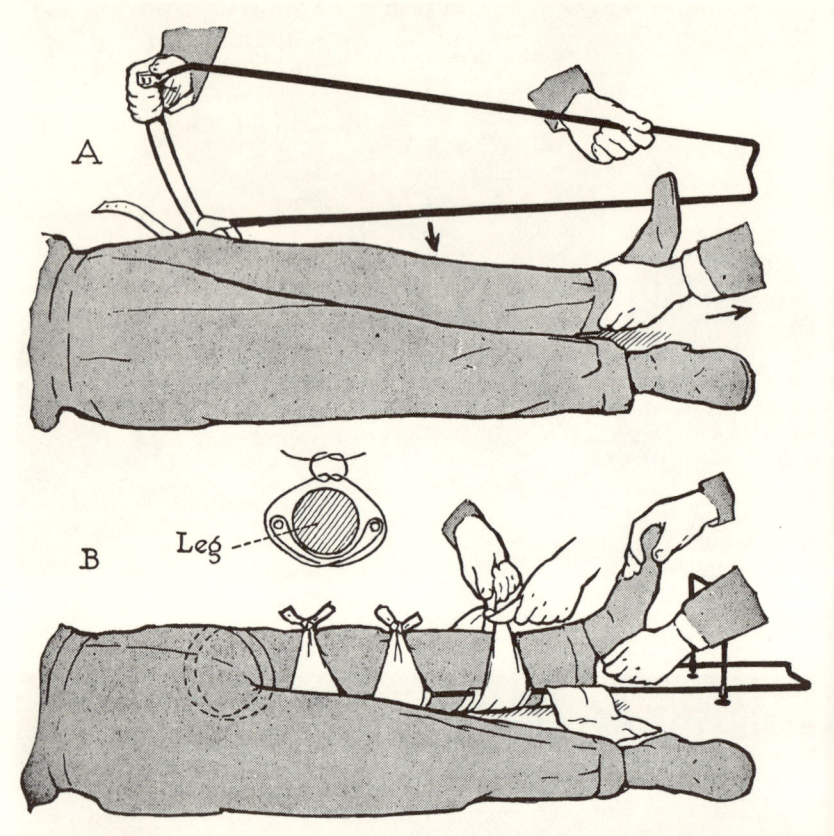

Fig. 6. Application of a half-ring (Keller-Blake) for fracture of the femoral shaft or a fracture of both bones of the leg in the upper two thirds. Traction splinting utilizing the half-ring splint is a two-man procedure. A, continuous manual traction is maintained by one man while the splint is applied by the other. B, multiple slings to support the extremity in the splint. The use of the triangular bandage is illustrated but slings or supports, now available commercially, offer many advantages.

fashion that supports the extremity in the splint. Continuous elevation of the distal end of the splint is a crucial part of traction splinting.

CLASSES OF SPLINTS. First aid splinting may be provided with either *standard* or *improvised* splints (Fig. 7). Standard splints, including inflatable splints, are not likely to be available at the site of the injury until after a well-equipped ambulance carrying splinting equipment and other equipment arrives on the scene or until the patient reaches a hospital. Undoubtedly first aid emergency splinting outside the hospital will be improvised in many instances. Various

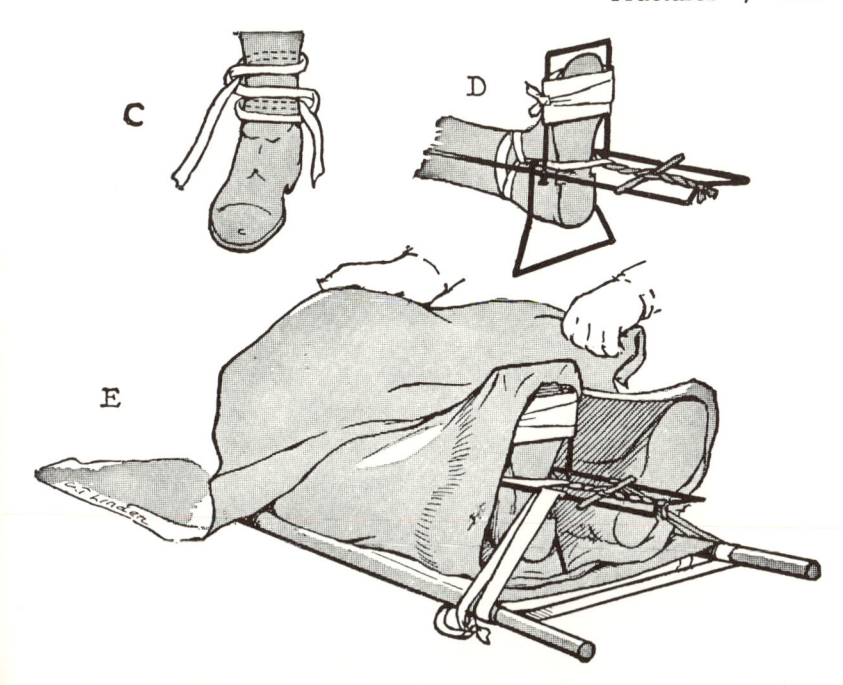

Fig. 6 (cont.) C, details of an improvised hitch utiliding a muslin bandage. Available commercial hitches simplify application of the hitch. D, windlass arrangement utilizing tongue depressors or an available short stick permit an increase in the traction. The right angle foot support and an additional support to keep the distal end of the splint elevated are shown. E, after patient is placed on stretcher, the distal portion of the splint is anchored to the stretcher and the patient covered with blankets.

materials which are likely to be available may be utilized to provide highly effective splinting albeit improvised.

SPLINTING FOR FRACTURES OF THE UPPER EXTREMITY.

THE SHOULDER REGION, ARM (HUMERUS), AND REGION OF THE ELBOW. (Fig. 8).

Standard Splinting. The extremity should be held with the elbow at a right angle and a sling applied (Fig. 7B). Merely the sling will afford considerable relief but if the arm and forearm are wrapped to the chest wall by means of a long roller bandage or another sling, better splinting will be obtained. If the patient has an injured elbow which has assumed an almost straight position and the patient resists any effort to bend the forearm at the elbow in order to place it at a right angle, all such efforts should be discontinued and the entire extremity, arm, elbow, and forearm should be bandaged to the body with the elbow in the position in which it was found. Patients with

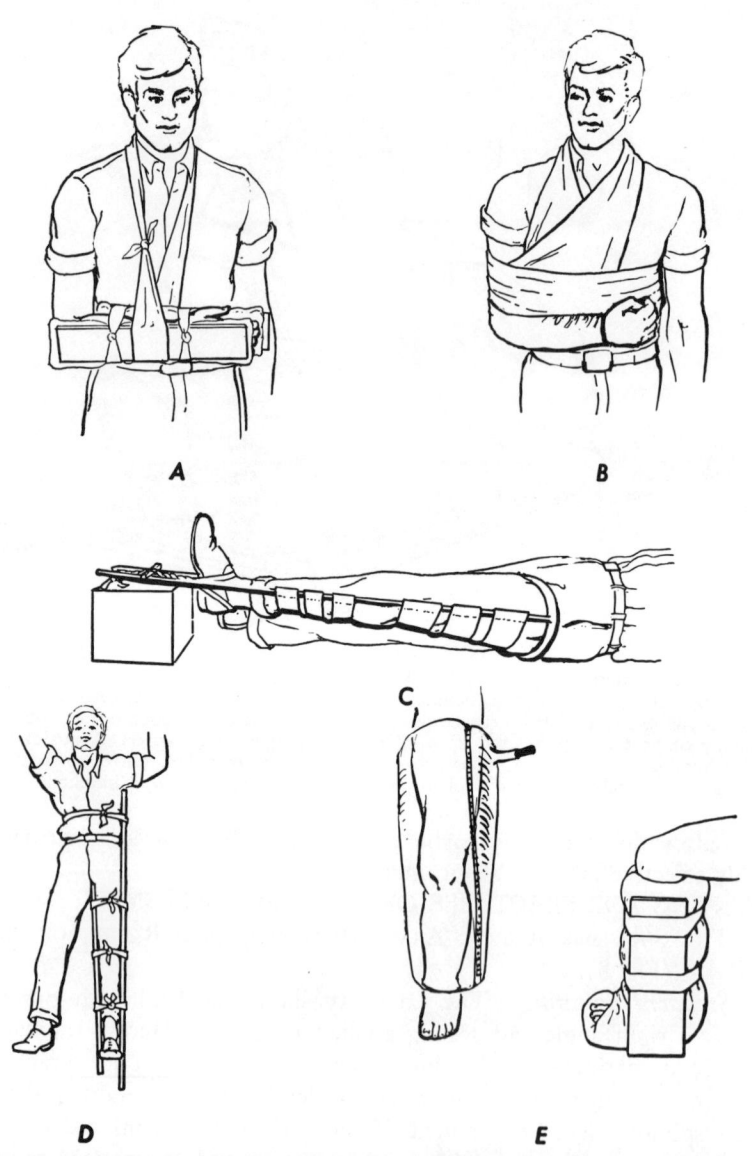

Fig. 7. Emergency splinting. A, coaptation splinting with padded boards for fractures of the forearm which is supported by sling. B, sling and swathe (circular bandage) about the thorax for fractures of the arm. Actually, the hand may be kept free. C, fixed traction in a Thomas full-ring splint for fracture of the femoral shaft. D, coaptation splinting with boards for a fracture of the femur. Note that the lateral board extends to near the axilla and is bound to the trunk, including the thorax. For fractures of the leg, the lateral board as well as the medial board need extend only to the hip, E, pillow splint reinforced by lateral boards for fractures about the ankle. (From Hampton and Fitts. **In** Rhoads et al. ed. **Surgery, Principles and Practice,** 3rd edition, 1965. Courtesy of J. B. Lippincott Company.)

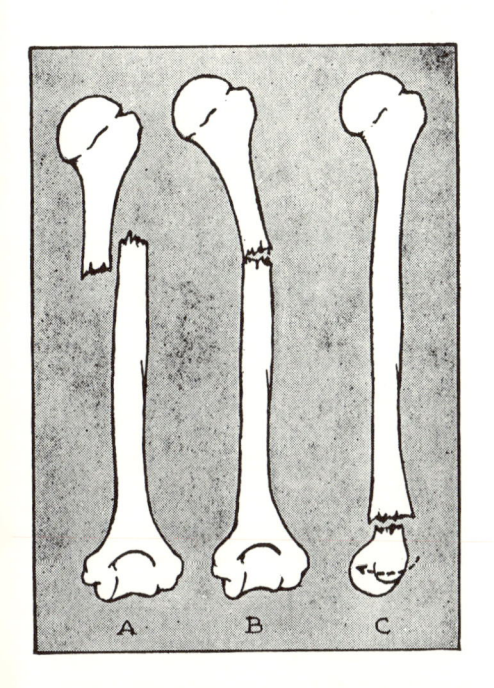

Fig. 8. Fractures of the arm (humerus). A, transverse fracture at the junction of the upper and middle thirds with complete displacement and overriding. B, transverse fracture in the same area as "A" with good apposition and, therefore, no overriding but with angulation. C, transverse fracture in the lower third in good apposition but with the lower fragment rotated 90°.

fractures about the shoulder, arm, or elbow are likely to be more comfortable in the sitting rather than the lying down position, and therefore, they should be allowed to sit up while being transported to medical care.

The splinting just described is known as a sling and swathe. At times, this splinting can be made more effective for fractures of the arm if first very short padded board splints are bandaged to the front and back of the arm. If a wire ladder splint is available, it can be bent to a right angle, and after being properly padded, can be applied to the arm, elbow, forearm, and hand with a bandage after which the sling and swathe are provided.

Improvised Splinting. An improvised sling may be obtained easily by turning up the front portion of the tail of the individual's shirt or blouse and pinning it to the shirt or blouse itself. More relief to the patient will be provided if some material such as strips of sheet can be found with which to bandage the extremity to the chest as described under standard splinting. Patients with fractures about the shoulder, arm, or elbow are likely to be more comfortable in the sitting rather than the lying-down position and, therefore, they should be allowed to sit up while being transported in an ambulance and about the hospital.

The full-ring, hinged arm traction splint is mentioned merely to condemn it. It has no place in the first aid splinting of fractures of the upper extremity. It is not recommended as standard equipment for an emergency ambulance.

FOREARM, WRIST AND HAND.

Standard splinting. Coaptation splinting utilizing a padded board or boards bandaged to the forearm and hand and with the forearm placed in a sling holding the elbow at a right angle provides effective first aid splinting (Fig. 7A).

Improvised splinting. Actually the standard splinting just described is, in a way, improvised splinting. Even when boards of the proper length are not available, however, fractures of the forearm and hand may be splinted adequately when a magazine or heavy newspaper is made to encircle the forearm and hand and is held in place with a bandage or adhesive tape. The application of some material as a sling is an important part of this splinting.

SPLINTING OF FRACTURES OF THE LOWER EXTREMITY.

HIP REGION, THIGH (FEMUR), AND REGION OF THE KNEE.

Standard Splinting. The most effective splinting of fractures in these regions is traction splinting utilizing the Thomas full-ring for a hinged half-ring splint (see Figs. 6 and 9). The application of such splinting is a two-man job. While one individual grasps the patient's ankle and makes continuous manual pull (traction) the other applies a traction hitch about the foot and ankle, preferably over a shoe (Fig. 6D). A shoe should never be removed before application of the hitch unless there are special indications, such as an associated injury in the region of the foot or ankle. Once the hitch is in place, the ends of the straps are tied to the end of the splint in a way that will provide moderate traction. Later, a short stick, perhaps several tongue depressors, may be entwined about the straps as a windlass which permits additional traction. Then the slings on which the thigh and leg will rest are arranged, after which continuous elevation of the end of the splint is provided by placing some object such as a brick, folded towel, or block of wood under the end of the splint. Then and only then is the manual traction released by the individual who first applied it.

Improvised Splinting. All splinting of fractures about the hip, thigh, or knee other than traction splinting is really improvised splinting. On the other hand, coaptation splinting using padded boards can be made quite effective. With this technique a long board is placed

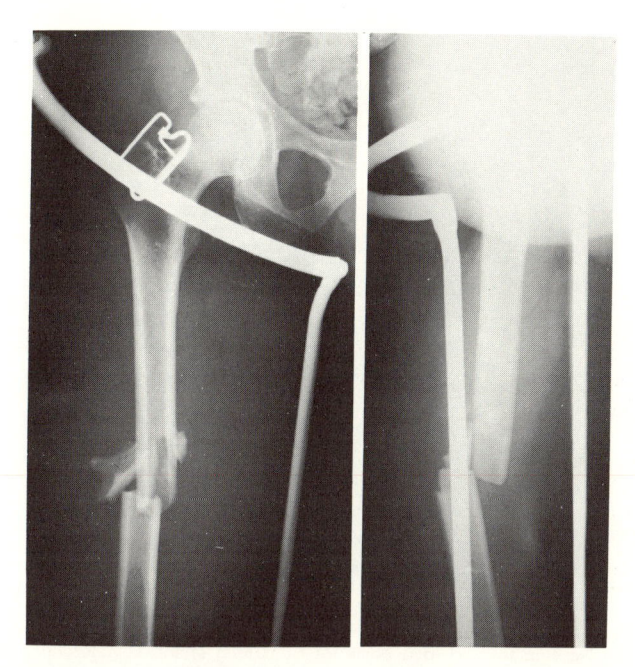

Fig. 9. X-ray films in the anterior posterior (front to back) and lateral (side to side) views of a somewhat comminuted fracture of the shaft of the femur in the upper portion of the middle third immobilized in fixed traction in a half-ring leg splint. (From Hampton and Fitts. **In** Rhoads et al. ed. **Surgery, Principles and Practice,** 3rd edition, 1965. Courtesy of J. B. Lippincott Company.)

on the lateral side of the extremity and trunk extending from below the foot to the lower thorax. Shorter boards are placed on the inner and back sides of the extremity. Then all three boards are bandaged to it, the long board also being bandaged to the trunk.

As a last resort, some degree of improvised splinting may be provided by bandaging the injured extremity to the uninjured extremity, preferably with folded towels or small blankets between them at pressure points such as the knee and ankle. The bandages should be made to encircle both thighs and both legs at several levels.

LEG (TIBIA AND FIBULA).

Standard splinting. Traction splinting as described for fractures above the knee may be utilized effectively for fractures of the upper two thirds of the leg (Fig. 6). Another form of standard splinting employs a posterior gutter splint made of metal, usually aluminum. The splint must be long enough to extend to the middle or upper

178 / Ch. 13: Fractures, Dislocations, and Sprains

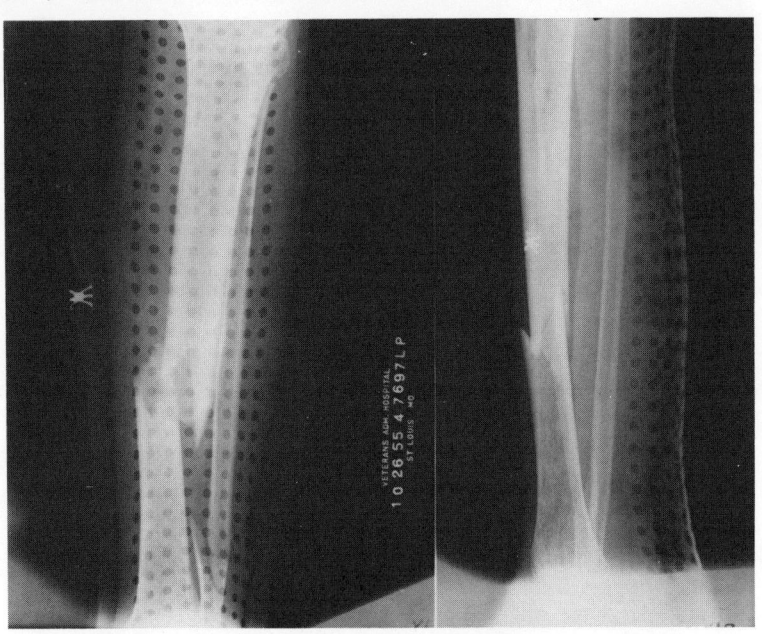

Fig. 10. X-ray films in the anterior posterior and lateral views of a fracture of both bones of the leg immobilized in a posterior aluminum splint, commercially available.

thigh. The leg and foot are placed in the splint, well-padded, and then the extremity is held in the splint by encircling bandages (Fig. 10).

Improvised splinting. The most common improvised splinting utilizes padded board splints, one on each side of the extremity (Figs. 7D and 11). At times three padded boards are used with the

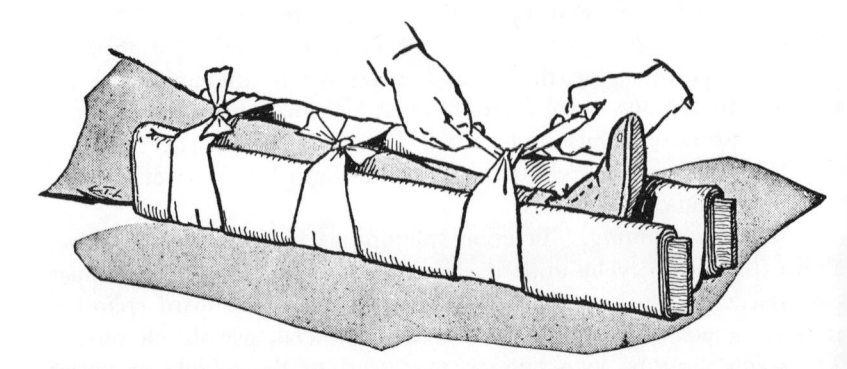

Fig. 11. Improvised splinting using a blanket roll to form a cradle reinforced by a board splint on each side of the extremity for fractures of both bones of the leg.

additional splint being placed along the back of the leg. The splinting is completed merely by bandaging the splints about the extremity.

A pillow splint is also a highly effective improvised splint for fractures of the lower third of the bones of the leg (Fig. 12). The extremity is merely placed on a pillow which is bandaged so that it encircles the leg from just above the knee to the point of the heel. Actually a board placed on each side of the pillow also to be encircled by the bandage reinforces the splinting and tends to make it more effective. Frequently the pillow is placed so that it extends

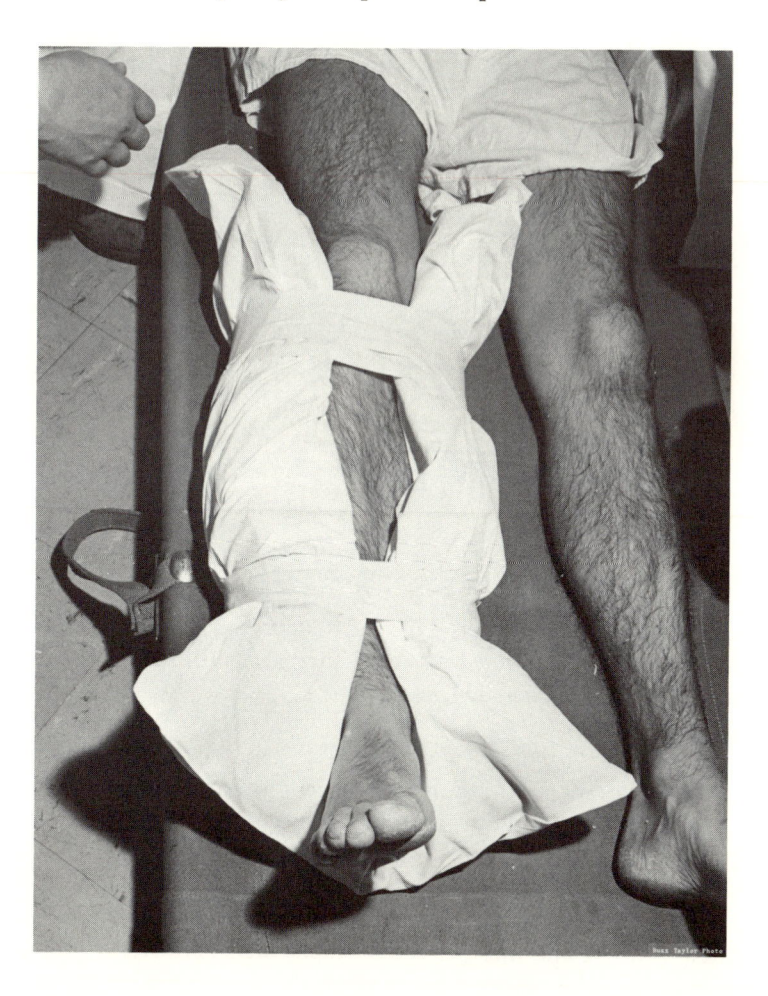

Fig. 12. Pillow splint as emergency splinting for fractures of both bones of the leg. Reinforcement by a medial and lateral board will improve the splinting.

180 / Ch. 13: Fractures, Dislocations, and Sprains

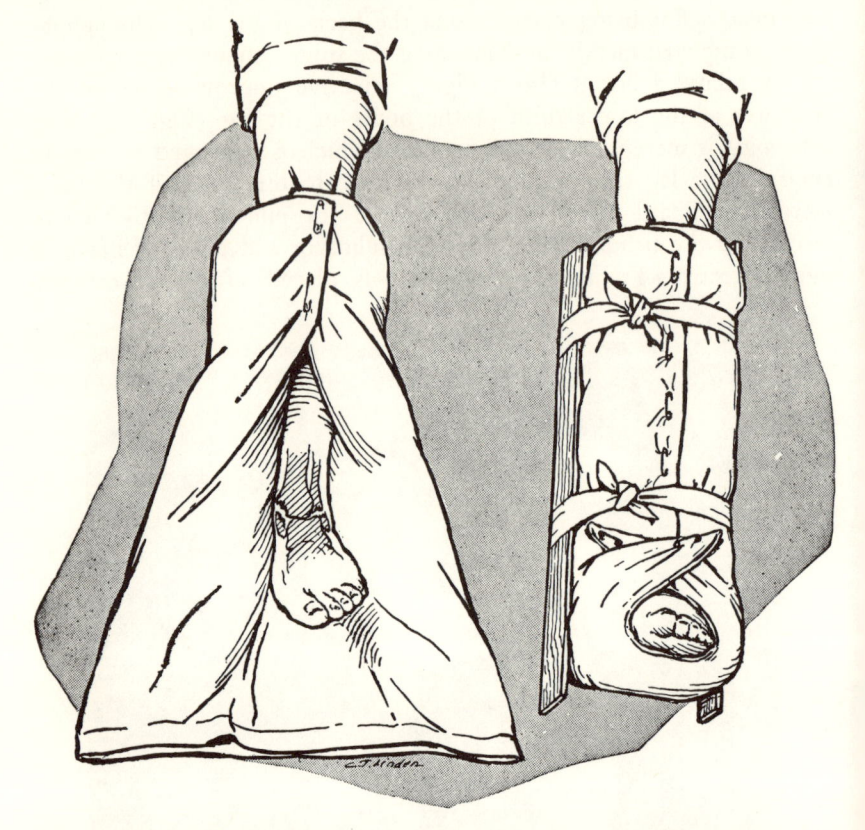

Fig. 13. Pillow splint with boards as emergency splinting for fractures about the ankle or foot. Note how the pillow has been pinned so as to support the foot.

several inches past the heel. This portion of the pillow preferably is turned upward and pinned to itself so that it affords some support to the foot (Figs. 7E and 13).

ANKLE AND FOOT.

Standard splinting. About the only standard splinting for these injuries is the use of a short posterior gutter splint of aluminum, well-padded particularly so that the point of the heel will not continuously rest against metal in a situation that would predispose to a pressure sore.

Improvised splinting. A pillow splint probably provides the simplest and yet the most effective improvised first aid splinting for these injuries. The pillow extends from the upper portion of the calf past the heel. After the pillow is bandaged to the leg, folding and pinning the portion which projects beyond the foot so that it supports the foot in a position close to a right angle is particularly important in first aid splinting of fractures about the ankle or foot (Fig. 7E).

Spine and Pelvis. The key words in first aid splinting of the spine and pelvis are *protection* and *immobilization*. These must be provided even during extrication of the patient from motor vehicles or from other situations in which the patient may be entrapped.

Cervical Spine (Neck). Protection and immobilization of the neck in a suspected fracture or dislocation of the cervical spine possibly is of greater importance than in other areas of the spine because of the great danger of damage to the spinal cord in the cervical region which may result in permanent, nearly total paralysis or in death.

When the emergency care worker first gains access to the patient the head should be grasped and supported. Gentle traction may be applied to the head as a means of support. If the head has dropped forward, usually it will be necessary to lift it gently into a neutral position in order to restore or maintain an adequate airway. A second worker should apply a supporting collar of a standard design if it is available or an improvised collar utilizing a folded large surgical dressing or bath towel (Fig. 14).

If the patient is being extricated from a motor vehicle, a short spine board should be utilized as shown in Figure 15, if one is available or can be improvised, perhaps utilizing a short door or short ironing board. Moreover, any available plank not too long and of sufficient width will serve the purpose. After protected extrication, the patient is placed face up on a stretcher or long board with sandbags or folded towels placed alongside the neck to help support it.

Key objectives throughout the handling of a patient with a suspected injury to the cervical spine are to avoid increased forward bending and all backward bending of the head unless it is necessary to restore the airway. Bending or turning of the head to either side also is to be avoided. If there appears to be danger of vomiting and aspiration, the entire person should be rolled onto the side rather than turning the head alone. This is facilitated if the patient, including his head, has been immobilized on a back board.

Dorsal and Lumbar Spine. Again the key words are *protection* and *immobilization*. Increasing flexion (forward bending) of the body

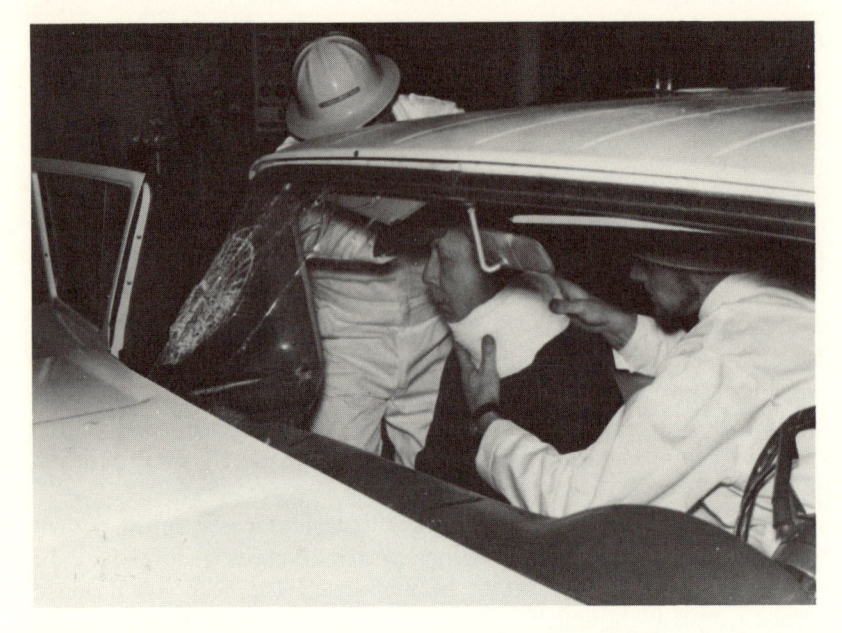

Fig. 14. Application of a supporting collar, of a standard design or improvised, to support the head with a suspected fracture or dislocation of the cervical spine. (Courtesy Dr. J. D. Ferrington.)

is to be avoided at all costs. The short spine board, standard or improvised as described above, should be utilized in extricating a patient from a motor vehicle. At the earliest feasible time, the patient should be placed upon a firm stretcher or a long spine board (a full-length door or broad board will suffice) (Fig. 15) with the short spine board still attached to the torso and head. Once he is upon something serving as a stretcher, it may be practical to unstrap the short board and slide it from beneath the patient.

In circumstances when extrication is not necessary, as when a patient has been thrown from a motor vehicle, the patient must be lifted in a manner that avoids flexion of the spine. When he is found face-down, he may be placed face-down on a stretcher or spine board which will serve as a stretcher. If, however, concurrent facial or chest injuries make the face-down position inadvisable, the patient should be rolled "in one piece" onto the backboard or stretcher so that he is placed in the face-up position (Fig. 16).

When the patient is found face-up, he should be placed on the stretcher or board face-up. Usually a small roll made from a bath

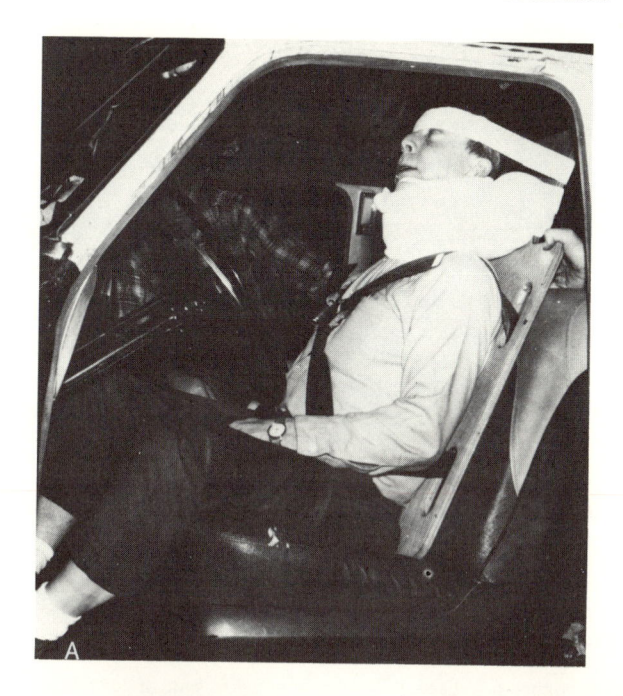

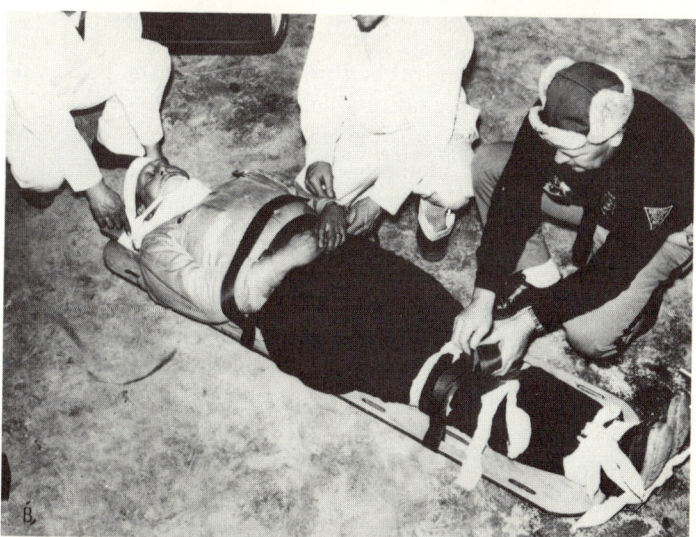

Fig. 15. A, application of the short spine board to permit extrication from a vehicle without the risk of further injury to the cervical spine and spinal cord. B, support of the patient on a long spine board after extrication from the vehicle. (Courtesy Dr. J. D. Farrington.)

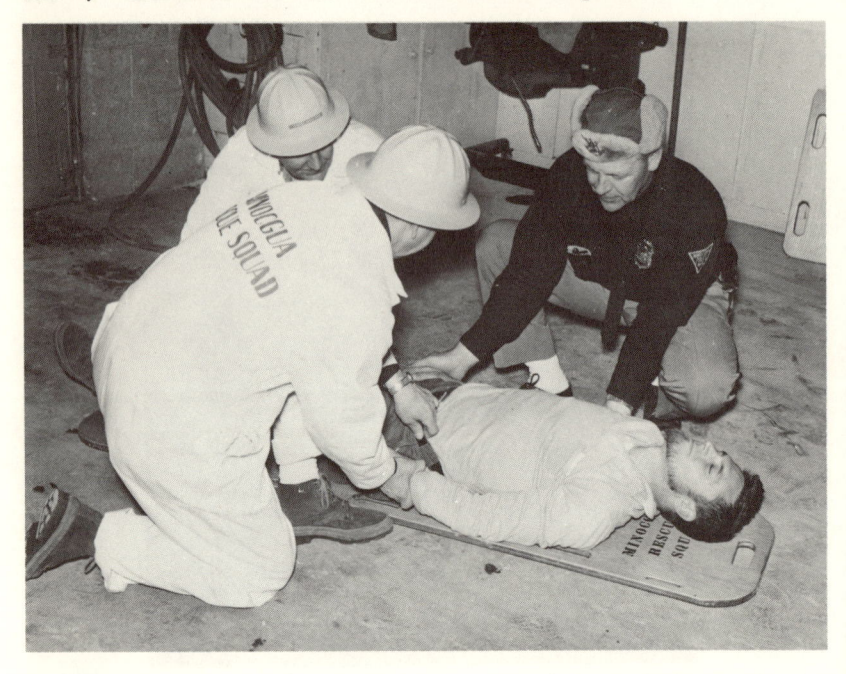

Fig. 16. The patient has been rolled 'in one piece' onto a long back board to be transported in the face-up position. (Courtesy Dr. J. D. Farrington.)

towel or folded blanket and placed in the small of the back will tend to make the patient more comfortable.

The on-the-side position is preferable, however, in every instance when there is danger of vomiting and aspiration in order that fluids will flow out the side of the patient's mouth. Regardless of the position in which the patient is found, transportation with him on his side may be advisable as a safeguard against aspiration.

Pelvis. Protection and support on a firm surface are the guiding principles of first aid for patients with suspected fractures of the pelvis. The same methods of careful extrication as for fractures of the lumbar spine are applicable. The patient will be most comfortable lying on his back on a padded, firm surface. He should be transported to and within a hospital in that position (Fig. 16).

Pelvic fractures are not infrequently complicated by injuries to the bladder. If the patient passes urine en route to the hospital, it should be observed for blood and the physician properly informed. In the hospital emergency department, the patient who has not voided should be asked to do so by the physician. If the patient cannot void or if bloody urine is passed, the physician should insert an indwelling catheter into the bladder through which a cystogram can be obtained while the patient is on the x-ray table for films of the fractured pelvis.

OPEN FRACTURES. An open fracture is more serious than a closed fracture, principally because of the dangers of severe hemorrhage and shock immediately following the injury and the danger of subsequent infection which could be so severe that it leads to amputation or even death. It is obvious, therefore, that precise and effective first aid measures are mandatory as the first effort to avoid such complications.

The first aid worker or physician should immediately apply a dressing of adequate size and thickness over the open wound and bandage it in place with adequate pressure to control the hemorrhage. The encircling bandage should not be so tight that it acts as a tourniquet. Handling an extremity properly for application of the compression dressing really requires two people, one to support the extremity while the other applies the dressing. Definitely antiseptics should not be applied to the wound.

Thereafter, splinting for an open fracture should be provided by the same method as would be selected for a closed fracture of the same region. An inflatable splint may be selected, rather than other splints, for an open fracture in a region where it is applicable (see p. 171).

At times in an open fracture, a fragment of bone will be protruding through the wound when the patient is first seen. It should not be replaced into the wound but, on the contrary, should be left protruding and the dressing applied over it. It follows that when fixed traction splinting is utilized for an open fracture of the femur or bones of the leg, the amount of traction should be held to that which will not pull the protruding fragment back into the depths of an open wound.

As stated above, severe hemorrhage and shock may occur with an open fracture. Control of hemorrhage is exceedingly important. If a compression dressing properly applied fails to control the hemorrhage adequately, the use of a tourniquet may appear necessary despite its inherent dangers (see p. 111). If shock appears imminent or established, those measures recommended as part of first aid for shock are indicated (see Chap. 8).

Dislocations

A dislocation is a disruption of a joint, including tears of many or all of its ligaments, and a displacement of the end of one of the bones making up the joint. Dislocations are *complete* when all contact of the articulating bones is lost, or *incomplete*, at times called a subluxation, when the ends of the bones remain partially in contact. Chip or even larger fractures may complicate complete or incomplete dislocations.

In injuries of the upper extremity the shoulder and elbow joints are most frequently dislocated. The wrist is rarely dislocated but a dislocation of a joint of a finger is rather common. In the lower extremity all of the major joints may be dislocated. Dislocations of the hip are the most common without an associated fracture. A fracture of the femoral head or the margin of the acetabulum (hip socket) at times does complicate such injuries. Dislocations of the knee, severe injuries, are uncommon. For a complete dislocation of the knee to occur, most and at times all of its supporting ligaments must be torn. Dislocations complicating fractures of the bony prominences of the ankle occur frequently. At times, a dislocation of joints in the foot or of a joint of a toe may occur.

Certain complete dislocations may cause injuries to major blood vessels and nerve trunks in the same manner as displaced fragments of a fracture. Dislocations of the knee particularly are likely to result in damage to the arteries and nerves behind the joint. Dislocations of the elbow to a lesser extent are associated with comparable injuries to arteries and nerves of the upper extremity. It is imperative, therefore, that anyone including a physician rendering first aid to a patient with a dislocation just as to one with a fracture, determine the status of the arterial pulsations and ability of the patient to move the digits distal to the injured joint. Lay first aid workers should be prepared to inform the physician who sees the patient of findings suggesting an arterial or nerve injury.

SYMPTOMS AND SIGNS OF A DISLOCATION OF A JOINT OF AN EXTREMITY. *Symptoms* of a dislocation are the same as those of a fracture, that is, pain at the site of the injury and loss of use of the involved extremity. *Signs* of a dislocation are more limited than those of a fracture. Deformity at a joint is the predominant sign. The area appears altered in contour with unusual bony prominences and is tender to even light pressure. Crepitus is not expected. Usually spasm of the muscles due to pain tends to prevent all active motion of the joint by the patient or passive motion by the first aid worker or physician. Therefore, false motion, at times an obvious finding with a fracture, is usually lacking with a dislocation.

SPLINTING FOR DISLOCATIONS. A guiding rule for splinting an extremity with a dislocated joint is to splint it in the position in which it is found. No effort should be made to straighten an angulation of the arm or leg with a dislocated joint. Rather, splinting for protection and to minimize pain should be applied and the services of a physician obtained promptly.

While the same type of splints and comparable methods of splinting may be utilized for dislocations as for fractures of the comparable region, usually some modifications or variations in technique are advisable. Special signs of dislocations of the major joints of the extremities and acceptable first aid splinting for them are described below.

DISLOCATIONS OF THE UPPER EXTREMITY.

SHOULDER. The most common dislocation of the shoulder is called an anterior dislocation (Fig. 17 A-B). It results from a fall on the outstretched arm, the leverage resulting in the upper end (head) of the bone being forced downward and forward until it tears the covering of the joint and becomes dislocated. The arm remains projecting away from the body, an important sign. The patient often supports the injured arm away from his body with the hand of the uninjured side, because even the weight of the arm tending to bring it downward toward the body is exceedingly painful. The shoulder appears square rather than rounded, another sign, because of the abnormal prominence of a bone on top of the shoulder (acromion). Occasionally a dislocated shoulder may be associated with an arterial or nerve injury.

Splinting. All splinting for a dislocated shoulder is in a way improvised. A pillow or folded blanket may be packed under the arm so as to support it in some abduction and a sling applied to support the weight of the forearm at or near a right angle. The patient at times may be more comfortable in the sitting position rather than lying down.

ELBOW. Dislocations of the elbow occur rather commonly although less frequently than those of the shoulder. The elbow becomes dislocated as a result of a force producing excessive straightening (hyperextension), such as may be created by a fall on the

188 / Ch. 13: Fractures, Dislocations, and Sprains

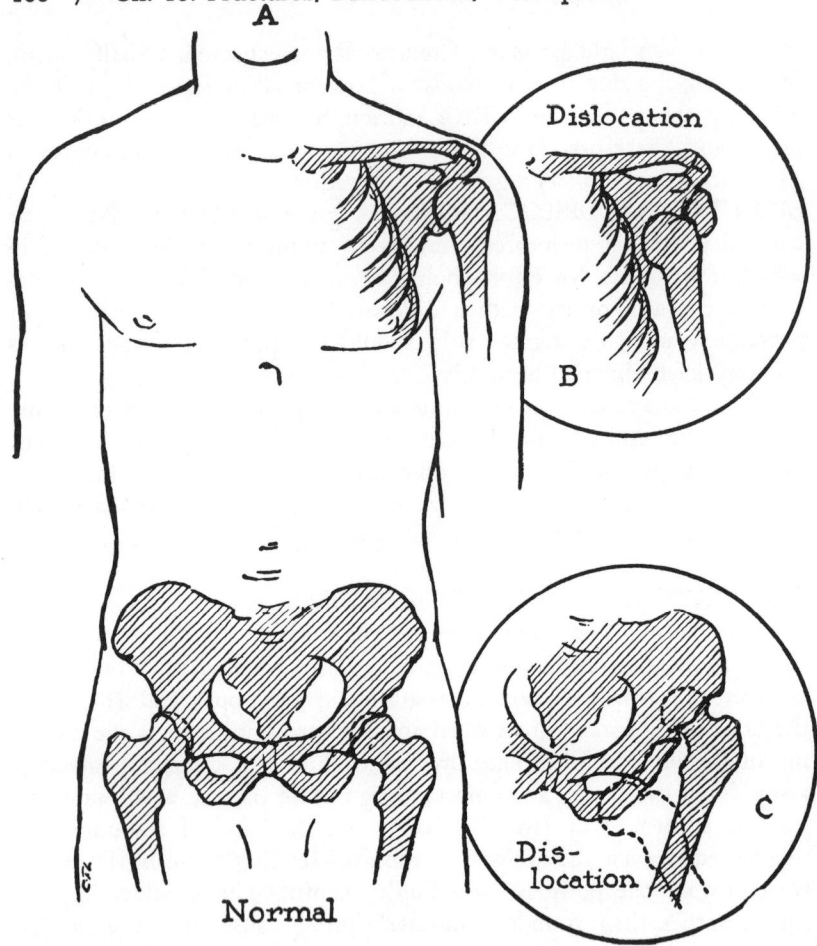

Fig. 17. Artist's sketches to illustrate dislocations of the shoulder and the hip. A, normal shoulder and normal hip. B, anterior dislocation of the shoulder, the most common type. C, posterior dislocation of the hip with the head of the femur displaced upward and backward. A posterior dislocation of the hip is the most common but occasionally an anterior dislocation, as indicated by the dotted line, occurs with forward and downward displacement of the head of the femur.

outstretched hand with the elbow extended. The upper end of the bones of the forearm (ulna and radius) are forced behind the lower end of the bone of the arm (humerus). They usually remain displaced backwards (posterior dislocation) although at times as the force continues they may assume a position to the side of distal humerus (lateral dislocation).

Pain and loss of use of the extremity constitute the symptoms which, of course, do not distinguish a dislocated elbow from a fracture near that joint. The patient may complain of numbness of the hand, particularly of the little and ring fingers due to trauma to the ulnar nerve. The elbow region appears deformed, an important sign. The point of the elbow (tip of the olecranon) creates an abnormal bony prominence. In a lateral dislocation, a portion of the lower end of the humerus also will assume an unusually prominent position. The forearm assumes a slightly flexed position (150°) in relation to the arm.

Splinting. No attempt should be made either to straighten or bend the elbow more. Splinting should be provided in the position in which the extremity is found. Standard splinting utilizes a "rigid" type of splint but one such as a wire ladder splint which may be bent so that it conforms to the position of the elbow. Properly padded, the splint is placed on the back of the arm and forearm and bandaged to them. Improvised splinting by bandaging the extremity to the body, will provide immobilization sufficient to permit the patient to be taken to a physician. Patients with dislocated elbows usually are more comfortable in the recumbent position.

WRIST JOINT. A true dislocation of the wrist without an associated fracture, for practical purposes, does not occur. Injuries which appear to be dislocations on examination are practically always displaced fractures close to the joint. A true dislocation of a small bone in the wrist (lunate) does occur rather frequently following an injury which produces excessive hyperextension of the hand, but even with this injury, a fracture is usually suspected before x-ray films are made. Pain, restricted use, and some deformity are present in most injuries about the wrist.

Splinting. Splinting for all injuries about the wrist consist of application of a padded rigid splint, a board or some firm supporting appliance, and a sling. An inflatable splint also may be utilized effectively.

JOINTS OF THE FINGERS AND THUMB. Any of the joints of the digits may be dislocated but the proximal and middle joints of the fingers and the proximal joint of the thumb are most susceptible to this injury. A force producing excessive hyperextension of a digit tends to cause a dislocation which is accompanied by a rather marked deformity.

Splinting. Splinting is really not required for these digital injuries but a splint will tend to minimize pain. Fortunately, reasonably strong traction usually leads to reduction which often may be accomplished without even local anesthesia.

Occasionally an operation is required for reduction of a dislocation because an extensor tendon has been trapped so that is passes through the joint and prevents reduction by strong traction.

DISLOCATIONS OF THE LOWER EXTREMITY.

Hip Joint (Fig. 17 A, C). Severe trauma is necessary to produce a dislocation of the hip. A dislocated hip may occur when strong adduction or abduction of the thigh levers the head of the femur (bone of the thigh) from the socket, particularly when the force includes strong internal or external rotation of the extremity. This injury also may result when a driver or a passenger in an automobile is thrown forward so that a knee forcibly strikes the dashboard usually with the thigh adducted at the hip. This impact tends to force the femoral head backward out of the joint and often produces an associated fracture of the back margin of the acetabulum (hip socket) (Fig. 18). The same mechanism exists when an exceedingly heavy weight falls onto the lower back of an individual who is standing with his trunk bent forward so that the hips are in some 90° of flexion. A dislocated hip can traumatize the sciatic nerve, therefore, its function should be determined when the patient is first seen.

The injury causes severe pain and totally incapacitates the patient. In the most common type of hip dislocation (posterior), the lower extremity assumes a position of flexion, adduction, and internal rotation in contrast to that of extension and external rotation with a fracture of the hip. The patient resists all efforts to straighten the hip and knee.

Splinting. Only some form of improvised splinting is possible. Fixed traction splinting is not applicable because the splint cannot be applied with the thigh and the knee in a flexed position.

Adequate improvised splinting consists of any measure which will immobilize the extremity in the position in which it is found. The patient may be placed on a stretcher, or a long board serving as a stretcher, after which pillows or blankets packed beneath the thigh and knee will afford some support for the extremity in the flexed position. At times the patient may be most comfortable if he remains in the sitting position during transportation to a hospital because the sitting position helps maintain the flexed position of the hip and knee.

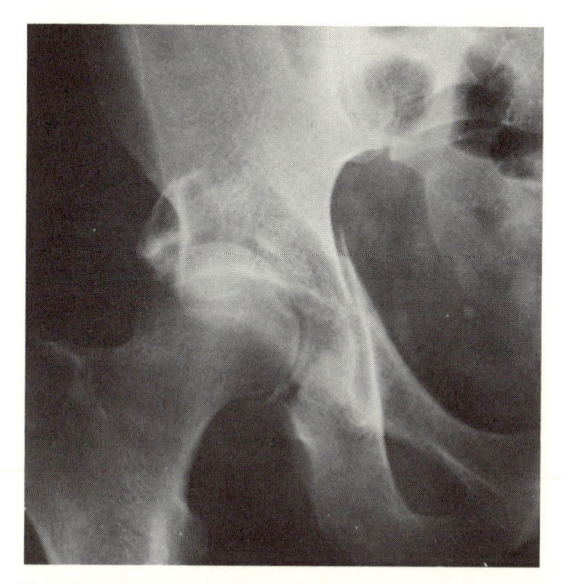

Fig. 18. X-ray film showing a dislocation of the hip, associated with a fracture of the posterior margin of the acetabulum (hip joint). (From Hampton and Fitts. **Open Reduction of Common Fractures,** 1959. Courtesy of Grune & Stratton, Inc.)

KNEE JOINT. A true complete dislocation of the knee is a more serious injury by far than that which the layman calls a dislocation of the knee. The latter is usually a torn semilunar cartilage within the knee joint or a complete or partial tear of one of the major supporting ligaments of the knee.

In a true complete dislocation of the knee, the upper end of the tibia (the large bone of the leg) is displaced forward or backward (usually) so that it no longer articulates with the lower end of the femur (thigh bone) and usually overrides it by one or two inches. What might be termed an incomplete dislocation of the knee in which the articulating surfaces of the femur and tibia remain in partial contact is really a severe injury to the major ligaments with resulting loss of the integrity of the joint.

A true dislocation of the knee, fortunately a rare injury, is produced by direct violence to the upper portion of the leg or the lower end of the thigh while the knee is completely extended or by forced hyperextension of the knee as might occur when a running individual steps into a deep hole causing the entire leg below the knee to be fixed as the running effort carries the body forward with great force. Possibly, momentary complete dislocation with spontaneous reduction occurs occasionally. In such instances, the knee is not dislocated when the patient is first seen but there is marked loss of stability of the joint in all directions because of torn ligaments.

Complications of a complete dislocation of the knee include damage to the popliteal artery or to one of the major nerve trunks about the knee, usually the peroneal nerve. The artery may be torn or its flow of blood merely obstructed by pressure. The importance of a prompt appraisal of the circulation to the leg and foot is obvious. The absence of the pulsations of arteries at the ankle and foot demands as prompt reduction of the dislocation as possible. Fortunately this often can be achieved without anesthesia. Because a complete dislocation of the knee may be recognized by a well-trained first aid worker from the obvious severe deformity, when the pulsations at the ankle and foot are absent the advantages of him applying strong manual pull on the lower leg in an effort to reduce the dislocation outweigh any disadvantages. Certainly under these circumstances, a physician should apply strong manual traction as soon as he verifies that the blood flow to the leg and foot has been interrupted. If after reduction of the dislocation, the normal pulsations at the ankle and foot do not return, then prompt surgical exploration of the popliteal fossa (back of the knee) is indicated with appropriate surgery to restore the circulation.

The only sign of a dislocation of the knee which fortunately and practically is enough to make the diagnosis is the marked deformity about the knee with the marked abnormal bony prominences both in front and in back of the region of the joint.

Splinting. The same methods of splinting as those recommended for fractures about the knee (see p. 176) are applicable to splinting of a dislocation of the knee. Either fixed traction splinting utilizing a half-ring or full-ring splint or the multiple padded board splints as recommended for improvised splinting for a fracture of the femoral shaft should be utilized. An inflatable splint may be effective if it reaches high on the thigh.

ANKLE JOINT. Dislocations of the ankle usually are complications of fractures about the joint although a partial dislocation (a spread between the lower ends of the bones of the leg accompanied by some shift of the talus) without fracture does occur. Only x-ray films will identify such an injury. A complete dislocation without a fracture is indeed a rarity. Fractures of one or both malleoli (the prominences on the sides of the ankle) are the basic injuries which frequently are accompanied by a complete or incomplete dislocation of the ankle (Fig. 19).

The mechanisms of injury producing fractures about the ankle and therefore complete or partial dislocations and the methods of splinting for these injuries are described on page 180.

JOINTS OF THE FOOT. Dislocations of the joints of the back part of the foot are not uncommon. They are produced by strong everting force on the foot. The injury is usually one described as a peritalar dislocation which means that the talus (the bone of the foot which articulates with the bones of the leg to form the ankle joint) remains in place, but those bones of the foot articulating with it are displaced. Rarely, the talus is completely dislocated (extruded) from the joint so that it no longer articulates in either the ankle or foot.

Dislocations of the joints of the foot produce an obvious deformity, usually so pronounced that it will not be masked by the swelling which takes place promptly. While the injury may be suspected from examination of the foot, the differential diagnosis between a dislocation and a fracture cannot be established until adequate x-ray films are made, usually in multiple views.

Splinting. The methods of splinting for all injuries of the foot or ankle are described on page 180.

JOINTS OF THE TOES. While each of the joints of the toes may be dislocated, those of the proximal joint of the great toe and the middle joint of the smaller toes are seen most frequently. They are produced by some force which produces hyperextension of the digit. Rather marked deformity is always present. True emergency splinting is not necessary. Strong traction is likely to reduce the dislocation although at times a tendon becomes trapped so that it passes through the joint preventing reduction without an operative procedure.

Sprains

Sprains are injuries to ligaments, structures which support, in full or in part, the joints of the body. These injuries vary in severity from mere stretchings to complete tears of the ligaments which may permit partial dislocation of the injured joint. Completely torn ligaments often accompany fractures about joints and become an integral part of the injury.

All joints are subject to sprains, but the knee joint is particularly

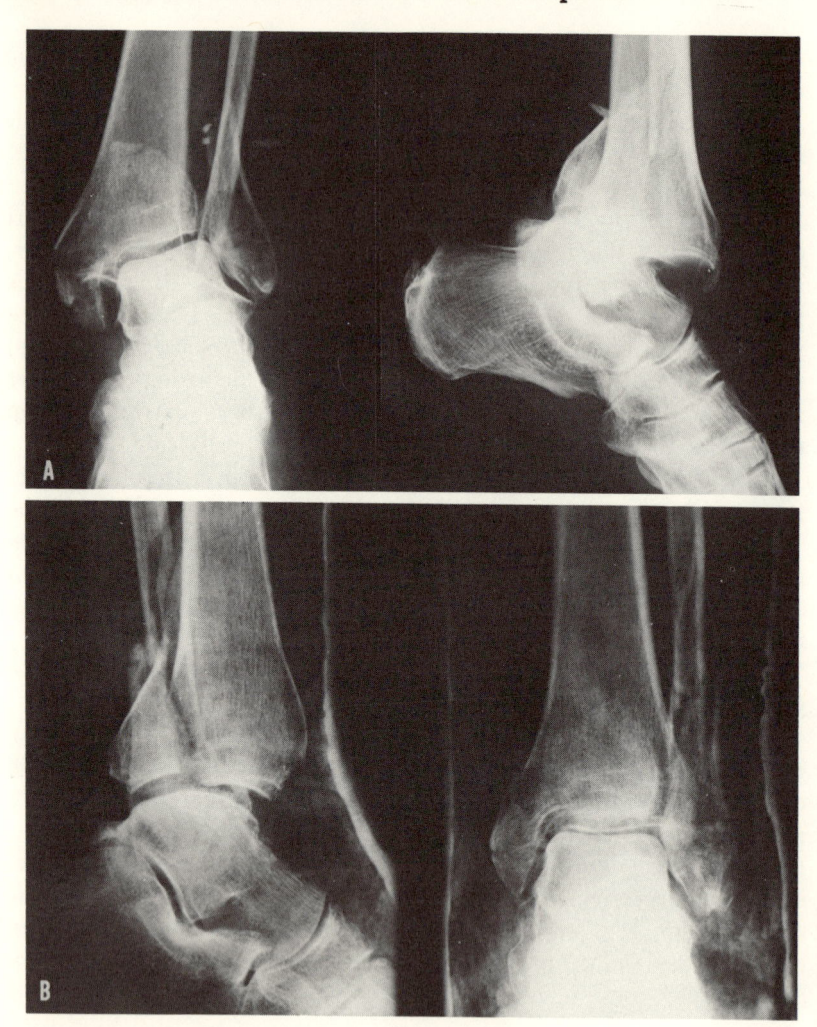

Fig. 19. Fracture dislocation of the ankle. Both the medial and lateral malleoli were fractured and there is a fracture of the posterior portion of the lower end of the tibia (sometimes called the posterior malleolus) with lateral and posterior dislocation of the foot. (From Hampton and Fitts. **Open Reduction of Common Fractures,** 1959. Courtesy of Grune & Stratton, Inc.)

prone to sprain. Injuries to the knee which appear to be sprains may be incomplete or complete tears of one or several major ligaments. The knee has two semilunar (half-moon in shape) cartilages which may be torn as part of an injury which includes a minor or major sprain. The first aid worker probably will be unable to determine the precise injury but he needs only to recognize that the knee has been injured and apply first aid measures for a sprain. The physician may test gently for the integrity of specific ligaments, especially in sprains of the knee. The ankle joint, supported to a large extent by ligaments, is also prone to sprain. Tears of particular ligaments may permit partial dislocation of the joint even without a fracture. Frequently, however, injuries particularly to the ankle or wrist which at first appear to be sprains turn out to be fractures. All sprains of any severity, therefore, should be considered as fractures until proven otherwise.

First aid for sprains includes recognition that the injury actually may be a fracture. Therefore, if there is the slightest doubt, splinting as for a fracture should be provided even in the emergency department of a hospital. Splinting can do no harm if, later after x-ray examination, the medical diagnosis is only a sprain; and it will provide some comfort to the patient.

First aid measures for sprains include application of a supporting bandage and ice bags or ice packs about the injured joint. Reasonable elevation, or at least avoiding the hanging position, of the injured extremity is advisable to help minimize swelling and to decrease pain. A sling should be provided for an individual with a sprain of a joint of the upper extremity (wrist, elbow, or shoulder). A person with a sprain of a joint of the lower extremity (ankle, knee, or hip) should be urged to keep the extremity somewhat elevated and to abstain from bearing weight on it and, to use crutches if they are available until a physician determines the extent of the injury. X-ray films are indicated to rule out fractures in all suspected sprains except for obviously trivial injuries as determined by a physician.

14 / Cardiorespiratory Emergencies

ARCHER S. GORDON

It is estimated that 95 percent of "time-dependent" emergencies are of a cardiorespiratory nature. They are the most urgent problems in first aid and medical rescue work. All medical and paramedical personnel, as well as professional rescuers, must be well-trained in the immediate diagnosis and effective treatment of these conditions in field and hospital situations. A slight delay in the restoration of breathing and/or circulation may mean the difference between life and death, whereas treatment of fractures, shock, burns, head injuries, and other wounds can be delayed for a short time without seriously affecting the ultimate prognosis. Only the control of massive external hemorrhage takes precedence over restoration of the cardiorespiratory functions.

Oxygen is the vital fuel of living tissues. It must be supplied and distributed constantly and in adequate amounts to these tissues. Its absence as a result of respiratory and/or circulatory failure for periods in excess of four minutes results in irreparable brain damage or death. Successful treatment of cardiorespiratory emergencies is directly related to the speed and efficiency with which it is applied (Fig. 1).

Normal Cardiorespiratory Mechanisms

Anatomically and physiologically, the heart and lungs are intimately and vitally connected. Under normal circumstances, the combined heart-lung system pumps and oxygenates the total blood volume every minute. We can restrict our discussion here almost exclusively to the mechanical functions of this system.

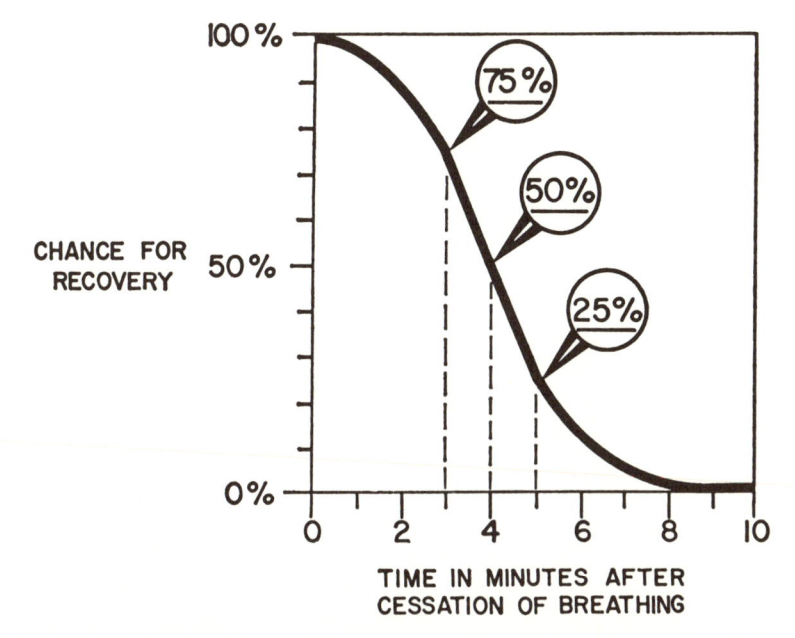

Fig. 1. Diagram illustrating the relationship between chance for recovery and time in minutes after cardiorespiratory arrest when effective resuscitation was started.

Quiet respiration has an active inspiratory and a passive expiratory phase. These result from the contraction and relaxation of two sets of muscles, the diaphragm and the intercostals. The diaphragm is a firm muscular dome which is attached to the borders of the lower ribs and separates the abdominal contents from the chest. During inspiration it contracts and descends to enlarge the thorax. This increase in chest volume increases the negative pressure in the closed pleural spaces and results in inflation of the lungs by drawing air in through the nose and mouth. During expiration the diaphragm relaxes and rises to its previous position. This reduces the size of the chest, and air is forced out of the lungs. The pistonlike action of the diaphragm is responsible for about 60 percent of normal ventilation. It is manifested clinically by the rise and fall of the abdomen during inspiration and expiration (Fig. 2A).

The action of the intercostal muscles accounts for the remaining 40 percent of normal ventilation. These muscles bridge the spaces between the ribs. Their contraction during inspiration lifts the ribs to give a bellows or gatelike action. This enlarges the chest in its

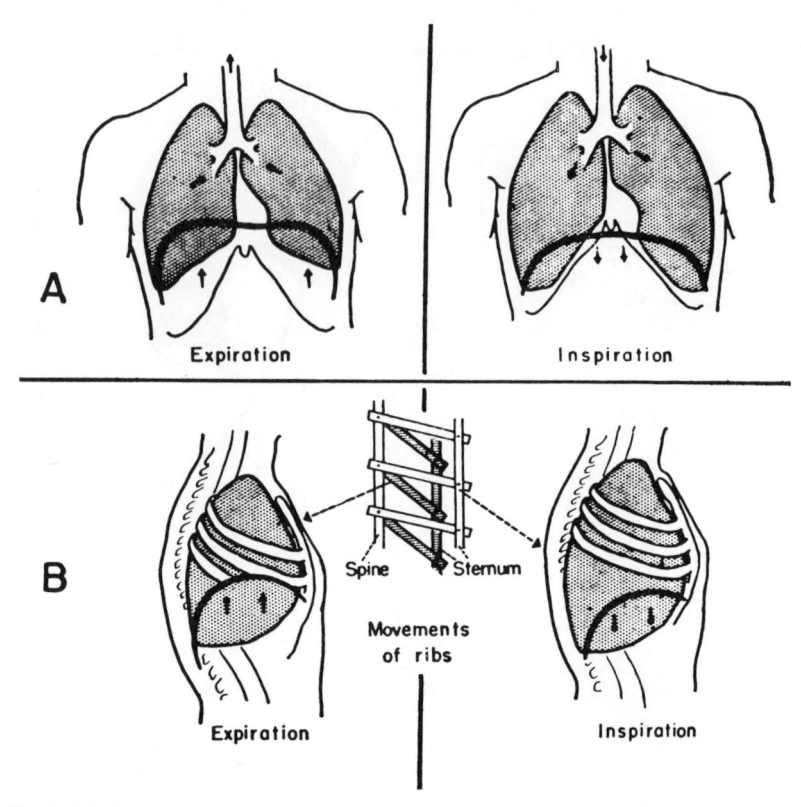

Fig. 2. Mechanisms of normal respiration. A, diaphragmatic—60 percent of ventilation. B, intercostal—40 percent of ventilation.

anteroposterior dimension and draws air into the lungs. During expiration, air is forced out of the lungs as the intercostals relax and the chest returns to its smaller resting volume (Fig. 2B).

The air drawn into the lungs contains approximately 21 percent oxygen and barely 0.04 percent carbon dioxide. The air passes through the nose and mouth, into the pharynx, between the vocal cords in the larynx, down the trachea, and into the bronchial tubes. These terminate in microscopic air sacs known as alveoli (Fig. 3).

The walls of the alveoli contain small pulmonary capillaries which carry desaturated venous blood from the body tissues. In its passage through the lungs this blood is separated from the oxygen in the alveoli by the thin capillary wall and the monocellular alveolar wall. The difference between the partial pressure of oxygen in the alveoli

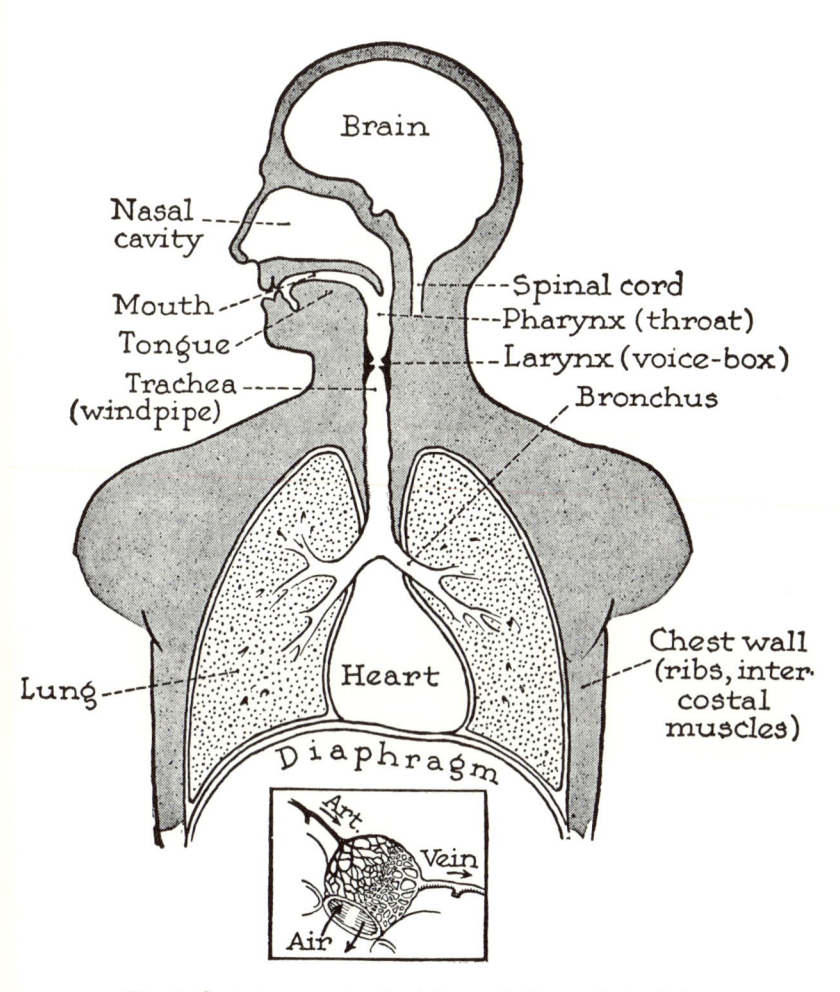

Fig. 3. Central organs involved in respiration and circulation.

and in the capillaries causes oxygen to diffuse readily into the blood. The huge surface provided by the millions of alveoli (estimated at 50 to 100 square meters) allows this exchange to occur in a fraction of a second (0.2 second).

Simultaneously with the uptake of oxygen, carbon dioxide is rapidly diffusing into the alveoli from the blood in the pulmonary capillaries. Thus, the blood returning to the left side of the heart from the lungs is enriched in oxygen and depleted of carbon dioxide.

The air exhaled from the lungs still contains approximately 16 percent oxygen plus 4 to 5 percent carbon dioxide. Oxygenation and carbon dioxide elimination occur only in the alveolar sacs, not in the bronchial tubes. These are merely conduits for the transport of air. The air which fills the mouth, pharynx, trachea, and bronchial tubes at the end of each breath is high in carbon dioxide, since it has just been exhaled from the alveoli. This is called dead space air, and the next breath must be large enough to flush this dead space volume in order to get fresh air into the alveoli. During exhalation the lung is not completely emptied. Even after a maximum expiratory effort, a residual volume of about one fourth of the total lung volume remains.

In the capillaries of the body tissues an exchange occurs which is the opposite of that just described for the alveoli. The partial pressure of oxygen is higher in the arterial blood than in the tissues, so oxygen diffuses out of the capillaries. The converse is true for carbon dioxide, and this gas passes from the tissues into the blood. The blood then is returned to the lungs to discharge its carbon dioxide and replenish its oxygen.

From the foregoing, it can be seen that the elimination of carbon dioxide is as important in the process of breathing as is the utilization of oxygen. Accumulation of carbon dioxide can be as deleterious as the inadequate uptake of oxygen. At concentrations of 8 to 10 percent carbon dioxide begins to act on the body as a depressant or anesthetic agent. This brief discussion also emphasizes the importance of an adequately functioning circulatory system in completing the process of respiration.

Respiration can be controlled voluntarily, but it is usually an involuntary act carried out automatically under the control of the central nervous system. The regular action of the diaphragm and intercostal muscles is mediated through the phrenic and intercostal nerves to these structures. The amount of oxygen and carbon dioxide in the blood exerts a strong chemical influence upon the automatic control of respiration by these higher centers.

The heart is a four-chambered pump which lies almost in the center of the chest between the sternum and the spine. It has two independent circuits, right and left. The right atrium receives desaturated venous blood under very low pressure from the caval and coronary systems. The right ventricle then pumps this blood through the lungs for oxygenation and carbon dioxide elimination. It returns to the left atrium and is ejected with much greater force (blood pressure) to the body by the left ventricle. The cardiac output in health and disease depends upon many factors. Important among these are adequate blood volume; adequate systemic and pulmonary venous return; adequate force of contraction; optimum and regular rate and rhythm; and absence from serious obstruction, regurgitation, shunts, or restriction (tamponade). The importance of these factors in cardiac resuscitation will become evident later.

The cardiac cycle has two phases, contraction (systole) and relaxation (diastole). Under normal conditions, ventricular systole occupies approximately 40 percent of each cardiac cycle and results in forceful ejection of blood to the lungs and to the body. Cardiac refill occurs as a more passive phenomenon during the longer diastole. The normal heart rate in adults varies between 60 and 80 beats per minute, each cardiac cycle requiring about one second. It is faster in children. Heart rate may be altered by exercise, emotion, stress, digestion, high environmental temperatures, and other factors which excite or depress the autonomic nervous system or upset the chemical, O_2-CO_2, acid-base, ionic, or hormonal regulatory mechanisms of the body. Disease, drug administration, blood loss, shock, fever, dehydration, sepsis, and many other conditions can affect the rate and rhythm of the heart.

Although the heart beat is regulated by nerve impulses and reflexes, it also has an inherent rhythmicity which maintains it in a beating state even after complete denervation. The quality of inherent rhythmicity also restores the heart beat after brief periods of cardiac standstill, or when the myocardium is electrically shocked into complete inactivity in the treatment of ventricular fibrillation.

TABLE 1. *Cardiopulmonary Arrest.*

Causes	
Pulmonary Arrest	*Cardiac Arrest*
1. Airway obstruction	1. Cardiovascular collapse
2. Respiratory depression	2. Ventricular fibrillation
3. Cardiac arrest	3. Cardiac standstill (Asystole)
Diagnosis	
Unconscious patient with deathlike appearance	
1. Absent breathing	1. Absent breathing
2. Cyanosis	2. Absent pulse
3. Widened pupils	3. Widened pupils

Pulmonary arrest is any condition in which there is absence or inadequacy of ventilation. It can be secondary to cardiac arrest or, if primary and persistent, it can lead to cardiac arrest. *Cardiac arrest* is any condition in which the circulation is absent or inadequate to maintain life.

When respiratory arrest is primary, the blood pressure and pulse gradually diminish and the pupils gradually dilate. Serious brain damage can occur in four to six minutes (Fig. 4A). When the precipitating cause of the emergency is circulatory arrest, the pulse and blood pressure disappear quickly, respiration ceases simultaneously or shortly thereafter, and the pupils become dilated rapidly. Severe brain damage can occur in two to four minutes under these circumstances (Fig. 4B).

PULMONARY ARREST. Pulmonary arrest occurs as a result of one or more of the three general causes listed in Table 1. Partial or

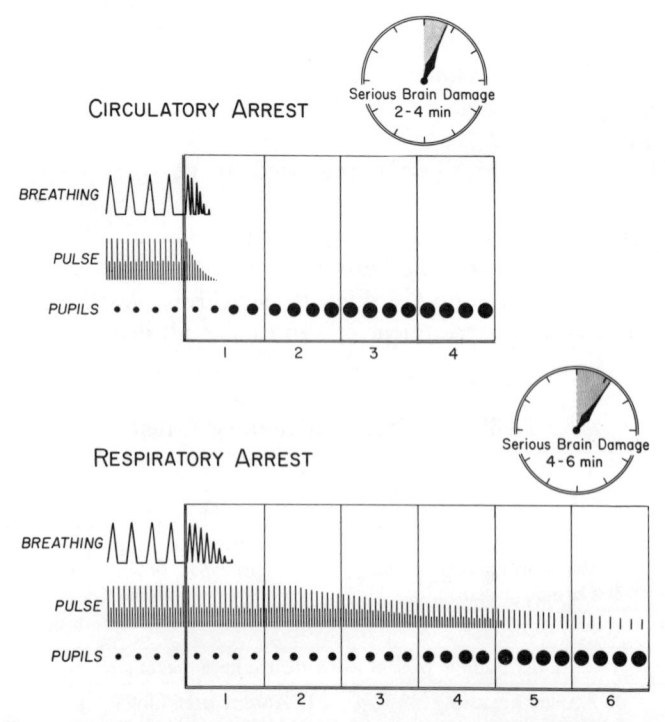

Fig. 4. Top, events following circulatory arrest. Bottom, events following respiratory arrest. (From Gordon. Cardiopulmonary Resuscitation: Conference Proceedings, National Academy of Sciences-National Research Council, Washington, D.C., 1967.)

complete airway obstruction may be: (1) Anatomic—due to the tongue blocking the pharynx. The tongue is attached to the lower jaw and floor of the mouth. In an unconscious person, relaxation of the lower jaw allows it to drop backward carrying the tongue with it to obstruct the pharynx. (2) Mechanical—due to foreign bodies, blood, mucous plugs, and so on, obstructing the pharynx, larynx, trachea, or major bronchi. (3) Pathologic—due to spasm or edema of the vocal cords or lower air passages, or to inflammation, constriction, or trauma to the tongue or lower air passages.

Injuries of the lung or chest wall may also interfere with normal ventilation. Such conditions as tension pneumothorax, crushed chest, or severe hemorrhage may threaten life by impairing ventilation and/or circulation. Their occurrence may require urgent treatment of a definitive nature. These and related conditions are covered in detail in Chapter 15.

Respiratory depression has many causes and leads to progressive anoxia and hypercarbia. In their early stages, anoxia and hypercarbia act as mild respiratory stimulants, but as they progress and deepen they produce increasing depression of the respiratory mechanisms. Respiratory depression may be caused by:

Factors acting on the central nervous system
  Overdosage of drugs—sedatives, narcotics, anesthetic agents
  Toxic gases—nerve gases, insecticides
  Disease or injury of the brain
  Disease or injury of the spinal cord

Factors acting on the respiratory system
  Submersion
  Strangulation
  Asphyxiation (smoke, smothering, and so on)
  Aspiration
  Chemicals

Factors acting on the blood and circulatory system
  Cardiac arrest
  Profound shock
  Carbon monoxide
  Cyanide poisoning
  Electrocution

CARDIAC ARREST. Cardiac arrest refers to any sudden, unexpected condition in which the circulation is absent or inadequate to maintain life. This includes three basic conditions: 1, cardiovascular collapse; 2, ventricular fibrillation; and 3, cardiac standstill (asystole).

Cardiovascular collapse occurs when there is a heart beat and usually a rhythmic electrocardiogram, but they are ineffectual in producing a peripheral pulse or blood pressure. Vasomotor collapse, syncope, profound hypothermia, central-nervous-system damage, secondary shock, serious hemorrhage, or an overdose of drugs or anesthetic agents can produce this condition. It is also known as electromechanical dissociation.

Ventricular fibrillation is uncoordinated, twitching contractions of the individual muscle fascicles of the heart. It is completely ineffectual and purposeless. When observed directly, the heart appears and feels like a "bag of worms," and there is no cardiac output. Ventricular fibrillation may occur as a primary or precipitating cause of cardiac arrest; or it may be secondary and represent a terminal or agonal state of the heart. Primary ventricular fibrillation is produced by factors which upset the delicate coordination and balance of the cardiac muscle and conduction system. This can result from low-voltage electric current (110 to 220 volts for 2 to 3 seconds duration); from sudden and severe ionic imbalance (especially potassium) such as occurs following hemolysis, fresh water drowning, or sympathetic stimulation of a myocardium sensitized by chemical or anesthetic agents (epinephrine, cyclopropane); from profound hypothermia; or from focal anoxia of the myocardium in conjunction with coronary artery spasm or obstruction.

Ventricular fibrillation which occurs as a terminal or agonal phenomenon may be noted with many conditions after a patient has been clinically dead for some time, and the myocardium may continue to fibrillate long after all body functions have ceased irreversibly. Terminal, secondary ventricular fibrillation should be distinguished from the sudden primary ventricular fibrillation described above, since only the latter can be effectively treated by emergency cardio-pulmonary (heart-lung) resuscitation.

When *Cardiac standstill (asystole)* occurs, the ventricles are essentially motionless and no blood is ejected from either the right or left heart. This is usually a manifestation of severe generalized anoxia or local myocardial anoxia resulting from any condition which impairs oxygenation of the blood.

When a sudden unexpected cardiac arrest occurs, it is not important initially to diagnose whether the cause is cardiovascular collapse, ventricular fibrillation, or cardiac standstill. When there is an unconscious patient with a deathlike appearance, absent pulse and widening pupils—do not waste time—begin external heart-lung resuscitation at once (also called cardiopulmonary resuscitation or CPR).

Principles of Emergency Heart-Lung Resuscitation (Cardiopulmonary Resuscitation—CPR)

A—Airway opened
B—Breathing restored
C—Circulation restored
D—Definitive therapy
   D—Diagnosis (ECG)
   D—Drugs
   D—Defibrillation

The basic principles and techniques for emergency heart-lung resuscitation are simple to comprehend, to practice, and to perform. The A-B-C-D order shown above is not just a mnemonic of convenience. These steps should be performed quickly, precisely, and in this specific order. Speed is vital. Do not waste time seeking an exact diagnosis, moving the victim, looking for help, or procuring adjunctive equipment. Begin these steps at once.

A—AIRWAY OPENED. Regardless of whether the cardiorespiratory emergency involves respiratory and/or cardiac arrest, ventilation of the lungs must be provided. This is dependent upon a patent airway.

In an unconscious patient the head flexes; the relaxed lower jaw drops backward; and the tongue, which is attached to the jaw and the floor of the mouth, obstructs the pharynx. This is the condition which has erroneously been termed "swallowing the tongue" (Fig. 5A).

This anatomic obstruction can be eliminated by anterior displacement of the lower jaw or by inserting an oropharyngeal airway. Such airways may not be available, spasm of the jaw muscles may prevent their insertion, or the rescuer may not be trained in their use. Therefore, for the emergency situation the air passage should be opened by manual positioning of the head. Various methods can be used for this. These include grasping the lower jaw between the

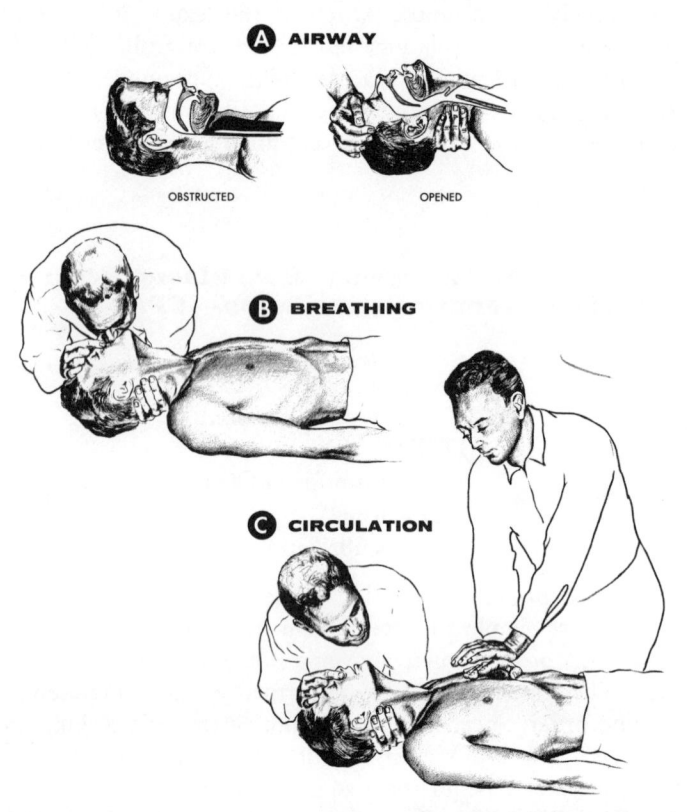

Fig. 5. ABC principles of emergency heart-lung resuscitation. (From Gordon. Cardiopulmonary Resuscitation, NAS-NRC Committee on CPR. **J.A.M.A.**, 198:4, 372-379, October, 1966.)

thumb and index finger and lifting the jaw upward, or placing the fingers behind the angles of the jaw and pushing it upward.

But the simplest, quickest, and best method for opening and maintaining the airway is maximum extension of the head. This stretches the neck and draws the jaw and tongue forward. Contrary to the popular notion, placing the victim in the prone position does not clear the air passage because the neck frequently remains flexed. In actual practice the proper way to open the airway is to lift the neck with one hand and tilt the head back with the other hand, so that the chin is pointing almost vertically upward.

B—BREATHING RESTORED, ARTIFICIAL RESPIRATION. (Mouth-to-Mouth Resuscitation; Mouth-to-Nose Resuscitation; Expired Air Inflation; Rescue Breathing). Mouth-to-mouth resuscitation has been proven experimentally and clinically to be the most effective technique for emergency artificial respiration. No adjuncts are required, and it can be started immediately. Since the victim is placed in the supine position and ventilation is accomplished by the rescuer's expired air, his hands are free at all times to maintain the patent airway achieved by the head-tilt method.

With the air passage maintained open by maximum extension of the head, as described above, the rescuer seals the victim's nose (to prevent the escape of air) by pinching it shut with his thumb and index finger. He takes a deep breath, opens his mouth widely, places it over the victim's mouth, and makes a tight seal. He then quickly blows a full breath into the victim's mouth until he feels the resistance of the expanding lung and sees the chest rise. The rescuer then removes his mouth and allows the victim to exhale passively (Fig. 5B).

For adult patients this cycle is repeated every five seconds, a rate of 12 times per minute. Each breath should provide at least 1,000 ml, or twice the normal resting tidal volume. Since expired air contains approximately 16 percent oxygen and 4 to 5 percent carbon dioxide, this degree of hyperventilation assures normal oxygenation and carbon-dioxide elimination of the victim's blood. If the rescuer develops hyperventilation alkalosis, as manifested by numbness, tingling, dizziness, paresthesias, or ringing in the ears, he should slow his rate or reduce the amplitude of each breath. With practice, it is possible to simplify the technique by the rescuer sealing the victim's nose with his cheek.

Effective artificial respiration can also be achieved by mouth-to-nose resuscitation. For this method, it is equally important for the rescuer to open his mouth widely and secure a tight seal about the victim's nose. He keeps the victim's head tilted back with one hand and uses his other hand to push the chin upward in order to close the mouth and seal the lips to prevent air leakage during inflation of the lungs via the nose.

The technique is essentially the same for infants and small children, with several exceptions. The rescuer places his mouth over the mouth and nose of these small faces and inflates the lungs about 20 to 30 times per minute, varying the amount according to the size of the child. This can be determined by watching the chest rise and fall and by feeling the resistance of the expanding lungs. Tiny babies only require small puffs of air from the rescuer's mouth and cheeks.

Practical studies and clinical experiences have shown that the three most common errors by rescuers in performing mouth-to-mouth resuscitation are 1, inadequate extension of the victim's head; 2, failure to open his own mouth widely; and 3, forgetting to seal the victim's nose or mouth. Special attention should be given to these points during practice sessions and during actual emergency resuscitation.

C—CIRCULATION RESTORED, ARTIFICIAL CIRCULATION. (External Cardiac Compression; Closed-Chest Cardiac Compression; External Cardiac Resuscitation). Until recently there was no emergency first aid treatment available when the diagnosis of cardiac arrest was made. In 1960, the development of external cardiac compression resolved this dilemma. This method is called external cardiac massage by some, but this is an unfortunate eponymic error. When the chest is opened and the heart is manually squeezed internally, this may correctly be called internal cardiac massage, since the squeezing of the myocardium is truly a massagelike action (although internal cardiac compression is a better term). However, external cardiac resuscitation accomplished by exerting pressure on the chest should be called external cardiac compression, or one of the alternate terms noted above.

Since the heart lies almost in the middle of the chest between the sternum and the spine, firm pressure over the lower sternum will compress the ventricles and produce a cardiac output during standstill, ventricular fibrillation, or circulatory collapse. In the human, lateral displacement of the heart is prevented during compression of the chest because it is relatively well-fixed by the mediastinum and the pericardial sac. External cardiac compression should be performed with careful attention to details in order to provide satisfactory blood flow and to avoid trauma (Figs. 6 and 7).

To assure compression of the heart, the victim must be on a firm surface. This can be the floor, a firm litter, operating table, or a board placed under the chest of a patient in bed. The operator can place one of his hands under the back to provide firm support for small children or babies.

The rescuer places the heel of one hand in the center of the

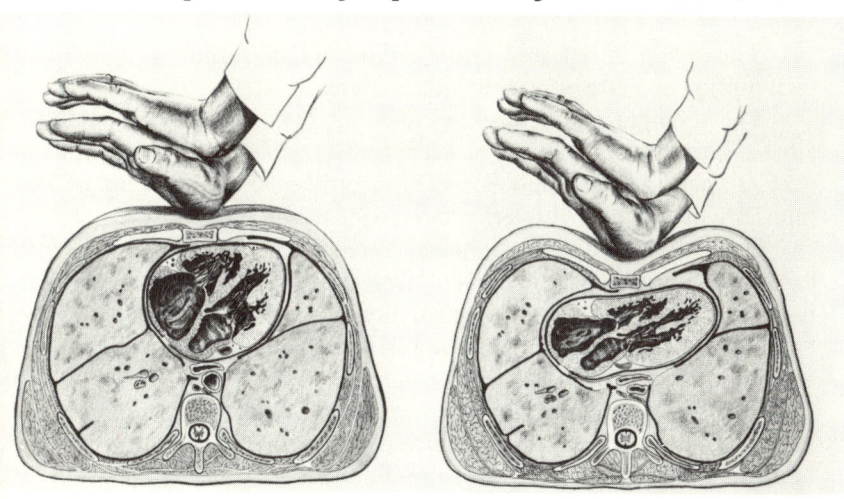

Principles of Emergency Heart-Lung Resuscitation / 209

Fig. 6. Thorax cross section showing placement of hands and movement of chest during external compression. (From Gordon. Cardiopulmonary Resuscitation: Conference Proceedings, National Academy of Sciences-National Research Council, Washington, D.C., 1967.)

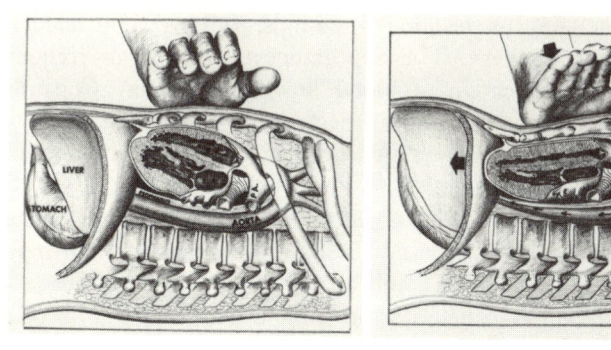

Fig. 7. Sagittal section of body showing placement of hands and movement of chest and abdomen during external cardiac compression. (From Gordon. Cardiopulmonary Resuscitation: Conference Proceedings, National Academy of Sciences-National Research Council, Washington, D.C., 1967.)

chest over the lower half of the body of the sternum (but not over the xiphoid process). The other hand is placed on top of this.

He then rocks forward keeping his arms straight and uses the weight of the upper part of his body to exert 80 to 120 pounds of pressure. This should move the sternum approximately one and one half to two inches. His hands are kept in place as he releases the pressure.

This cycle is repeated once per second uniformly and without interruption at a rate of 60 times per minute.

The compression:relaxation ratio (systole:diastole) should be 50:50. This smooth and regular rhythm provides satisfactory blood flow, allows adequate time for cardiac refill, and avoids some of the injuries which occur with jerky and irregular ratios.

Only the heel of one hand is required to perform external cardiac compression on children under eight years of age. The other hand can be used to provide firm support beneath the chest. Only two fingers are required to compress the center of the sternum on a baby or very small child.

Properly performed external cardiac compression produces a blood pressure with systolic peaks of 100 mm of Hg, or over, in humans and experimental animals. This will frequently produce a carotid or femoral pulse and provides evidence of effective artificial circulation. However, measured blood flow to the brain with this method seldom exceeds 25 to 30 percent of the normal flow (Fig. 8). Experimental studies and clinical experiences have shown that this amount is adequate for prolonged periods, followed by successful resuscitation and recovery. The appearance of the pupils frequently provides the best indication of blood flow to the brain. Constricted pupils indicate adequate cerebral perfusion; widely dilated pupils are evidence of inadequate oxygenation of the brain and imminent death.

External cardiac compression alone does not produce adequate ventilation of the lungs. It must be used in conjunction with mouth-to-mouth resuscitation. This combination of artificial respiration and artificial circulation is called Cardiopulmonary Resuscitation (CPR) or Heart-Lung Resuscitation (HLR). Optimum performance and effectiveness is achieved when there are two rescuers using a 5 to 1 ratio of compression to ventilation.

One rescuer at the side of the victim compresses the chest rhythmically, smoothly, and with no interruptions at a rate of once a second, 60 times per minute, as described above. The other rescuer "interposes" one breath between every five chest compressions. A series of chest compressions followed by a pause during which the lungs are inflated should be avoided. The 5 to 1 technique with "interposed" breaths allows the external cardiac compression to continue at a uniform, uninterrupted rate of 60 times per minute with full lung inflation 12 times per minute between each five compres-

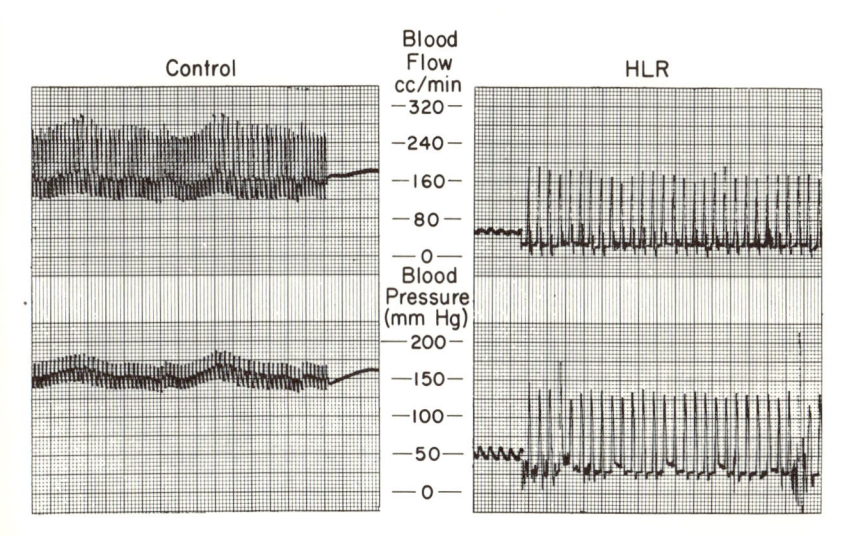

Fig. 8. Blood flow and blood pressure in the carotid artery during well-performed, uninterrupted heart-lung resuscitation. Breaths are "interposed" between each five external cardiac compressions.

sions. The "interposed" technique produces the best oxygenation, blood flow, and blood pressure. When there is a pause for inflation between each series of compressions, the compression and ventilation rates are reduced, the mean arterial blood pressure and blood flow are reduced, and the oxygen saturation and carbon-dioxide elimination are reduced.

When heart-lung resuscitation must be performed by only one rescuer, the best technique is to compress the chest 15 times and then quickly extend the head and inflate the lungs two times. Then quickly repeat this 15 to 2 cycle of compression and ventilation. Since there is only one rescuer, he must interrupt the chest compressions in order to ventilate the lungs. These pauses make it impossible to achieve a chest compression rate of 60 per minute when a rate of once a second is used. Therefore, it is necessary for the single rescuer to compress the chest somewhat faster—at a rate which would provide 80 compressions per minute if continued without interruptions—in order to compensate for the ventilatory pauses and produce an actual chest compression rate of 60 per minute.

Heart-lung resuscitation can and should be continued for long periods of time when necessary. Full recovery has occurred in humans following immediate and effective cardiopulmonary resuscitation without interruption for periods in excess of one hour. When artificial respiration and artificial circulation are prolonged, careful attention must be directed to performing them urgently, uniformly, and uninterruptedly. When facilities become available for airway intubation, intravenous fluids, drugs, electrocardiography and external defibrillation, these should be instituted without any interruption of heart-lung resuscitation.

One of the most important rules to follow is:

> **NEVER INTERRUPT HEART-LUNG RESUSCITATION FOR MORE THAN 5 SECONDS FOR ANY REASON**

Complications of CPR

Injuries can occur as a result of external cardiac compression. Costochondral separation and rib fractures are a common occurrence and sometimes cannot be avoided when external cardiac compression is performed with adequate vigor to produce a peripheral pulse. This type of injury is a small price to pay for a successful resuscitation. Careful attention to details will help to minimize these and other injuries. The rescuer must constantly remind himself 1, keep only the heel of one hand on the sternum; 2, do not press on the chest with the fingers or the rest of the palm; 3, keep the hand over the lower half of the sternum only; 4, do not compress over the xiphoid process; 5, press vertically downward so that pressure is not exerted laterally on the rib cage; and 6, use a smooth 50:50 compression:relaxation ratio in order to avoid sudden and jerky movements.

Bone-marrow emboli have been found in the lungs of victims expiring after the application of external cardiac compression. However, it is worthy of note that bone-marrow emboli are also found post-mortem in the lungs of a significant number of people who have not received external cardiac compression, and it has never been proved that these minute emboli were the cause of death in any of these cases. Furthermore, it is obvious that during a cardiorespiratory emergency, these patients would have had no opportunity for survival without external cardiac compression.

Serious damage to the heart does not result from external cardiac compression, unless there is a ventricular aneurysm secondary to a previous myocardial infarction. It has been shown that under ordinary circumstances, external cardiac compression is less traumatic to the heart than is internal cardiac massage. Since ventricular aneurysms are not a common occurrence, since their presence cannot be diagnosed at the time of the cardiorespiratory emergency, since rupture of the heart may occur in their presence with either external or internal cardiac compression, and since this is the only treatment available when death is imminent from cardiac arrest, external cardiac compression is justified even where this lesion exists.

Damage to the lungs can occur secondary to rib fractures, but this is seldom of a serious nature. Forceful inflation of the lungs simultaneously with compression of the chest may create enough intrathoracic force to rupture pulmonary blebs or bullae. This possibility is another reason for "interposing" breaths between chest compressions.

The most serious and lethal complication of external cardiac compression is laceration of the liver. This can usually be attributed to placement of the hands too low. This is the reason for stressing the importance of compressing only the lower half of the body of the sternum, not over the xiphoid process or the epigastrium. Proper training should help to avoid this complication.

External cardiac compression is preferable to internal cardiac compression for the treatment of cardiac arrest both inside and outside of the hospital, when personnel trained in its use are available. There are few advocates of open-chest cardiac resuscitation outside of the hospital. Most authorities feel that internal cardiac compression should be restricted to the operating room and/or hospital, and then only in specific situations, e.g., (1) when cardiac arrest occurs in the operating room and the chest is already open; (2) multiple serious rib fractures, or crushed chest syndrome; (3) inadequate knowledge, training, or experience with external cardiac resuscitation; and (4) in cases where the rescuer feels that he is not getting adequate circulation and/or ventilation with the closed method. This last would particularly include such lesions as tension pneumothorax, cardiac tamponade, and cardiac lacerations, injuries, and aneurysms.

Training in Heart-Lung Resuscitation

The foregoing A-B-C principles of heart-lung resuscitation are relatively simple. However, for medical and paramedical personnel and professional rescuers, proper performance should be assured by actual training and practice. This is now possible through the use of life-size and lifelike resuscitation training manikins. These are constructed specifically so that the rescuer can practice opening the air passage by extending the head, inflating the lungs by mouth-to-mouth and mouth-to-nose resuscitation, and producing artificial circulation by external cardiac compression. Proper head extension and ventilation cause the chest to rise and fall; proper external cardiac compression provides a palpable pulse in the neck and a measurable systolic blood pressure of 100 mm of Hg, or over. These devices should be a part of every good training program in emergency first aid and heart-lung resuscitation (Fig. 9).

Other Considerations

CPR FOR INFANTS AND SMALL CHILDREN (Fig. 10). The technique of cardiopulmonary resuscitation is basically the same for infants and small children. However, there are a few major differences.

For infants and small children the rescuer need only compress the chest with two fingers, the index and middle fingers of one hand. The other hand should be placed under the thorax to provide firm support. This is the preferred method, but two alternate techniques are recommended by some: (1) the rescuer's hands can encircle the infant's chest and pressure is exerted with the two thumbs over the sternum; (2) the infant is turned on his side, one hand encircles the upper hemithorax and the index and middle finger are used to compress the sternum.

The fingers are placed higher on the chest, at about the midsternum. This is at the nipple line of an infant. The infant's chest is shorter from neck to diaphragm and the liver is proportionately larger and more cephalad. Special care must be used to avoid pressure over the liver.

The compression rate should be faster, about 100 to 120 per

Other Considerations / 215

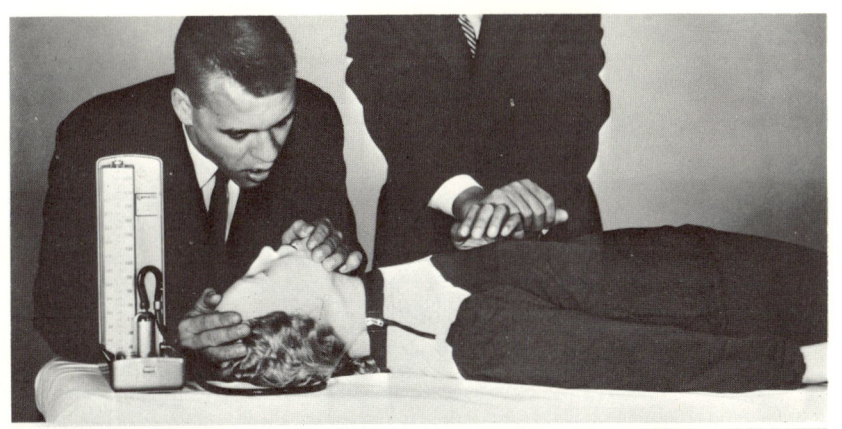

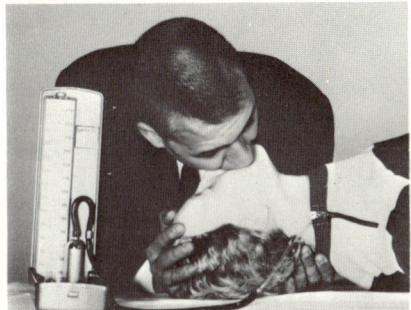

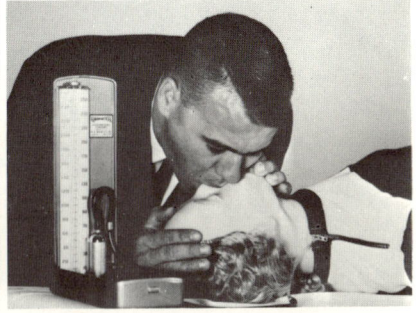

Fig. 9. Practice and training in heart-lung resuscitation using a lifelike and lifesize Resusci-Anne training manikin. Top, external cardiac compression and artificial respiration. Bottom left, mouth-to-mouth resuscitation. Bottom right, mouth-to-nose resuscitation. (Courtesy of Laerdal Medical Corporation, Tuckahoe, N.Y.)

minute. The amount of pressure used should be gauged to compress the sternum about 20 percent of the anteroposterior diameter of the chest.

For artificial respiration, the rescuer covers the mouth and nose of the victim with his mouth. He interposes breaths between each five compressions keeping the head in maximum extension as described previously. Infants and small children only require small breaths from the rescuer's mouth and cheeks to provide adequate lung inflation. Excessive volume tends to force air into the stomach and can produce serious gastric distension.

Larger children only require chest compression by the heel of one hand of the rescuer. This should also be at the mid-sternum and the other hand can be used to provide support beneath the thorax.

FIRM BLOW TO THE CHEST. It has been recommended by some that the first action in any cardiac arrest should be a firm blow (or

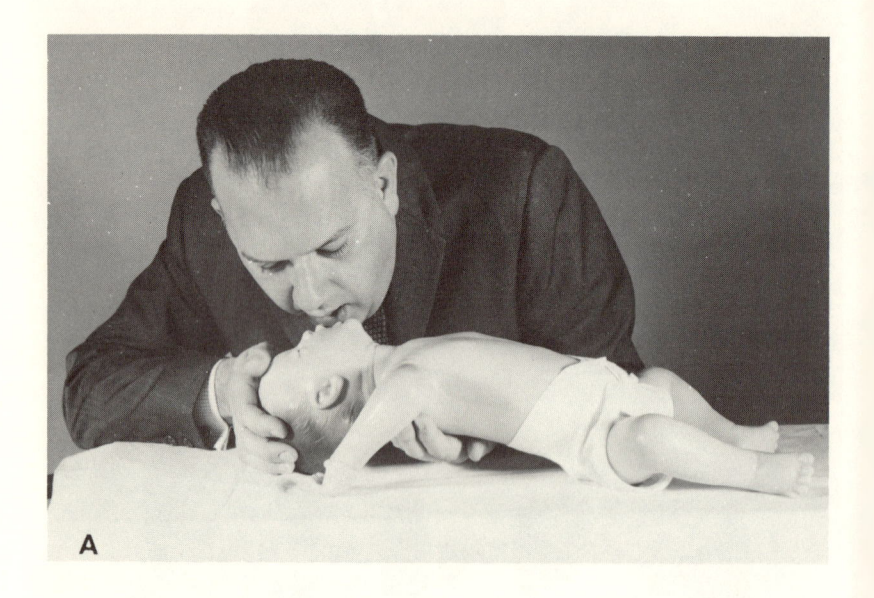

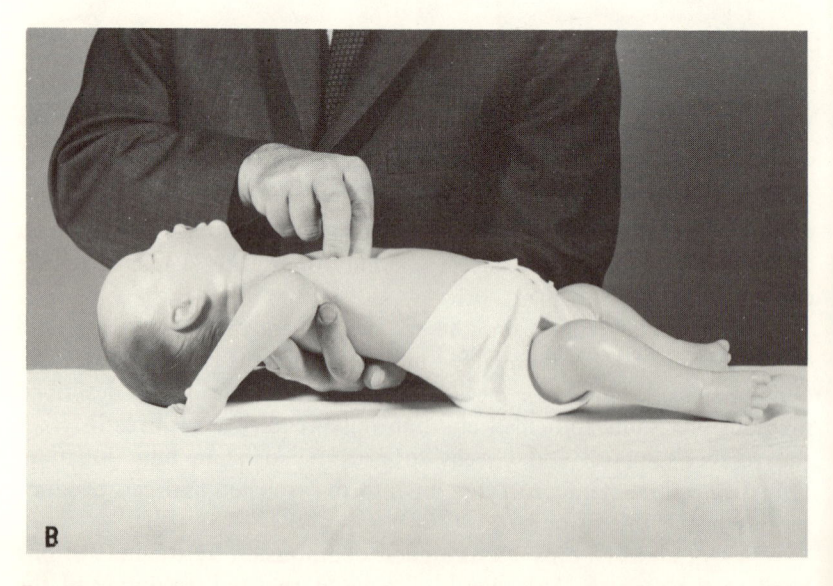

Fig. 10. A, technique of mouth-to-mouth resuscitation for infants and small children. B, technique of external cardiac compression for infants and small children. (From Gordon. Cardiopulmonary Resuscitation: Conference Proceedings, National Academy of Sciences-National Research Council, Washington, D.C., 1967. Courtesy of Laedral Medical Corp., Tuckahoe, N.Y.)

series of blows) on the sternum. This is an erroneous concept that has been promoted widely.

It has been known for many years that patients with heart-block (Stokes-Adams Disease) suffer from periodic episodes of asystole which can frequently be restored to a rhythmic beat by any stimulus to the heart, including a blow over the sternum or precordium. When such patients are being monitored on an ECG or oscilloscope and a cardiac standstill is noted, a blow to the chest is a quick and appropriate action to try to restore a heart beat. If it restores rhythmic electric activity and a peripheral pulse, this is a successful resuscitation. If not, the A-B-C's of emergency heart-lung resuscitation must be started at once.

However, the so-called firm blow to the chest only provides an adequate stimulus for the patient with heart-block. It should be reserved only for monitored patients who are suspected of having this condition. Actual studies show that, at best, it only provides as much blood flow and blood pressure in the coronary and carotid arteries as effectively performed heart-lung resuscitation. It is ineffectual as a treatment for ventricular fibrillation or other forms of cardiac standstill. If used routinely as the first step in resuscitation emergencies, much valuable time is lost in frantically delivering repeated blows to the chest and trying to determine if a peripheral pulse has been restored. Therefore, in all other resuscitation emergencies, always start cardiopulmonary resuscitation immediately and only use the blow-to-the-chest technique for monitored Stokes-Adams patients.

GASTRIC DISTENSION AND VOMITING. Excessive airway pressure applied during any form of mouth-to-mouth or mouth-to-adjunct resuscitation can result in gastric distension. This occurs very frequently in children whose stomachs sometimes become massively distended. It is also common in adults. Gastric distension is deleterious in several ways. The enlarged stomach elevates the diaphragm and reduces ventilation of the lungs. Massive gastric distension increases intraabdominal pressure which reduces venous return to the heart, thereby reducing cardiac output. It may also promote vomiting with subsequent aspiration of gastric contents into the lung.

Gastric distension should be prevented, if possible, by avoiding excessive inflation pressure or volume. When it occurs, it should be relieved as soon as feasible. Endotracheal intubation is the best measure since the use of a cuffed endotracheal tube prevents gas from entering the stomach and eliminates the hazard of vomited material being aspirated into the lungs. However, since it must be performed quickly and correctly to avoid delays in CPR, its application is limited to anesthesiologists, anesthetists, and other highly trained persons.

Another technique which has been recommended is the blind passage of a cuffed esophageal tube down to the mid-esophagus. Inflation of the cuff prevents air from entering the stomach, or gastric contents from leaving it. This should be easier to perform than endotracheal intubation, but there has been inadequate experience to recommend this technique at this time.

There are several emergency measures which can be taken to relieve gastric distension and prevent aspiration. In the unconscious patient, manual decompression of the stomach is the simplest and most expedient maneuver for both children and adults (Figs. 11A and B). They should be turned up onto their side with the head rotated further to the side. The rescuer then exerts firm pressure with one hand over the victim's epigastrium. In the unconscious patient this will eliminate both gas and liquid. This pressure should be maintained, if possible, or repeated periodically in order to avoid recurrence. If available, a nasogastric tube can be passed without interrupting resuscitation and can be used to keep the stomach decompressed.

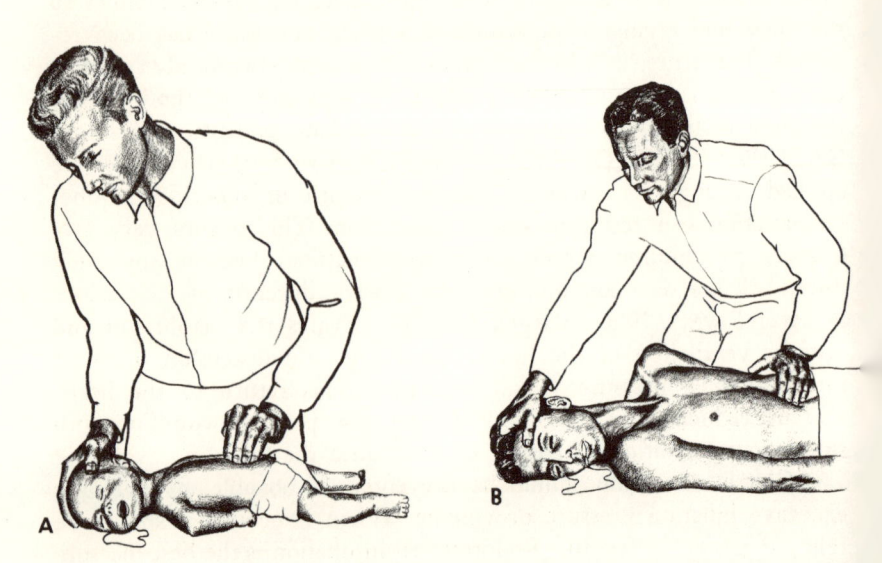

Fig. 11 A and B. Gastric decompression of infant and adult by turning head to side and exerting moderate pressure over epigastrium.

It has also been recommended that firm pressure on the cricoid cartilage will cause it to compress the upper esophagus, thereby preventing air from passing into the stomach or fluids from being regurgitated.

AIRWAY OBSTRUCTION. Another critical consideration in emergency resuscitation is obstruction of the airway by foreign material.

The exact incidence of foreign body obstruction of the airway is unknown, and it varies significantly under specific circumstances. In most resuscitation emergencies first tilt back the head and begin mouth-to-mouth resuscitation. Then if unable to inflate the lungs when the victim's head is in the proper position, quickly seek some obstruction by sweeping your fingers deeply into the upper air passages. Following drowning there will usually be aspirated material in the airway. Much of this can be cleared with the fingers, sometimes covered with a clean cloth or handkerchief. Dental plates and bridges should be removed whenever found.

The most serious airway obstructions result from food or other objects which are aspirated into the larynx. This is more common in children but also occurs frequently in adults. When this occurs, the victim usually coughs and chokes, sometimes violently, in an effort to expel the object. Back slapping at this stage is contraindicated. If unsuccessful in expelling the foreign body, the victim becomes anoxic, with progressive cyanosis and unconsciousness.

Attempts to reach and extricate the foreign body are usually fruitless. The reason for this is that they are usually impacted by the glottic musculature. The normal defense mechanism of the glottis results in severe spasm of its muscles and the vocal chords. This keeps the foreign body from passing into the trachea and also keeps it from being expelled. At this stage, the best emergency measure is to invert a child or roll an adult onto his side and deliver repeated firm blows with the heel of your hand directly over the spine between the shoulder blades. This will sometimes jar the obstruction loose (Figs. 12A and B).

After a quick series of blows again place the victim on his back and attempt to ventilate his lungs by mouth-to-mouth resuscitation. Blow hard and slowly. Sometimes you can get enough air past the obstruction to keep the patient alive until some more definitive action can be taken. Do not be concerned about forcing a foreign body deeper into the lungs. These are usually supralaryngeal and do not pass

220 / Ch. 14: Cardiorespiratory Emergencies

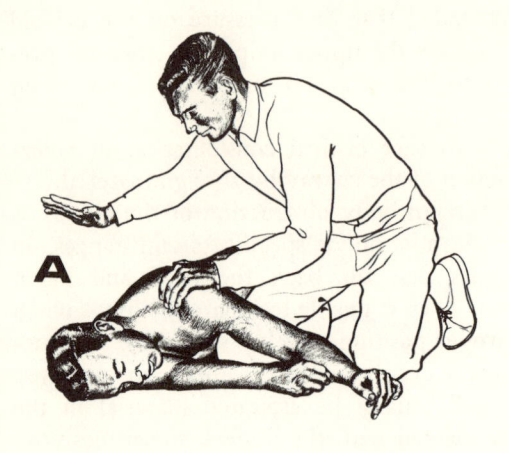

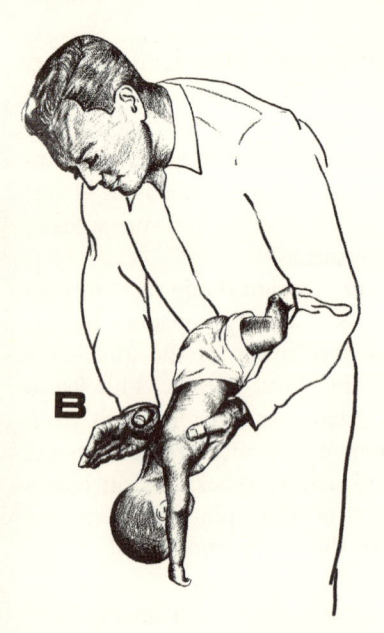

Fig. 12. Deliver firm blows over the spine between the shoulder blades to dislodge a foreign body: (A) in the airway of an adult, or (B) in the airway of a child.

through the chords. If below the chords, you can only hope to force the object down the trachea and into one major bronchus so the patient can breathe or be ventilated through the other one.

Repeat the blows on the back. Then try to ventilate him again. Persist. As the patient becomes more anoxic, the muscular spasm begins to relax. Now your chances of dislodging the foreign body are improved. Do not give up too soon.

In situations where partial ventilation cannot be achieved by artificial ventilation, or where foreign bodies cannot be dislodged by firm blows on the back, or where trained personnel are not available to visualize and remove the object, or where injury, swelling, or edema have caused the upper airway problem, it may be necessary to resort to other methods. These include the use of needle tracheostomy, tracheotomes, cricothyrotomy, and tracheostomy.

Needle tracheostomy has been recommended by some as the simplest and quickest method for establishing an opening in the trachea when the upper air passages are blocked (Fig. 13). The rescuer feels and fixes the trachea with one hand. He then takes a #12 gauge needle and advances it into the trachea. Although this will establish a channel for ventilation, it is not usually adequate to sustain an adult patient. Furthermore, its introduction is fraught with hazards to surrounding structures, particularly in children. A variant of this technique is provided by the *tracheotome*. This instrument has a slotted needle which is introduced as detailed above. A blade is inserted into the slot in the needle and forced through the skin and tracheal wall carrying a tracheostomy tube into place in the trachea. This concept is logical and unique. However, the force required to thrust the blade and tube into place has resulted in such dire complications as tracheoesophageal fistulae, bilateral pneumothorax, hemo-

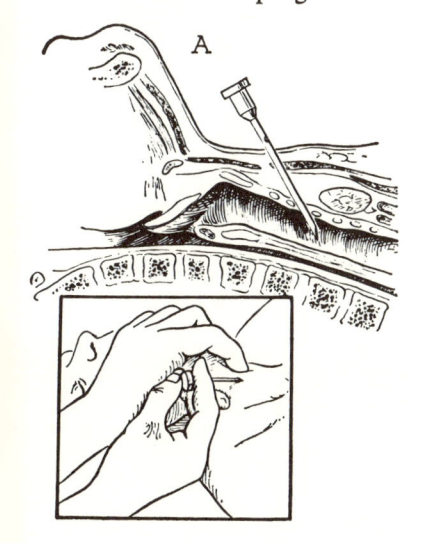

Fig. 13. Large-caliber needle in the trachea to establish an emergency airway.

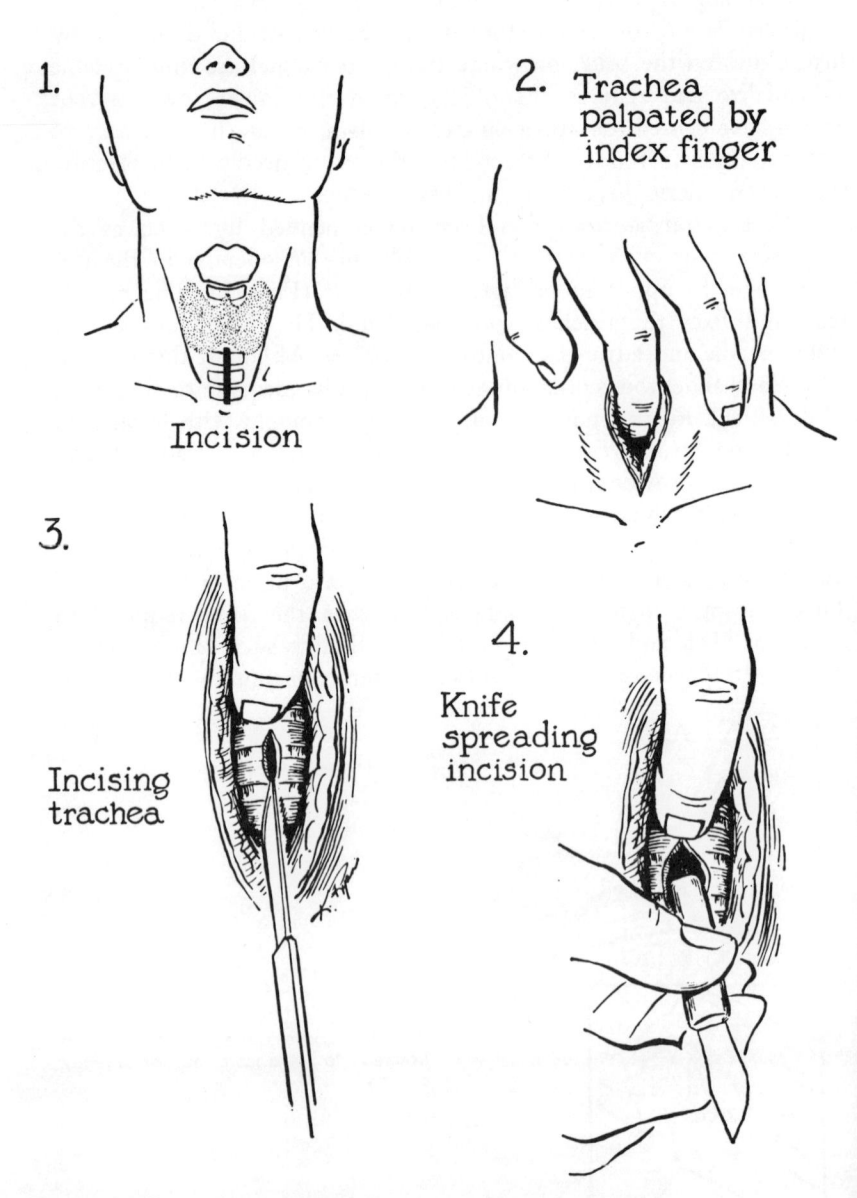

Fig. 14. Technique for emergency tracheostomy.

pneumomediastinum, and carotid artery laceration. Accordingly, the use of tracheotomes and needle tracheostomies is not recommended.

Tracheostomy can be a life-assuring procedure for numerous conditions which require by-pass of the upper airway, reduction of the respiratory dead space, or relief of the work of breathing. Under the usual circumstances, it is a routine procedure carried out electively or on a semiemergency basis. However, emergency tracheostomy performed as a life-saving measure in a resuscitation emergency can be a harrowing experience. Special instruments and medical personnel are usually required for this, although it has occasionally been accomplished by relatively untrained individuals using a pocketknife. The technique for emergency tracheostomy is shown in Figure 14. With the neck extended, the operator spreads the skin over the trachea to make it tense. He then makes a single vertical incision, which is extended in the midline down to the trachea after palpating it with his finger. Several tracheal rings are then incised and the knife handle or some other blunt instrument is used to spread the edges of the tracheal incision.

As indicated above, the use of needle tracheotomy, tracheotome, and emergency tracheostomy have inadequacies and hazards in emergency resuscitation situations. Unless adequate time, trained personnel and proper equipment are available to perform a proper tracheostomy, the fastest, simplest, and most effective technique for establishing an emergency airway is *cricothyrotomy* (Fig. 15). The neck is extended and a knife, blade or razor is used to make a short puncture-incision between the thyroid and cricoid cartilages. This is the area where the airway is closest to the surface, being covered only by skin, subcutaneous tissue, and cricothyroid membrane. After the incision is made it can be held open with a blunt instrument, or a tube or cannula can be inserted. However, incisions in the cricothyroid membrane are prone to leave an internal scar which can cause stenosis of the airway. Therefore, the cricothyrotomy should be converted to a routine tracheotomy as soon as possible.

Equipment for Resuscitation

AIRWAY ADJUNCTS. Esthetic considerations have resulted in the development of a wide assortment of mechanical airway adjuncts which avoid direct mouth-to-mouth contact during emergency resuscitation. Some of these are useful, some of them are not. In no case

224 / Ch. 14: Cardiorespiratory Emergencies

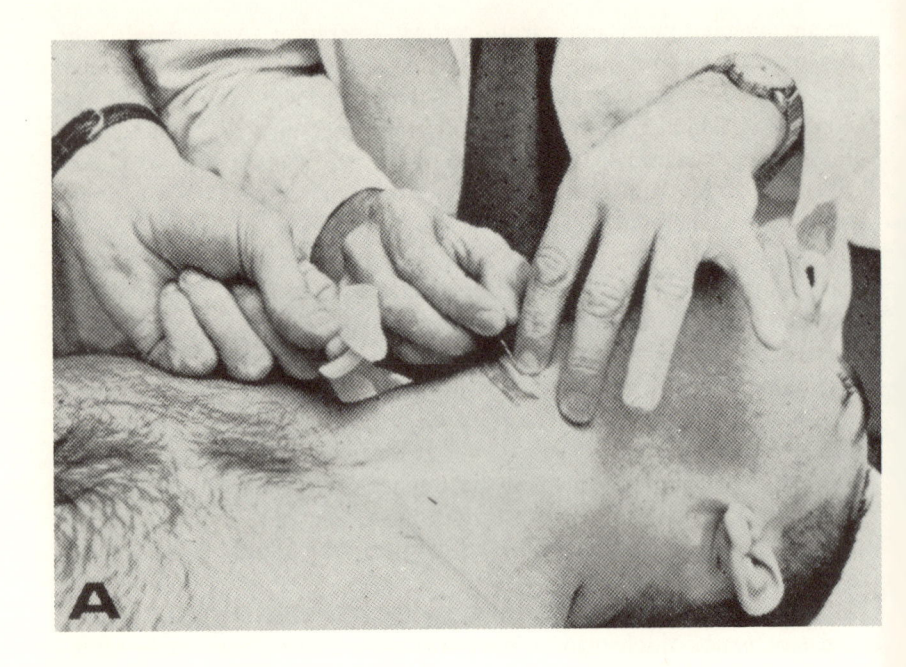

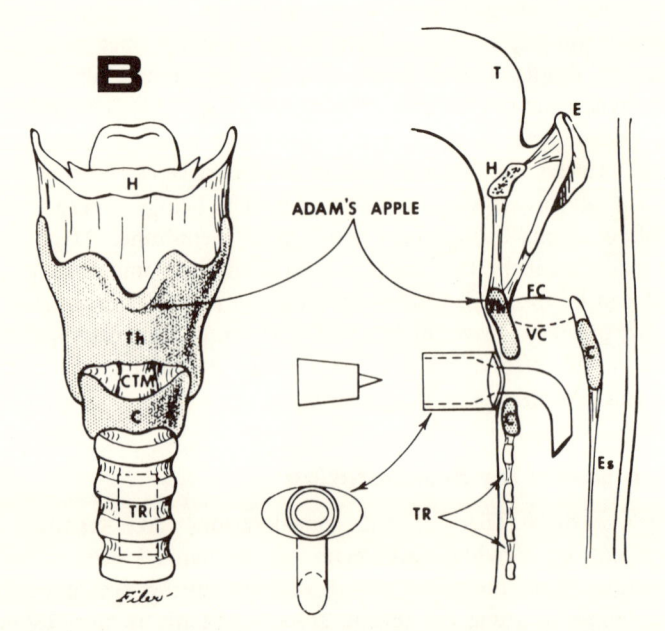

Fig. 15. A and B. Technique and anatomy for emergency cricothyrotomy.

does use of such equipment improve the method. Valuable time must never be lost in seeking such devices. Direct mouth-to-mouth or mouth-to-nose resuscitation must be started at once. Adjunctive equipment is useful only when it becomes available and if the rescuer has adequate knowledge of its performance. For emergency use, the simpler such devices are, the better. A clean handkerchief or gauze square frequently provides the best and most readily available adjunct when it is desired to avoid direct contact. This imposes no serious impediment to easy inflation of the lungs.

Emergency airway adjuncts can be divided into two basic types, oral or oropharyngeal airways and face masks (Figs. 16A and B). These are available as simple devices with no valves, or in combination with valving mechanisms. In all instances the simpler devices are easier and more effective to use. A simple transparent plastic mask with a well-fitting inflatable cuff provides the most effective adjunctive device. It is readily available, allows the rescuer to use both hands to provide a good seal and keep the head tilted back, shows the victim's exhalation by condensation on the mask and permits visualization of the lips for cyanosis and the mouth for vomitus. Medical, nursing, and paramedical personnel can use it to provide good pulmonary ventilation with minimal training. The S-tube or double oropharyngeal airway is almost equally effective. Other airway adjuncts are not recommended.

BAG/VALVE/MASK DEVICES (Fig. 16C). A wide assortment of bag/valve/mask devices has become available commercially to medical and paramedical personnel. Although their general design is similar, most of them have serious defects. There are three major

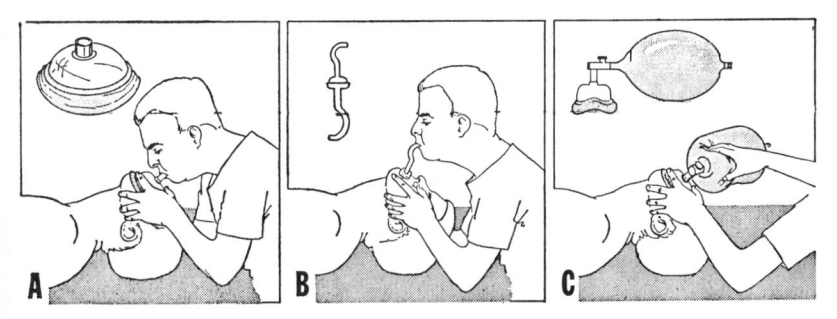

Fig. 16. Adjunctive equipment for inflation of the lungs. A, ordinary face mask. B, double oropharyngeal airway. C, mask with self-inflating bag and nonrebreathing valve.

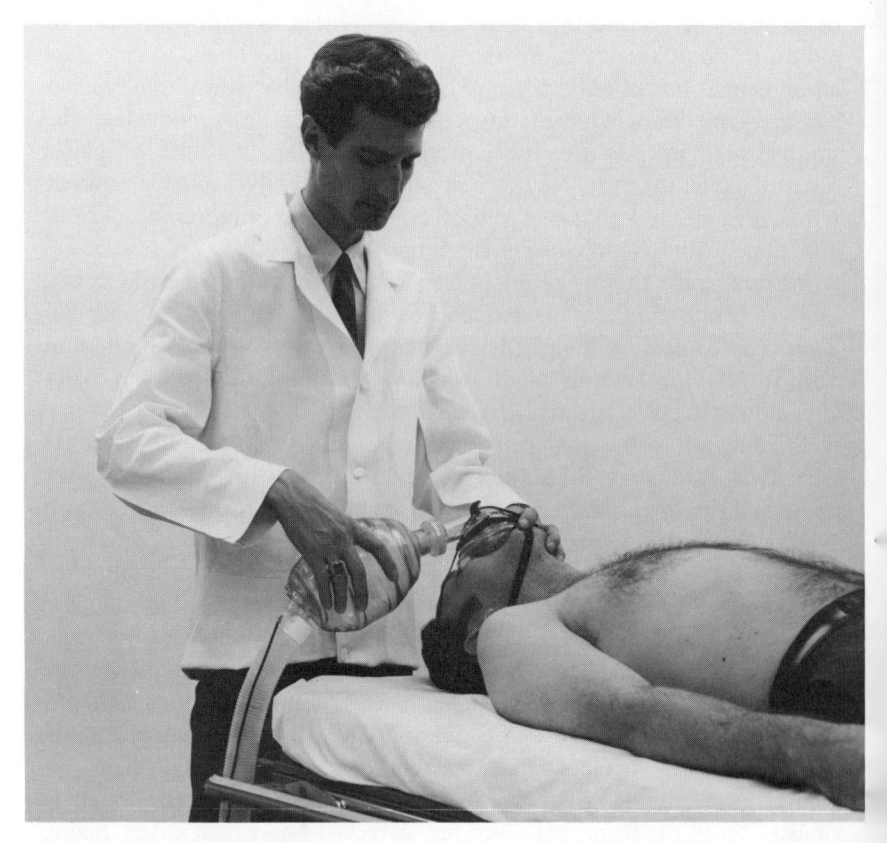

Fig. 17. Use of properly designed bag/valve/mask unit. (Courtesy of Laerdal Medical Corporation, Tuckahoe, N.Y.)

areas of concern: 1, basic design characteristics; 2, component design characteristics; and 3, performance characteristics.

There are two basic designs for bag/valve/mask devices, either a bellows bag which must be pumped up and down manually, or a plastic or rubber bag which is squeezed manually and then self-inflates. The bellows design should be condemned unequivocally. Some are poorly engineered and all of them pose serious performance problems in that the rescuer is attempting to hold the chin up and the head back with one hand and is forcing the head and chin down with the other hand. Ventilation is usually inadequate and bellows type resuscitators should not be used.

For optimal ventilation, the self-inflating bag/valve/mask units should include specific design components (Fig. 17). The *mask* should be transparent and must be provided with a facially contoured inflatable cuff which assures a tight seal. A standard pharyngeal airway should always be used in order to assist in keeping the tongue from obstructing the air passage. Mask straps should be used—not to provide a tight seal, but rather to hold the mask in the proper position so the operator is free to adjust his hand to assure a leakproof fit and retain the head in maximum extension. The *valve* must be truly nonrebreathing in order to avoid the accumulation of carbon dioxide in the bag and system. Many so-called nonrebreathing valves are not truly unidirectional. In addition, the design must be simple so that the valve can be unscrewed, disassembled, and thoroughly cleaned between use on patients. The *bag* must have a volume which allows 1,000 to 1,200 cc to be delivered to the patient on each compression. Ideally, it should be transparent and there must be no foam or sponge lining since this cannot be cleaned and becomes an ideal culture media. The bag must be cleaned and disinfected or sterilized between use.

Bag/valve/mask units do not provide better ventilation than direct mouth-to-mouth or mouth-to-adjunct resuscitation. They are more esthetic and allow the rescuer to stand back and better appraise the patient and situation. However, their primary purpose is to deliver an oxygen-enriched atmosphere to the victim, and adequate provisions should be made for this. This should include an oxygen inlet which fills from the back of the bag and an oxygen reservoir which also empties into the back of the bag. With this arrangement, when the bag is released, the initial filling is 100 percent oxygen followed by some room air. At 10 to 12 liters-per-minute flow in the oxygen line, the patient can be given 60 percent oxygen inhalation with each breath.

Performance of bag/valve/mask resuscitation is somewhat dependent on the design of the unit but primarily depends on the training and experience of the user. It is ideal when used in conjunction with an endotracheal tube. However, when used with a mask, it is only effective in the hands of experienced anesthetists, anesthesiologists, or other specially trained persons. Most doctors, nurses, and paramedical personnel cannot deliver adequate ventilatory volumes because of the difficulties involved in simultaneously lifting the chin, tilting the head, holding the mask, and assuring a tight seal with one hand while holding and squeezing the bag with the other hand. Unless they have extensive training, retraining, and continuing experience with bag/valve/mask units, most of these people can assure better ventilation of the victim's lungs with mouth-to-mouth or mouth-to-adjunct resuscitation.

AUTOMATIC VENTILATORS AND RESUSCITATORS. Automatic breathing devices and inhalation therapy units are now widely available both in hospitals and in emergency and rescue vehicles. Most of these are highly specialized pieces of equipment which are designed for specific purposes and their use is restricted to definitive therapy by specially trained personnel.

Automatic ventilators and resuscitators are not available initially during cardiopulmonary emergencies. They are only useful if some other form of emergency artificial respiration has previously been started and if the correct type of device is used properly. These devices are useful where prolonged resuscitation, transportation of the victim, or oxygen therapy is required. They are usually equipped with an aspirator for removing mucus, blood, or vomitus from the airway. With such units it is equally important to keep the air passage open by tilting the head back, extending the jaw, and/or inserting an oropharyngeal airway. In addition to resuscitation, these devices can be used to amplify depressed respiration and for oxygen administration after normal spontaneous respiration has been reestablished. The use of automatic breathing devices for cardiopulmonary resuscitation depends upon their specific type. There are three basic types and these are based upon the mechanism which is used to cycle the unit: 1, pressure-cycled; 2, time-cycled; and 3, volume-cycled.

Pressure-cycled ventilators are used in hospitals to provide intermittent positive pressure breathing (I.P.P.B.) to patients who require respiratory assistance. They are also used by rescue groups to provide positive and negative pressure for resuscitation of nonbreathing patients. Although both of these types of pressure-cycled ventilators may be useful for cases requiring ventilation only, **they must never be used in conjunction with external cardiac compression.** The reason for this is that every compression of the chest raises the airway pressure in the patient and unit and causes it to cycle into exhalation. The patient never receives a full inflation of his lungs, oxygen saturation falls dramatically, and carbon dioxide is retained. Therefore, it is of critical importance to remember:

NEVER USE PRESSURE-CYCLED VENTILATORS IN CONJUNCTION WITH CARDIOPULMONARY RESUSCITATION.

Time-cycled ventilators are usually manually triggered (Fig. 18). The rescuer inflates the patient's lungs by pressing a button or lever which allows oxygen to flow in for as long as he holds it. When he releases the lever the patient exhales passively. A pressure-limiting valve prevents excessive pressure build-up and a high instantaneous flow rate provides rapid filling of the lungs. Breaths can be interposed between chest compressions making such devices useful for CPR as well as artificial ventilation alone. Sometimes a demand valve is also included and the device can also be used for inhalation therapy.

Volume-cycled ventilators are of two types depending upon the specific purpose for which they are designed. Some are complicated units engineered to deliver adjustable tidal volumes, minute volumes and/or respiratory rates to be used on patients in controlled respiration for respiratory insufficiency associated with severe respiratory

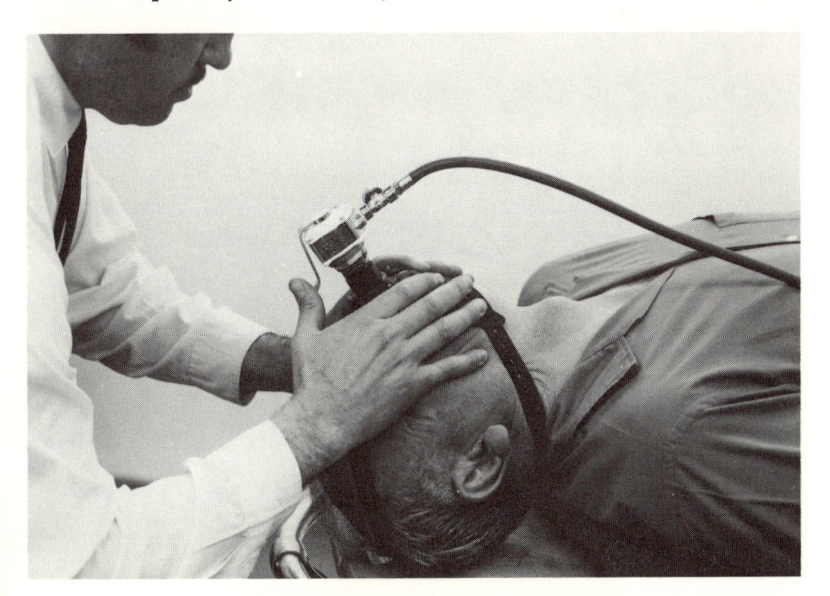

Fig. 18. Manually-triggered, time-cycled ventilator (Elder Valve) which is effective for demand inhalation, artificial respiration, and cardiopulmonary resuscitation.

disease, postoperative cardiac surgery, crushed chest, and so on. These are not applicable in cardiopulmonary resuscitation emergencies.

The other type of volume-cycled device is designed to provide adjustable volumes of oxygen interposed quickly between external chest compressions. This automatic volume-cycled ventilator is usually combined with an automatic mechanical chest compressor as discussed in the following section.

MECHANICAL HEART-LUNG RESUSCITATOR (HLR). An ideal Heart-Lung Resuscitator (HLR) should provide for all three of the A-B-C's of emergency resuscitation. This has been achieved in the device shown in Figure 19.

The HLR is lightweight and portable and can be actuated by a portable oxygen pack, large oxygen cylinders, or wall oxygen lines. It can be applied to a victim who is already receiving heart-lung resuscitation with only two interruptions of five seconds each. The HLR provides a shoulder lift which tilts the head back into a position

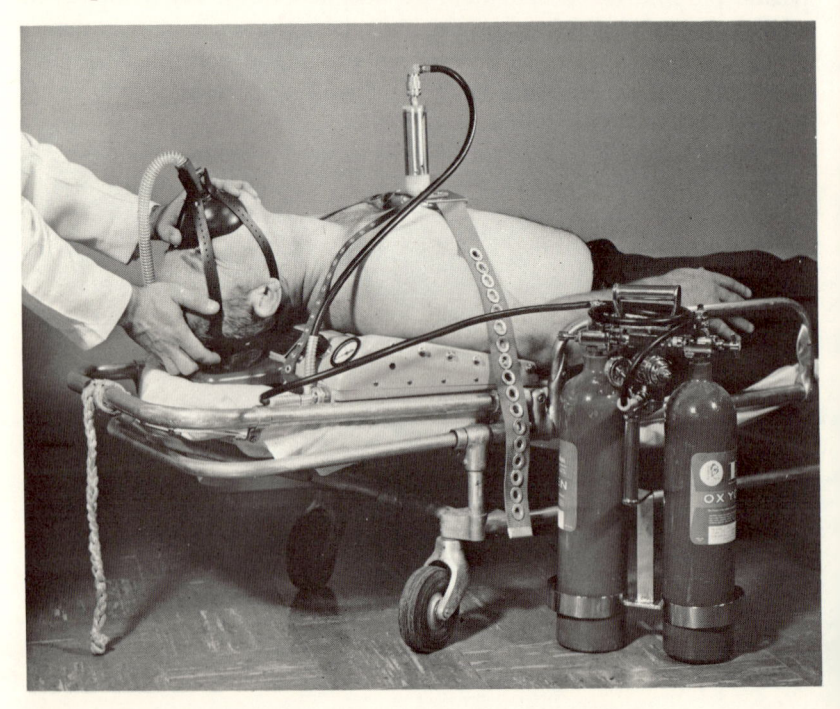

Fig. 19. Mechanical Heart-Lung Resuscitator (HLR) for prolonged, uniform, uninterrupted resuscitation, or resuscitation of victim during transportation. (Courtesy of Travenol/Brunswick.)

of extension to assist in opening the air passage; a ventilation line providing adjustable volume-cycled artificial respiration which can be used alone or "interposed" between each five chest compressions; and an adjustable pneumatic external chest compressor which provides artificial circulation at a rate of 60 times per minute with a 50:50 ratio of compression:relaxation.

Such equipment is very useful for uniform, uninterrupted heart-lung resuscitation when prolonged resuscitation is required, or when it is necessary to continue resuscitation during transportation of a victim for definitive treatment. One rescuer must always remain at the patient's head. Here he maintains the head in extension to keep the air passage open; holds the mask to assure a tight seal; removes the mask and turns the patient's head to avoid aspiration if regurgitation occurs; observes the chest compressor to be sure it is in the proper place and providing the proper movement of the sternum; periodically observes the patient's pupils and checks the carotid pulse; and regulates the controls. External defibrillation can be accomplished without interrupting the use of such a unit, since it is insulated from the patient.

Definitive Therapy

The A-B-C's of emergency resuscitation should be continued until the patient recovers, until he is pronounced dead, or until definitive treatment can be instituted. Recovery frequently depends upon such definitive treatment. This applies to all cases of cardiac arrest but particularly those in which ventricular fibrillation occurs. In this instance, emergency heart-lung resuscitation must be continued until the heart is defibrillated and has resumed a rhythmic beat capable of producing a peripheral pulse.

Definitive therapy should be started as soon as possible. However, at the present time this is only possible in the hospital, except in special situations where mobile coronary care units or ambulances with doctors or nurses are available. Although definitive therapy currently is not part of first aid, the basic aspects of diagnosis, drugs, and defibrillation will be discussed here.

The diagnosis of ventricular fibrillation can be made with assurance only from an electrocardiographic or oscilloscopic tracing. When this has been obtained, preparations should be made for the intravenous administration of drugs and for external defibrillation. The most useful drugs in cardiorespiratory emergencies involving ventricular fibrillation are epinephrine and sodium bicarbonate. The pH of the blood rapidly becomes severely acidotic following cardiac arrest. This inaugurates a vicious cycle, since acidosis weakens the myocardium which leads to further circulatory inadequacy and further depression of the pH. Even the most effective heart-lung resuscitation fails to prevent or to correct this acidosis. Intravenous sodium bicarbonate (1 ampule contains 50 ml, 3.75 g, 44.6 mEq) is a relatively innocuous drug which can be used to reverse this process, thereby improving the myocardial status and assisting in defibrillation and restoration of a normal heart beat and cardiac output. This dose should be given as quickly as possible and repeated empirically every five to ten minutes until an effective rhythmic beat is restored.

Epinephrine chloride acts like other vasopressors to increase vasomotor tone and improve blood pressure. It also has a direct inotropic effect which improves myocardial tone and the quality of the fibrillation, enhances electric defibrillation and assures an improved cardiac output following defibrillation. It should be administered in doses of 0.5 to 1.0 mg (0.5 to 1.0 ml of 1:1,000 concentration) every five to ten minutes. Many other drugs are recommended for special conditions during the cardiorespiratory emergency, but these two are the most important.

Ventricular fibrillation is best terminated by the use of external DC defibrillators. These can be battery-powered portable units, or they can be actuated by AC line voltage. For external termination of ventricular fibrillation large (9 cm), well-insulated electrode paddles should be used. Electrode jelly or well-soaked saline pads serve as a conductor between the skin and the electrodes. The least resistance to flow and the greatest current flow through the heart itself is achieved by placing one electrode just to the right of the upper sternum and the other over the apex of the heart. Firm pressure must be exerted to prevent skin burns and voltage loss when the shock is delivered. Ideally, the shock should be monophasic and provide 100 to 400 watt seconds of energy. Following defibrillation, the rescuer cannot rely on a satisfactory electrocardiogram or oscilloscopic tracing as an indication of adequate cardiac output. A peripheral blood pressure or pulse must be obtainable. Sometimes it is necessary to resume and continue heart-lung resuscitation for variable periods of time after defibrillation until breathing and peripheral pulse and blood pressure indicate a properly restored cardiorespiratory system.

Special Considerations

The preceding A-B-C-D principles can be applied to most cardiorespiratory emergencies. They are not all-encompassing, but the individual rescuer should be able to adapt them to special rescue situations. Always start with the A-B-C's immediately, and get the victim to a hospital as quickly as possible so that definitive treatment can be administered.

In the presence of noxious fumes, smoke, or carbon monoxide, the victim should always be removed from this environment as soon as possible and before resuscitation is started. This may require breaking of windows or doors, seeking and eliminating the source of the agent, or using a gas mask to evacuate the victim.

Never perform external cardiac compression on a victim who is in the vertical position. Careful studies have shown that in this position there is no blood flow to the brain during external compression of the chest in the presence of cardiac arrest. Artificial respiration is effective in either the horizontal or vertical position, but the patient must be horizontal for effective cardiopulmonary resuscitation. If sitting up, lay him down. If in a dental chair, straighten out the chair or place him on the floor. If propped up in bed, remove the pillows or lower the top half of the bed. For linemen requiring resuscitation on a telephone pole, start with mouth-to-mouth resuscitation, lower the victim quickly and then start heart-lung resuscitation on the ground.

When a mechanical HLR is not available to provide continuous resuscitation during movement of the patient, the following routine should be used to assure uninterrupted heart-lung resuscitation during movement.

Start the A-B-C's immediately using one or two rescuers as available.

Place the victim on a spine board with only a brief interruption in resuscitation. Then continue CPR.

Place the spine board and patient on a stretcher which has a high and low position. Use the low position while moving him to an ambulance. One rescuer remains at the head and performs artificial respiration; one rescuer walks alongside and performs external cardiac compression. A third rescuer or bystander helps move the stretcher to the ambulance.

If it is necessary to move the stretcher either up or down stairs, stop at the top, bottom, and each landing to perform effective CPR, then move quickly up or down the stairs. Do not attempt CPR during movement on the stairs.

In the ambulance continue CPR with one or two rescuers, as available. Be sure the rescuer is above the victim so he can press straight downward on the sternum.

Drowning is merely a special form of asphyxia wherein anoxia has resulted either from laryngospasm or from flooding of the airway. In experimental mammals, fresh water submersion results in a high incidence of ventricular fibrillation, whereas, sea water submersion results in cardiac standstill or circulatory collapse. In either case the most effective emergency treatment is cardiopulmonary resuscitation.

Water in the lungs cannot be "poured out" and valuable time should not be lost in attempting to empty anything but the upper airway. Resuscitation should be started at once. If further obstruction seems to be present, the victim should be rolled over and/or inverted. Frequently, the stomach of a drowning victim is massively distended with swallowed water following submersion. In such cases, after effective resuscitation has been started, it is helpful to roll the victim into a prone position, place your hands under his waist, and lift. This tends to compress and empty the stomach, which facilitates breathing, circulation, and recovery.

15 / Injuries of the Chest

*HIRAM T. LANGSTON, WALTER L. BARKER, AND
BERNARD J. LEININGER*

Anatomy and Physiology

In its simplest terms, the chest can be pictured as an airtight, cone-shaped box, the walls of which are made up of a bony (rib) cage covered by muscles and skin. These walls are movable and by moving increase the size of the chest cavity (inspiration) or decrease it (expiration). The chest cavity is further separated by a median partition, the mediastinum, wherein lie the heart, great vessels, esophagus (gullet), and trachea (windpipe). The floor of each half is formed by a powerful and domed muscular sheet (diaphragm) whose contraction draws it down, flattening its contour and thereby greatly increasing the capacity of the corresponding chest cavity.

The two halves of the chest cavity contain the lungs, which normally lie free within the chest cavity, except for the area of the lung root (hilum). Through this area pass the air conduits (bronchi) to the lung and also the blood vessels that carry blood to and from the lungs for the purpose of oxygenation.

Air passes in and out of the lungs from the nose or mouth by way of the trachea, which divides into a right and left bronchus to supply the corresponding lung (Fig. 1).

In the phases of respiration, the lungs follow the chest wall. In inspiration, as the chest cavity is enlarged, air is drawn into the corresponding enlarged lung. In expiration, air flows out of the lung as it keeps pace with the decreased volume of the chest cavity.

The derangements that alter the mechanics of this bellows function are the principal items to be discussed in this chapter.

Inspiration   Expiration

PARADOXICAL MOTION

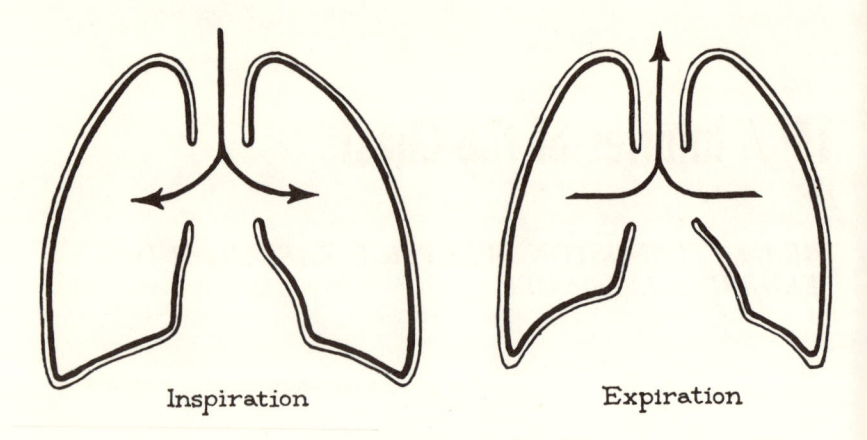

Inspiration   Expiration

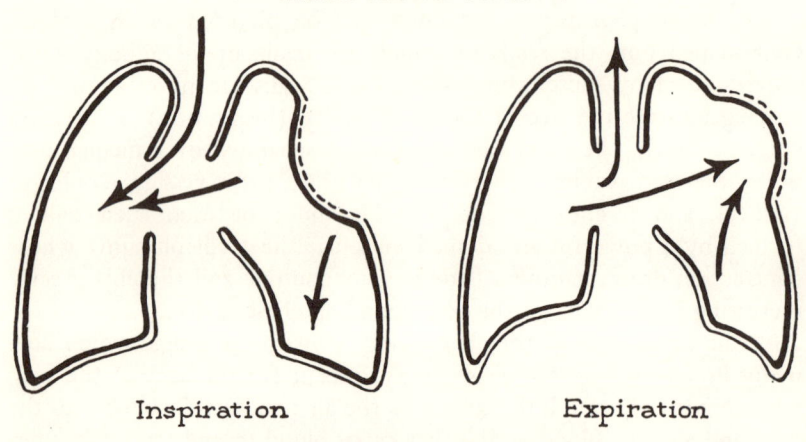

Fig. 1. Diagram showing normal respiratory movements and paradoxical motion when the solidity of the thoracic cage is destroyed by trauma.

General Considerations of Management

Interference with the function of these organs presents a serious situation. Shock is a common accompaniment of such injuries. The principal factors that tend to perpetuate the state of shock are pain and derangements that reduce the volume of the lungs, thereby reducing their efficiency as ventilatory organs. The circulatory system will become affected in consequence of the above.

PAIN. Whatever its cause (lacerated soft tissues or fractured ribs), pain is a more serious problem here than elsewhere because it not only is unpleasant but also can affect very seriously vital body functions. Thus, since the pain tends to be reproduced with each respiratory movement, especially when ribs are fractured, splinting of the chest occurs on the injured side, restricting its effectiveness in ventilation. As bad as this may be, if uncurbed, pain can reach such intensity as to cause limitation of motion, even on the opposite side, producing a truly critical situation. Oxygenation will then be deficient with cyanosis (blueness) of the patient and rapid, shallow, grunting respiration. Bronchial secretions will be retained in the tracheobronchial tree, leading to further decrease in efficient oxygenation and ultimately resulting in progressive deterioration of the patient's condition.

There are three principal methods of combating this problem. These are judicious use of narcotics, intercostal nerve block by procaine, and general supportive measures.

Narcotics can be harmful by virtue of their side effects, particularly in depressing respiration and cough. If used in carefully adjusted dosage to allay pain but not depress, advantage can be taken of this effect to insist on having the subject cough in order to clear the airway and avoid the dangers of sputum retention. Narcotics also help greatly in allaying the fear and apprehension often experienced by those persons who have had such a vital part of their body affected.

Injection of procaine into the intercostal nerves lateral to the spine will interrupt the intercostal innervation, relieve pain, and likewise stop spasm of the intercostal muscles, freeing chest wall motion and removing much of the hesitation to breathing and coughing. This is the ideal method of controlling severe pain and can be repeated as often as indicated.

Whereas the two preceding methods require skill and equipment for their performance, certain general and simple measures should not be forgotten.

The subject's position should be looked into. A semirecumbent position is a favored attitude when shortness of breath is a problem, unless there are other injuries to contraindicate this position. Lying on the injured side may help splint the moving chest cage and thereby improve respiratory exchange.

A snug binder about the chest with added padding over the painful area may be acceptable. It should not, of course, be so constricting as to interfere with adequate excursion of the uninjured side.

Adhesive strapping is likewise effective but should not be encircling. It is preferably placed while the chest is in deep expiration and should not go very far beyond the midline, front or back. It is most effective when placed in strips horizontally about the lower rib cage.

Clothing should be loosened and cool fresh air should be assured as this is comforting even though it does not contain any increased oxygen. Supplemental oxygen is, of course, often necessary and as a temporary means of decreasing the rate of respiration is useful. Like narcotics, however, it can render more tolerable the retention of secretions and therefore lead to unwanted side effects.

DERANGEMENTS OF LUNG VOLUME AND FUNCTION. The recognition of the various situations which make up this category of injury is difficult, unless an x-ray picture of the chest can be obtained. Even though by physical examination alone a diagnosis is generally possible, confirmation by an x-ray is advisable except under the worst circumstances.

Alluding again to the previous discussion, it is to be recalled that the lungs are not a source of painful sensations. Thus, except for deep-seated discomfort, breathlessness, and so on, complaints of pain must be ascribed to injuries of the chest wall. Fractured ribs, contusions, lacerations, and other injuries will produce pain and are to be managed according to the prior discussion. The derangements that we are about to discuss generally do not produce pain per se.

FLAIL CHEST. When multiple ribs are fractured at multiple points, the portion of chest wall lying between these areas of fracture will not move in unison with the rest of the rib cage and, therefore, it can be said to be flail (Fig. 1). Crushing injuries, such as are seen in today's high speed automobile accidents, account for many if not most of these injuries.

The seriousness of this accident depends on the relative size of the segment which is rendered flail. Its mechanical importance lies in the fact that on inspiration, when the rib cage expands outwardly, this functionally detached portion of the chest wall sinks. On expiration the reverse occurs. Not only does this paradoxical motion repeat the pain at the fracture site, but air tends to be shuttled back and forth between the area of the lung under the flail segment and the rest of the same lung or, if extensive enough, actually from one lung to the other. This latter factor leads to retention of CO_2 and lessened oxygenation as a result of rebreathing. These factors obviously deepen any shock that may be present or may actually produce shock.

Further, as a result of the severe injury, increased bronchial secretions are to be expected. Since respiration is hampered and cough is ineffective, retention of these is a consequence and leads to further reduced respiratory efficiency. This succession of events accounts for the morbidity and mortality attendant upon such injuries.

Emergency treatment of a patient with a flail chest requires a basic understanding of the established modalities of therapy. The paradoxical movements of a flail chest can be stabilized either by internal or external fixation. Internal stabilization consists in splinting the unstable chest wall by applying positive pressure to the tracheobronchial tree. Usually this is accomplished by use of a volume-controlled ventilator through a cuffed tracheostomy tube. The work of breathing is completely taken over by the ventilator requiring no muscular effort on the part of the patient. In this manner the inflated lung cushions the unstable chest wall on its surface. Thus the need for negative intrathoracic pressure to effect inspiration is eliminated. Such patients are maintained on a ventilator until there is sufficient healing and fixation of the chest wall to permit satisfactory ventilation by the patient. This usually requires from one to several weeks of support mechanical ventilation.

External stabilization, on the other hand, consists in either holding the unstable segment of the chest wall out with traction or in by compression. Towel clips placed into the ribs or sternum are attached to weights by a rope and pulley system. This holds the flail segment out thereby giving fixation of the chest wall and allowing negative pressure to develop within the thorax. This allows the patient to breathe on his own. External stabilization by holding the chest wall in can be effected by compression dressings, binders, taping, sand bags, or having the patient lie on the affected side. Many authors have mentioned these methods only to condemn them. Admittedly, some of the basic principles of respiratory physiology are violated (the total lung volume is reduced), yet it can be an effective emergency maneuver. For example, if one side of the chest is crushed, respiratory efforts by the patient may result in moving the flail segment in a paradoxical manner. Ventilation thus is rendered ineffective until stability of the chest wall is achieved.

Use of the Ambu bag with a face mask is the simplest and most effective way to assist the patient's own ventilatory motions. If such equipment is not available external stabilization with compression bandages or traction should be considered particularly if transportation of the injured patient is necessary.

In small children dramatic changes in effective ventilation can be accomplished by simply grasping the skin and suspending the flail segment manually.

Finally, the work of ventilation in a normal chest as reflected in changes in intrathoracic pressures are very minimal (minus 5 cm H_2O inspiration to minus 1 cm H_2O expiration). In the immediate post-trauma period the work of ventilation may remain close to normal by hypoventilation and splinting. However, as secretions accumulate edema of injured lung tissue develops, and associated injuries increase oxygen consumption. The patient is forced to ventilate probably in response to a rising carbon-dioxide level. Thus the work of ventilation increases. If this increase in negative intrathoracic pressure exceeds the stability of the chest wall paradoxical motions result, ventilation becomes ineffective, more secretions are retained, and hypercarbia becomes more pronounced thus creating a vicious cycle. Thus because of conpensatory mechanisms initially, ventilation may be normal only to deteriorate rapidly later as oxygen demands and carbon-dioxide elevation force an increased ventilatory effort in a patient with an unstable chest. This latent period is one in which the patient must be watched very closely and corrective measures instituted early.

Control of pain as outlined before is basic, and assisted cough is required even before evidence of retained secretions is noted. Failing adequate control of the situation by these methods, intratracheal suction by catheter or bronchoscopy is in order, and a tracheotomy (an opening into the windpipe) may ultimately be required as a portal through which secretions may be aspirated. It also will tend to relieve paradoxical motion. It is necessary for the use of some of the mechanical respirators.

PNEUMOTHORAX. This situation can be defined as the presence of air in the pleural cavity (space between the lung and the chest wall) (Fig. 2).

Air enters this space from defects of the chest wall or defects of the lung.

Defects of the Chest Wall. When the continuity of the chest wall is disrupted, air will rush in through the defect on inspiration, and the lung, which is inherently elastic, will collapse space with the

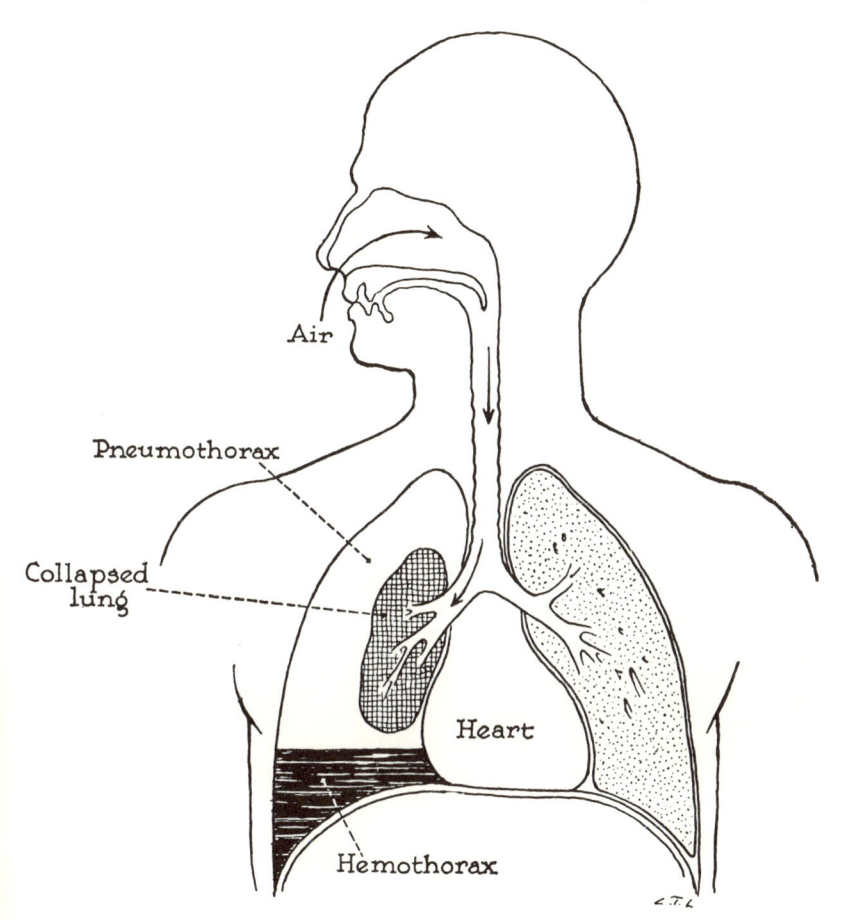

Fig. 2. Complications which may arise following wounds of the chest. Note the pneumothorax (air in the pleural cavity), collapsed lung, and hemothorax (blood in the pleural cavity).

amount of air admitted. The lung may become totally airless. If the defect in the chest wall is widely patent, air will flow in and out synchronously with respiration. This is called a *sucking wound*. This situation is obviously serious in that the function of one lung is lost by collapse. Worse yet, however, is the fact that the uninjured side is affected very materially as well, because the midline portion between the two lungs (the mediastinum) tends to be pulled toward the good side during inspiration, since it is not of itself rigid. This partition, therefore, being nonrigid tends to follow the lung rather than oppose it, as it would were it more resistant to displacement.

The size of opening that a person can survive varies, but for short periods of time robust and muscular people can survive openings of remarkable size, certainly much larger than the cross section of the trachea (windpipe).

The prime requisite of treatment is, of course, to seal this defect by suitable occlusive dressings. If these are placed at the end of an expiratory effort, maximum use of the underlying lung will presumably be preserved. Debridement and surgical closure under an anesthetic are to be carried out at the earliest opportunity.

If the defect in the chest wall is transient, there being no replacement of the pneumothorax air, aspiration of this air by needle or continuous decompression by a catheter passed intercostally into the pleural cavity and connected to a water seal will correct the situation. Small amounts of retained air will be absorbed and require no specifically directed treatment.

Defects of the Lung. The source of air here is, of course, from the bronchial tree, i.e., air which leaks into the chest cavity through a tear in the pleural covering of the lung. Small amounts of air in this location may be merely watched, may be aspirated, or if greater in volume, decompressed by catheter as referred to above. The amount of air present and the extent of lung collapse under these circumstances will require an x-ray for proper evaluation.

At times, however, due to a peculiar ball-valve type of arrangement at the lung defect or pleural tear, more air escapes into the pleural cavity with each expiratory cycle than escapes back from the pleural cavity through the defect. This leads to progressive collapse of the lung, progressive displacement of the mediastinum and consequent encroachment on the other side. This condition is termed *tension pneumothorax* and can become fatal rapidly. The absence of breath sounds over one side (as determined by listening with the stethoscope or unaided ear) or a highly resonant sound when percussion is carried out on this side suggests tension pneumothorax and may justify insertion of a needle for the aspiration of air before the availability of an x-ray. Such patients are usually severely dyspneic. If air under pressure is present, the needle may then be connected to a tube whose end is placed in water, or better yet an intercostal catheter should be inserted and this connected to a water-seal (Fig. 3). In the absence of a water-seal or for the purpose of transportation, a fish-mouthed, rubber finger-cot tied over the end of the rubber tubing can be used to permit the egress of air but impede its ingress at the

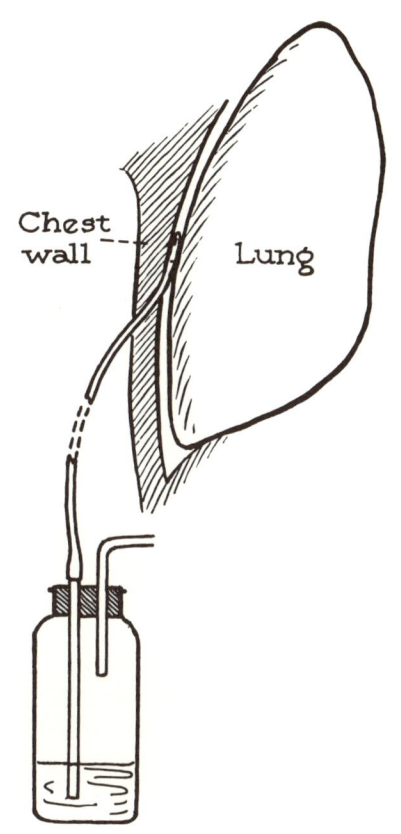

Fig. 3. Diagram of the principles utilized in the water-seal mechanism often used in the treatment of pneumothorax and after operation on the chest.

next inspiratory effort. Such devices, however, are less reliable than the simple expedient of leading the tube under water in a container placed two to three feet below the patient's chest.

HEMOTHORAX. This condition is defined as the presence of blood in the pleural cavity. The usual source of blood is some injured vessel in the chest wall. Wounds of the lung rarely produce bleeding of any great amount because the spongy nature of the organ itself and the relatively low pressure of the pulmonary circulation tend to limit it. The spitting of blood (hemoptysis) may be alarming though usually it will be self-limited, ultimately ceasing and generally will not be great in total volume. The source of blood in hemoptysis is the lung. Sedation and rest are the principal approaches to treatment for hemoptysis.

In most patients with injury to the chest, a variable amount of blood will escape into the chest cavity at the time of an injury. Even though it may be small in amount initially, it will evoke an outpouring of pleural fluid within the next 24 to 48 hours. An x-ray will show this clearly, but when there are diminished or absent breath sounds over the injured side with dullness to percussion, and when the mediastinum is displaced away from the injured side as determined by the point of maximum impulse of the heart, presumption of fluid in the chest is justified. The proper immediate therapy is its removal by needle as necessary for comfort; within a few days all should be removed.

The diagnosis of continued bleeding into the pleural cavity is often difficult to establish but if suspected calls for prompt and active operative intervention to control the bleeding point. This surgical procedure is beyond the scope of this book.

At times, and contrary to former opinion, clotting of intrapleural blood does occur. This renders aspiration difficult or impossible and calls for special management by the instillation of lysing enzymes, such as Varidase, or surgical decortication at an elective time later.

There is little that can be done to control bleeding short of operative exposure, preferably under anesthesia. Packing of a chest-wall wound may control the bleeding from the muscles or a severed intercostal vessel, but generally there can be no assurance that bleeding into the pleural cavity is effectively stopped by this maneuver. Blood replacement is in order but no time should be lost in providing for secure control of the bleeding source.

SUBCUTANEOUS EMPHYSEMA. This condition may be defined as swelling of the soft tissues due to the presence of air. This occurs most frequently about the chest wall, neck, and face.

Air can find its way into the planes of the chest wall or mediastinum where it distends the tissue. This presupposes a break in anatomic continuity of the lung surface or bronchi at some point. Once started, this air tends to spread along any of the cleavage planes of the body tissues as it is fed from its source. If small in amount, its presence may be recognized only by a crackling sensation when the hand is run over the involved area, but if the volume is greater, it will produce swelling and bloating of all areas affected. It may result in a frighteningly grotesque appearance where the eyes are closed, the girth is greatly increased, the scrotum is voluminous, and the neck is massive. The legs, feet, and scalp may even become involved.

The presence of the air itself is innocuous beyond the alarm and discomfort to the victim. The important consideration is the source. Usually this is from a leak in the lung accompanied by some disruption of tissue planes (pleura usually), permitting the air to migrate. Contrary to prior opinions, death from emphysema alone probably does not occur, and all attention should be directed toward controlling the source as in pneumothorax above. In its most massive forms following immediately on injury, particularly one without external wound, emphysema results from the disruption of the bronchus itself. This situation should be handled by prompt surgical intervention, but decompression of the pleural space by one or more catheters may allow time to arrive at the proper diagnosis and surgical correction.

INJURIES TO THE HEART. These are obviously serious in nature and until recently, much pessimism has overshadowed them. It is, however, increasingly true that many of these are compatible with recovery by well-directed treatment. The possibility that the heart may be contused in crushing injuries to the chest must always be remembered. This type of injury has become relatively common as a result of high-speed automobile accidents.

The manifestations of such an occurrence may be ill-defined and may be made known only through abnormalities seen in electrocardiographic tracings. Symptoms are varied and may even be absent. At the present time, rest and protection of the heart from the demands of physical exertion form the basis of medical management, which in many respects is similar to the treatment of myocardial infarction.

Much more dramatic are the lacerations which enter the heart chambers. These permit the escape of blood from the heart into the pericardial sac. From here the blood escapes into the chest cavity. Less often the blood will escape directly from the chamber into the chest cavity or directly to the outside through the wound track.

Unimpeded escape of blood leads to death promptly by exsanguination. Blood filling the pericardial sac, however, quickly leads to compression of the heart and reduced cardiac function by its choking effect on heart action, resulting in cardiac tamponade, which is of itself capable of producing death. Those victims whose hearts continue rhythmic beating and are not stopped or thrown into disordered action (fibrillation) by the original physical insult, and who therefore survive to come under observation, generally have established a balance between the amount of blood lost from the circulation on the one hand, and the degree of tamponade on the other.

Thus, tamponade may be beneficial in preventing death by exsanguination because of its compressive effect on the heart laceration and yet, the pericardial sac being slow to stretch, may bring about death if the amount of blood forced into the sac is excessive. Escape of blood from the pericardial sac into the chest cavity or to the outside will relieve the tamponade but swings the problem now toward one of exsanguination.

If the degree of tamponade required to stop the flow of blood from the heart is compatible with life, nonoperative management (aspiration) can be considered. If aspiration of blood from the pericardial sac can keep an acceptable level of tamponade without bringing on fresh bleeding from the heart wound, conservative management may succeed. There is obviously a very narrow margin of safety, and if tamponade recurs after aspiration, or if there is suggestion that blood is being lost in spite of tamponade, open operation, evacuating the intrapericardial blood and suturing the lacerated myocardium, should be carried out immediately.

The recognition of a wound of the heart is generally not difficult. The point of wounding and the presumed course of the wounding instrument generally suggest it as a possibility. A state of shock, with low blood pressure particularly in the systolic level, distention of veins (neck and arms), distant or inaudible heart tones, an enlarged cardiac silhouette seen on an upright x-ray (if possible) or this same picture at the fluoroscopic screen, where reduced cardiac activity is also recognized, should lead to puncture of the pericardial sac with the recovery of blood on aspiration. The presence of inaspirable clots in the pericardium must be considered if free blood is not obtained on puncture when the usual manifestations of tamponade are present. This situation strengthens the indication for operative intervention.

The transportation to the hospital of such a victim must be accomplished with upmost dispatch. The surgical facilities should be mobilized and made available even while the decision for operative intervention is being reached. Elevation of the head (semirecumbent position) is usually gratifying to these persons, because venous distention created by the poor cardiac filling (tamponade) is partially relieved by this position.

Removal of the wounding instrument (if it remains in site) is accomplished with maximum safety only under direct vision at operation. The duller instruments (e.g., ice pick) may by their presence minimize the escape of blood from the heart; pulling them out before ready access to the wound is achieved in the operating room may initiate serious active bleeding. However, serious bleeding can take place around a blunt object in the heart wall; accordingly the indications for operation may not be altered by the type of object penetrating the heart.

HICCOUGH. This is caused by a sudden spasm of the diaphragm It is observed very commonly, but only rarely is it serious. Occasionally it develops with moderate severity in patients who have had abdominal operations, but it may develop in healthy people. If it does not disappear after a few minutes, numerous home remedies may be tried. In the mild forms usually seen in healthy people, these remedies should suffice. Often swallowing a glass of cold water slowly will stop the hiccough. At times, pulling out the tongue, hitting the affected person on the back, or surprising him in some way will cause the hiccoughts to disappear. Rebreathing into a paper bag is effective sometimes. If these procedures do not help, a physician should be called. Occasionally, however, nasopharyngeal stimulation with a small (No. 12 or No. 14 F) plastic or rubber catheter will reflexly stop intractable singultis.

CARDIAC ARREST. Much has been written glamorizing the heroic aspects of cardiac massage through the open chest when sudden cessation of heart action is believed to have occurred.

The emphasis tends to have been centered on the heart as the focal organ in this endeavor. It is true that if heart action is not restored, death is certain and in fact can be said to have actually occurred. It is nonetheless true that the tissue quickest to suffer irreversible damage from lack of oxygen is the brain and that mechanical activation of the heart as a mere pump will bring a flow of blood to the brain as well as to other important areas, such as the heart itself. Oxygen is the commodity that the blood must transport if success is to be achieved.

Without more or less complex diagnostic equipment, certainty that heart action has ceased is difficult to achieve, since some reversible states may well mimic this picture of profound collapse. Thus, unless it is certain that cardiac arrest has occurred, and unless adequate means for resuscitation are at hand, a conservative attitude is by far the wiser course. Management as outlined for syncope should be instituted (Chap. 22).

If revival does not occur promptly, and it seems reasonable that cardiac standstill has occurred or that totally ineffectual heart action (ventricular fibrillation) is taking place, prompt action is justified in the hope of maintaining blood flow to vital organs.

In the absence of more sophisticated equipment, this can be accomplished by mouth-to-mouth ventilation and closed cardiac massage as follows (see also Chap. 14).

With the victim supine and on a firm, hard surface the heel of one hand is placed on the lower one third of the sternum (breastbone). The other hand is placed over this, and the sternum is pushed quickly and deeply toward the back followed by sudden release of pressure, allowing the chest to spring back to normal contour. This maneuver is rhythmically repeated approximately 60 times per minute, while forceful insufflation of the lungs is carried out synchronously using the mouth-to-mouth technique (Chap. 14). These maneuvers are preferably carried out by two separate operators.

If effective in establishing circulation, a return of the pulse at the thigh (femoral) or neck (carotid) should be noted. If the recognized pulse beat is produced directly by the chest compression not being maintained otherwise, the maneuver should be continued until the victim can be placed in the hands of physicians equipped to deal with such emergencies.

Although much safer than the more dramatic maintenance of cardiac pumping action by direct massage through the open chest, fractures of the ribs and rupture of such organs as the liver have occurred as complications of this method of cardiac massage.

The control of ventricular fibrillation calls for such armamentarium as does not come within the scope of this chapter. Often the establishment of circulation will bring about return to normal rhythmicity simply by improving oxygenation within the heart itself.

When such a catastrophe takes place in an environment that offers adequate equipment for resuscitation and likewise makes rather certain that cardiac arrest has actually occurred (e.g., during surgical operations or anesthesia), preservation of cerebral blood flow by open cardiac massage is justifiable. Obviously, this should be carried out only by physicians.

This is accomplished by a rapid incision over the left chest below the nipple, carrying it into the chest cavity. (If cessation of heart action has actually occurred, no bleeding should be seen from this incision. If, however, active bleeding does occur, the incision should not be carried into the pleural cavity, since heart action is still present.)

The heart is then grasped and rhythmically massaged so as to propel blood through it while all other supportive measures are instituted.

Since the brain can survive oxygen deprivation for only four minutes on an average, no delay can be countenanced if such action is required.

Management of Cardiac Arrest Associated with Chest Injuries

Cardiac arrest occurring in patients with chest injuries requires primary attention to the A-B-C's of resuscitation (Chap. 14), i.e., airway patency and breathing and circulatory restoration. Dynamic changes associated with chest injuries can quite easily lead to cardiac arrest. Cardiac tamponade, tension pneumothorax, bleeding into the tracheobronchial tree and pleural space, paradoxical respirations, and direct myocardial injury represent mechanical problems that must be corrected as the usual resuscitative measures are carried out.

Closed chest massage combined with mouth-to-mouth ventilation is the keystone of cardiac resuscitation; however, in the presence of associated chest injuries with mechanical defects additional measures are frequently necessary. There is little benefit to be gained in closed chest massage of a patient whose pericardium is distended with blood thereby preventing adequate cardiac filling, or in administering positive pressure ventilation to a patient whose lung is collapsed by a tension pneumothorax. Closed chest massage administered to patients with a crushed chest injury may not only be ineffective but could compound existing injuries. It becomes readily apparent then that a certain amount of clinical judgment may be needed for resuscitation of patients with associated chest injuries.

With the excitement of resuscitation, simple and obvious observations of clinical significance may be completely missed. For example, the patient who is cyanotic (blue) prior to cardiac arrest suggests that the heart continued to pump in the absence of oxygenation. Therefore airway obstruction and fluid or blood in the tracheobronchial tree must be considered. Sucking wounds of the chest, tension pneumothorax, flail chest with severe paradoxical motion, and massive hemothorax are all potentially correctable causes of hypoxia. Usually the skin is pale and white when the heart stops concomitantly with or before spontaneous respirations cease.

Distended neck veins alert one to the possibility of cardiac tamponade; however, internal bleeding into the pleural or peritoneal space can easily go undetected. Simple aspiration of one or more of these spaces with a 19-gauge needle and a 10-cc syringe may establish the need for massive and rapid volume (blood) replacement.

Another maneuver that has repeatedly proved to be life saving is the insertion of a large bore central venous cannula through a percutaneous puncture of the common femoral vein. Valuable time is frequently lost by doing a cutdown on a peripheral vein only to find that fluid will not run through it because of venous spasm associated with shock. By placing a finger on the femoral artery and palpating the pulse effected by closed massage, the needle can be directed medially into the common femoral vein. It is then passed into the right atrium where volume replacement and/or intracardiac medication can be administered with ease.

In summary, if cardiac arrest occurs and the airway is controlled with an endotracheal tube, mechanical defects must be corrected concomitantly with other resuscitative measures. If closed cardiac massage is then thought to be ineffective, open massage should be carried out.

Summary

It is obvious that chest injuries and wounds are severe in nature and often very complex in character. All aspects herein discussed may occur to varying extents and in varying combinations. An analytic approach is, however, to be cultivated because by so doing, a logical method of treatment will emerge. Thus, for example, when confronted by air and blood in the chest resulting from an open defect in the chest wall, closure of the hole and aspiration of the blood and air result in the mechanical restoration to normal. Time for ultimate healing is all that is further required.

The treatment of chest injuries is basically conservative. Operative intervention other than to debride wounds is reserved for: 1, wounds involving the mediastinum—the posterior mediastinum in particular; 2, wounds involving the diaphragm; 3, tension pneumothorax not controlled by catheter decompression; 4, continued intrapleural bleeding not controlled by debridement of the chest wall wound; and 5, wounds of the heart.

The factors that militate against successful survival following important chest wounds are: 1, pain—this is true because of its widespread restriction of ventilatory motion; and 2, derangements which reduce the efficiency of the lungs as respiratory organs and thereby adversely affect the circulation as well. These factors include collapse of the lung by air, blood, or both in the pleural space, or inability to reexpand the lung by virtue of continued air leaks. This circumstance often becomes manifest as extensive and extending subcutaneous emphysema. The lungs may also be unable to act efficiently as respiratory organs due to the retention of secretions within the bronchial tree.

16 / Abdominal Emergencies

CHARLES B. PUESTOW AND SAM F. SEELEY

The tremendous advancements in power and mechanization in both civilian and military life have increased the severity of personal injuries in spite of the developments of precautions to prevent them. The potentials of modern warfare jeopardize civilians as well as combat forces. Accidents at home, at work, on the highways, or while engaged in sports claim many thousands of lives and injure millions each year. Traumatic injuries now account for a high percentage of all surgical patients. Injuries are frequently multiple and present complex first aid problems as well as therapeutic problems in definitive care. Although abdominal injuries are encountered less frequently than those of other portions of the body, they usually are more difficult to diagnose and their symptoms may be masked by other associated trauma. Their symptoms are less likely to be apparent and may be delayed in their manifestations. Injuries to the extremities usually are obvious. Fractures of the bones of the arms or legs cause deformity and superficial wounds are apparent. Injuries to the head and to the chest, likewise, usually present physical findings and symptoms which may attract more attention to underlying damage while equally hazardous injury to the abdominal contents may not be recognized. In order to recognize and evaluate symptoms of abdominal injury, one must have a fundamental knowledge of the anatomy and physiology of this portion of the body.

The nature of injuries to the abdomen is influenced not only by the contents of its cavities but also by the nature of its protective coverings. The upper portion of the abdomen is protected by the lower rib cage. The back of the abdomen is protected by the spine and its associated muscles. The lateral and anterior portions of the abdomen have the support of relatively thin and flexible muscle structures. The lower or pelvic portion of the abdomen is protected by the lower spine and the bony pelvic girdle. Thus, the abdomen has relatively little protection on its anterior and lateral surfaces between the lower border of the ribs and the superior border of the pelvis.

The nature of the organs of the abdominal cavity greatly influence their vulnerability to injury. The abdominal contents may be divided into solid organs, such as the liver, spleen, pancreas, and kidneys, and hollow organs, which include the stomach, small and large intestines, gallbladder and bile ducts, and the urinary bladder. Injuries to solid organs may result in hemorrhage from them into the general peritoneal cavity as well as a loss of their secretions into surrounding tissues or cavities. Hollow organs, when injured, may spill contents whose danger is dependent upon bacterial flora as well as chemical composition. Distended hollow organs are more easily traumatized and their contents may be more dangerous than the contents of the same organs injured when empty. It is difficult to rupture an empty stomach, yet a distended stomach filled with food and gas can be easily torn and its contents poured into the peritoneal cavity. This can be serious but does not carry with it as great a danger as a ruptured colon, which can disseminate its far more lethal contents and produce a more severe peritonitis. An empty urinary bladder is seldom injured. A distended bladder is frequently ruptured in abdominal injuries, especially those involving the pelvis. These points are emphasized to show the importance of determining the time before injury of the ingestion of food or liquids and of the emptying of the patient's bladder. A knowledge of the activities of the patient prior to his accident is most valuable. Drinking of alcoholic beverages before an accident is likely to increase the contents of hollow viscera as well as diminish the sensations of the patient.

The location and fixation of organs within the abdomen are important in their susceptibility to injury. The liver and the spleen, although protected by the lower ribs, are vulnerable to injuries which cause fractures of the overlying ribs, while the small intestine, though poorly protected anteriorly and laterally, is seldom injured because of its free mobility within the abdominal cavity. The portions of the small intestine which are most frequently injured are those which are more firmly fixed, such as the duodenum and upper jejunum and the terminal ileum. Thus, it is important in abdominal injuries to consider the anatomy of the area involved and to determine from the history the probable contents of hollow viscera.

Classification and Types of Abdominal Injuries

Abdominal injuries usually are divided into two classes, penetrating and nonpenetrating wounds (Fig. 1). Penetrating wounds are more obvious and more likely to receive prompt first aid as well as early definitive care. However, severe damage may occur to internal organs with no evidence of external abdominal injury. This is of great importance to the person administering first aid. He should remember that signs of external violence are not essential to intraabdominal injury. This is of increasing importance in our modern age of nuclear energy and other high explosives which can produce blast injuries causing severe intraabdominal damage with no external evidence of injury.

PENETRATING WOUNDS. Penetrating wounds of the abdomen are encountered frequently in both military and civilian life. Most penetrating wounds of the abdomen sustained during war by troops are due to bullets, shell fragments, and flying missiles and fragments of various types. If there is a wound of entrance and exit, one may conjecture the probable course of the missile and the organs which lie in its path. Most high-velocity missiles will travel in a comparatively straight line through the body. However, bullets and foreign bodies propelled by explosives may travel devious routes even though they both enter and leave the body, and one is never entirely sure of their course. One cannot be complacent in believing that because the wounds of entrance and exit apparently do not involve a vital structure no serious damage has resulted. Bullets and foreign bodies often will be deflected even by soft tissues and cause damage which cannot be interpreted by a logical, supposed course of their trajectory.

In civilian life many abdominal injuries of penetrating type are encountered both as a result of gunfire and of sharp weapons. These include razors, knives, ice picks, and other penetrating objects. It is well to attempt to determine the direction of the missile from the history given by the patient. Often this is erroneous. One can only conclude that from the depth the missile is able to penetrate, it may have traversed in any direction, and he can then interpret what damage may have occurred. Lacerated wounds produced by knives and razors usually cause more damage to the abdominal wall than to the contained viscera. Stab wounds are likely to produce varying de-

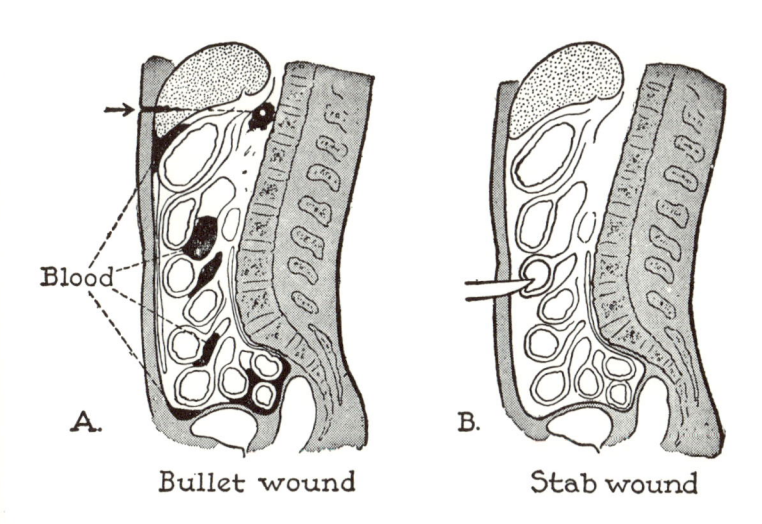

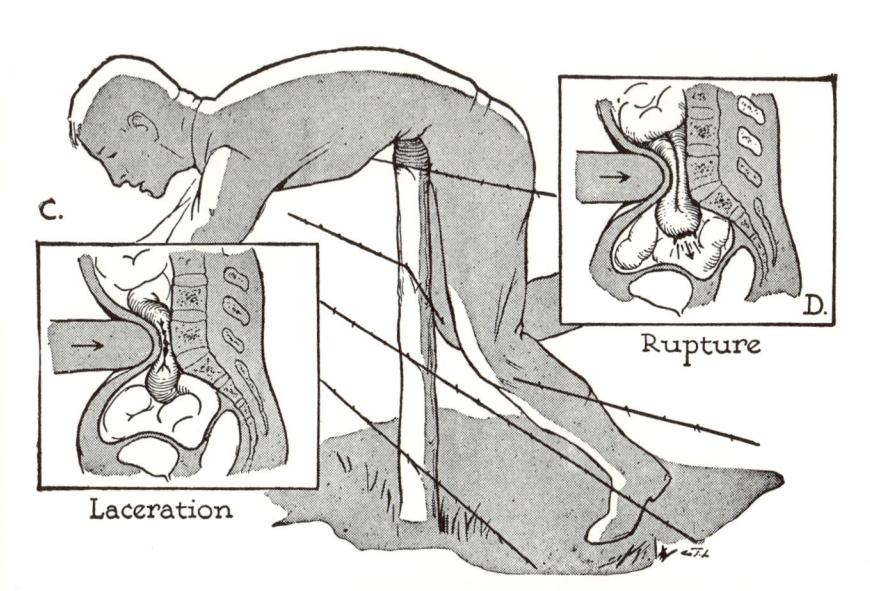

Classification and Types of Abdominal Injuries / 255

Fig. 1. Mechanisms of injuries to organs in the peritoneal cavity. A, gunshot wound of the liver has given rise to severe hemorrhage. B, stab wound has injured the intestine. C, crushing of the intestinal loop between the object and vertebral column (as illustrated by the man falling on the fencepost) may produce a laceration of the intestine. D, injury inflicted as in C may produce a rupture because of sudden pressure exerted on gas in a loop of intestine.

grees of intraabdominal injury. *It is imperative that patients with penetrating wounds of the abdomen, whether they have only a wound of entrance or of entrance and exit, be transported to a hospital as soon as possible* where immediate surgical therapy can be instituted if it is deemed advisable. Every penetrating wound of the abdomen should be considered a surgical emergency irrespective of how minimal are the symptoms which the patient may present.

Symptoms produced by penetrating wounds of solid viscera, such as the liver, spleen, pancreas, and kidneys, may develop slowly. They result from the loss of blood into the peritoneal cavity or surrounding tissues or from the spread of secretion from these organs, such as bile, digestive ferments from the pancreas, or urine from the kidneys. Bleeding from these organs may be slow but may continue for hours or days. Therefore, it is important that the patient be kept under careful observation in order to recognize such hemorrhage and the development of evidences of peritonitis and shock. The effects of secretions from these organs, although accompanied by little bleeding, will produce marked tissue reaction and a possible chemical peritonitis and shock.

Penetrating wounds of the gastrointestinal tract permitting an escape of contents into the peritoneal cavity will be slow in producing symptoms of peritonitis, but the severity of the symptoms and the prognosis will depend upon the portion of the bowel which is perforated. Leakage from the stomach and the upper small bowel will produce a chemical peritonitis which results in rigidity of the abdomen, pain, an elevated white count, and fever. However, because of the low virulence of the bacterial content of these organs, a serious bacterial peritonitis will be delayed. Rupture or perforation of the lower small bowel or colon may be slow in producing symptoms, but highly virulent organisms may be liberated into the peritoneal cavity, which can produce a rapidly fulminating and possibly fatal peritonitis. Because of the uncertainty of the consequences of any type of penetrating abdominal wound, it is most important that a patient with such a wound be transported to a hospital as soon as possible where emergency surgical care can be rendered.

Many penetrating wounds of the abdominal cavity are associated with wounds of adjacent portions of the body. This is particularly true of wounds of the chest. Because the diaphragm arches well into the chest, bullets or other missiles may enter the chest, penetrate the diaphragm, and injure intraabdominal structures. These are called thoracoabdominal wounds. The possibility of such combined injuries must always be kept in mind. Wounds of the buttocks may likewise result in missiles entering the abdominal cavity. Such complications could prove very serious if overlooked.

NONPENETRATING WOUNDS. The effects of nonpenetrating injuries to the abdomen can be fairly accurately determined by the nature of the force, the location of its impact, and a knowledge of the anatomy involved. An upper abdominal injury can cause serious trauma to fixed organs both hollow and solid, whereas a midabdominal injury is less likely to cause serious intraabdominal damage. Injury to organs of the lower abdomen usually results from trauma to the surrounding structures, especially the bony pelvis.

The symptoms produced by intraabdominal injury often are masked by injury to protective structures. Thus, injury to the liver or spleen may be masked by the symptoms produced by fractures of overlying ribs. When injury is confined to the abdomen, the symptoms usually begin in a local area. There may be pain, tenderness, and rigidity of the overlying muscles. If intraperitoneal contamination results, there is usually a progressive spread of these symptoms expanding in the involved quadrant and then extending to the adjacent quadrants until the entire abdomen is involved. This may be followed by a rise in temperature, an increase of leukocyte count, and increasing rigidity and distention. These symptoms and findings are described for the first aid worker only to emphasize the importance of early care of abdominal injuries. Patients with such injuries demand early transportation to the hospital and priority over most other injuries. However, because abdominal injuries are frequently associated with injuries of other parts of the body, one must first and always consider the injured patient as a whole. Shock or impending shock must be treated. Hemorrhage must be controlled.

In the presence of trauma to other structures abdominal injuries may be easily overlooked because of the severity of injuries to the chest or the extremities, or because of unconsciousness. External evidence of abdominal injury may be minimal. Blunt trauma to the abdomen, always difficult to evaluate, requires good diagnostic acumen, very careful observation, frequent examination of the patient and sound judgment. One must carefully analyze the nature of the injury and anticipate what damage may exist within the abdominal cavity.

Symptoms and Signs of Abdominal Injuries

Injuries to the abdomen often are difficult to diagnose, even by well-trained physicians. Therefore, they present an unusual challenge to the first aid worker. He must be aware of the fact that abdominal injuries often are slow to develop manifestations and frequently are masked by the symptoms of associated injuries. He must be aware of these difficulties and should have them in mind if the patient is responsive and can be carefully questioned as to the nature of his injury. Much can be learned from a carefully taken history. Diagnostic problems are particularly difficult in those injuries in which there is no external evidence of abdominal trauma. Crushing and blast injuries often produce intraabdominal trauma which is masked by lack of external trauma as well as by other associated injuries.

Symptoms manifested by the patient are of great value. *Nausea* and *vomiting*, especially if the vomitus contains blood, should immediately alert the first aid worker to the possibility of intraabdominal injury. Pain in the abdomen is another symptom of trauma to its contents. Pain, however, may be minimal in the first few hours following injury and often is disregarded because of the predominance of other symptoms. It may likewise be masked by unconsciousness, somnolence, shock, or mental confusion. The signs of abdominal injury may be elicited by careful abdominal examination. *Tenderness* is a common finding. Its location and intensity may be a guide to the location of the organ involved and the severity of the damage to it. *Muscle spasm* (a stiffening or rigidity of the abdominal muscles) suggests an irritation of the peritoneum (lining of the abdominal cavity beneath the spastic muscles) and aids in localizing the injury. Such peritoneal irritation can result from contamination by blood, secretion of abdominal organs, or infection. These complications produce peritonitis, which is inflammation of the peritoneal cavity and usually requires urgent surgery.

Shock often follows peritonitis, whether it be on a chemical, bacterial, or hemorrhagic basis. The patient will develop not only abdominal symptoms consisting of pain, distention, tenderness, and rigidity but will show evidence of pallor, a cold and clammy skin, a rapid pulse, and low blood pressure. If the patient's condition is too critical to withstand prolonged transportation to the hospital, blood expanders or blood plasma should be administered intravenously to support the patient until he can receive definitive care (see Chap. 8).

First Aid Treatment of Abdominal Injuries

It is most important for the first aid worker to be cognizant of the dangers of abdominal injuries and to examine the patient for the possibility of their existence. Open wounds of the abdomen (penetrating wounds) are easily recognized. Intraabdominal wounds due to blunt force (nonpenetrating wounds) may show little external evidence of injury but may be equally serious. Wounds of the abdomen, along with those of the head and chest, should be given priority in transportation to the hospital or to qualified medical care. The death rate from abdominal injuries is greatly influenced by the length of time between injury and administration of definitive treatment. This fact is of great importance in mass casualties where the first aid worker should give priority to patients with abdominal injuries over those with injuries of the extremities, even though the latter may appear to be more severe.

Because of the possibility of intraabdominal hemorrhage in abdominal wounds whether penetrating or nonpenetrating, a bandage compressing the abdomen may help suppress hemorrhage. This is best accomplished by a *scultetus* or many-tailed binder. Such binders consist of a 12-inch square of heavy material, such as flannel, with tails extending out from each side, 3 inches in width and 18 inches in length. The square is placed under the back of the patient and the tails are folded across the abdomen, beginning at either the top or the bottom and overlapping each preceding tail, pulling them fairly snug. They may be fixed in position by multiple safety pins. If such a binder is not available, a clean bath towel, pillow case, or portion of a sheet may be wrapped about the patient, pulled tightly, and secured with safety pins. Binders should not be extended far upward onto the chest as they will interfere with breathing.

If a wound of the abdomen is present, it should be covered with a sterile, or at least clean, dressing over which is placed a compression binder. In lacerated wounds of the abdomen through which the bowel or other abdominal organs protrude, *the first aid worker should not attempt to replace these structures.* They should be left on the surface of the abdomen and covered with large sterile or clean cloths, plastic wrap, or aluminum foil (Fig. 2). Only if delivery of the patient to a hospital is delayed for an hour or more should moist dressings be applied to prevent drying of the bowel. Cloths or pads may be moistened with any sterile, nonirritating solution, such as water,

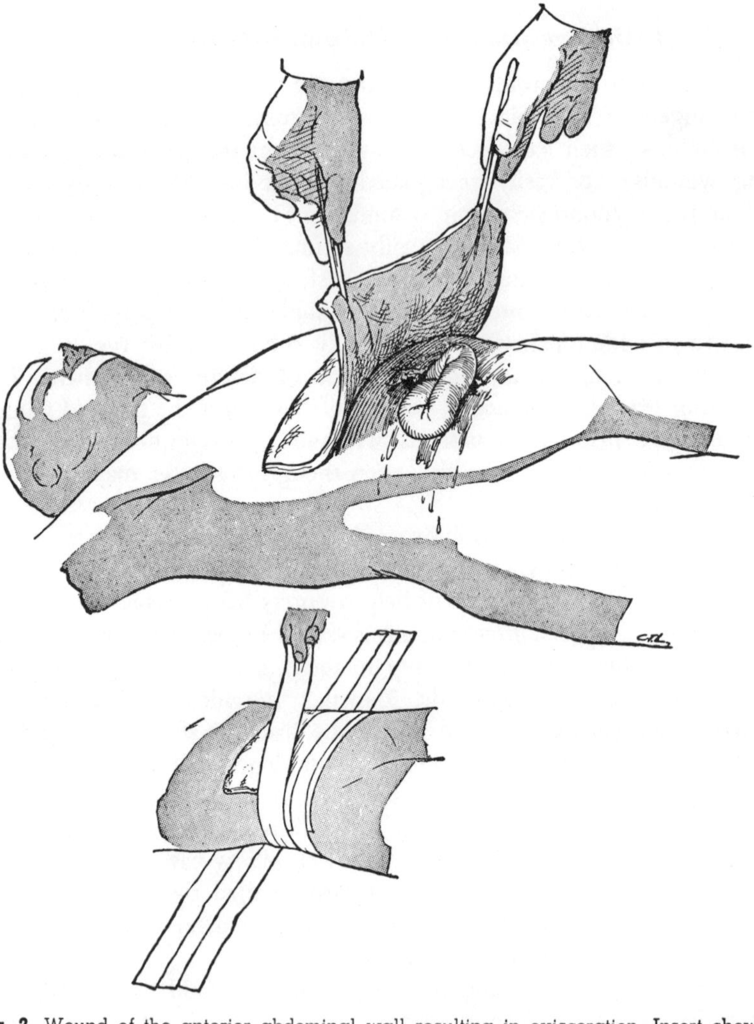

260 / Ch. 16: Abdominal Emergencies

Fig. 2. Wound of the anterior abdominal wall resulting in evisceration. Insert shows method of applying a scultetus binder to afford fixation of dressing. It is applied tightly for hemorrhage, but loosely when prolapsed intestine is present, lest the pressure jeopardize the blood supply to the prolapsed loop.

saline solution, or plasma. If sterile solutions are not available but water can be sterilized by boiling, this should be used to moisten the dressings. However, the water should be cooled sufficiently so as not to damage the tissues. After covering the exposed organs with wet dressings a compression bandage should be applied over them, snugly but not tight enough to interfere with circulation. *The first aid worker should remember not to administer anything by mouth* to the patient with an abdominal injury. This is especially true for irritating solutions, such as whiskey, which can produce severe inflammation if they leak into the peritoneal cavity.

Abdominal Pain

Abdominal pain frequently is encountered in individuals who have been involved in an accident. It may be a steady pain, varying in intensity, which often accompanies some form of inflammatory process. If the pain is severe and intermittent (colicky), it generally is produced by obstruction of some tubelike structure, such as the intestines, bile ducts, or ureters. Nausea and vomiting often are associated with abdominal pain. Tenderness and rigidity (tightening of the abdominal muscles) may accompany the pain if the lining of the abdominal cavity becomes irritated by a leakage of intestinal contents, bile or urine, or by infection. The patient may or may not have an elevated temperature. The abdomen may become markedly distended if peritonitis or bowel obstruction has been present for many hours, and this is a grave sign that calls for medical care. Abdominal pain often is serious and needs urgent medical attention.

These few "don'ts" should be remembered by the layman. *Never give a cathartic. Do not give food, fluids, or drugs by mouth.* These may not only aggravate serious abdominal disease but if retained in the stomach, increase the danger of vomiting and inhalation of stomach contents on the administration of an anesthetic and the possible development of postoperative pneumonia. A small low enema is permissible when symptoms are not severe, if constipation is suspected and tenderness does not exist. The patient should be kept at rest and if the pain persists, he should be seen by a doctor or sent to a hospital as soon as possible. Some of the more common abdominal diseases producing pain will be briefly described.

ACUTE APPENDICITIS. In former years many deaths resulted from acute appendicitis because patients were given strong cathartics such as castor oil or epsom salts. This disease usually produces pain which begins in the region of the navel and gradually shifts to the right lower portion of the abdomen. Tenderness over the appendix usually can be noted, but the muscles do not become rigid until the disease has irritated the peritoneum. Early in the disease the patient's temperature usually is normal. Where this disease is suspected, it is most important that no cathartic be given and that all food and fluids be withheld. A doctor should be called as soon as possible.

PERFORATED PEPTIC ULCER. When a peptic ulcer perforates, stomach and duodenal contents are liberated into the peritoneal cavity producing immediate and severe symptoms. The pain is steady and intense. The entire abdomen rapidly becomes rigid. The skin may become cold and clammy, and the patient may present a picture similar to shock, although the blood pressure is seldom below normal. Any movement of the patient intensifies his pain, and he will object to being examined or to having his position changed. It is most important that these patients be given nothing by mouth, as anything received in the stomach is likely to cause greater spillage into the peritoneal cavity. *Such a patient should be transported to a hospital by ambulance as soon as possible.*

GALLBLADDER COLIC. This is usually produced by a gallstone blocking a bile duct. The pain is in the upper abdomen, usually on the right, and radiates to the right shoulder blade. It is intense, but abdominal tenderness usually is confined to the upper abdomen on the right and rigidity is not marked if present. A doctor should see the patient as soon as possible to determine if hospitalization is indicated and to give the patient relief.

INTESTINAL OBSTRUCTION. Intestinal obstruction is most commonly due to adhesions within the abdomen following surgical procedures. In infants and young children, however, some birth abnormalities may cause obstruction. Tumorous growths, a twisted loop of bowel, some intestinal diseases, or inflammation following perforation of the bowel may also produce obstruction.

Intestinal obstruction is manifest by recurring colicky pain which may be very severe. Nausea and vomiting may appear early in obstructions high in the intestinal tract. Although, at the height of pain, there may be an urgency to pass gas or have a bowel movement, inability to do so should be looked upon as a danger signal. Large amounts of fluid elements of the circulation and of body tissues accumulate above the point of obstruction which may produce severe shock and intravenous fluids and blood transfusion must be administered without delay.

Even though the symptoms of obstruction may subside completely, the patient may be in the stage of greatest danger since there remains the possibility that obstruction to circulation of a loop of bowel may have caused death to the tissues and pain signals can no longer be generated. On suspicion of intestinal obstruction, the patient should seek medical advice as soon as possible, because delay to the point of abdominal distention, vomiting of fecal material, shock, fever, and increased white blood cell count complicate surgical procedures and greatly increase mortality.

RENAL COLIC. Stones blocking the ureter (tube leading from the kidney to the bladder) likewise can produce severe pain. The pain usually is located in the kidney area and radiates down toward the bladder. It may be very intense, colicky in nature but has little associated abdominal tenderness or rigidity. This is discussed in the chapter dealing with emergencies of the genitourinary tract (Chap. 20).

STRANGULATED HERNIA. A hernia is a protrusion of some anatomic structure through a natural or unnatural opening in the wall of its natural cavity. Hernias are most commonly seen in the inguinal region (groin) or in the scar of a previous abdominal operation where the deeper layers have partially separated. A bulging or mass protrudes due to the contents of the abdominal cavity which are forced into the hernial sac. The omentum or a portion of the intestine are most commonly found in hernias. If they do not become blocked off and if the blood supply is not impaired, they may not produce symptoms. However, if these complications arise, the hernia becomes strangulated and pain and tenderness rapidly develop. The intestine becomes obstructed and nausea and vomiting frequently occur. When such symptoms develop and the mass cannot readily be replaced, urgent surgery is frequently necessary and delay may prove fatal. Therefore, early medical or surgical care is imperative.

SWALLOWED FOREIGN BODIES. Emergencies arising from swallowed foreign bodies occur much more commonly in children than in adults, because children so commonly insert various objects in their mouth during play. While swallowed chicken bones or fish bones may lodge in the esophagus and not cause abdominal symptoms, perforation of the esophagus is highly dangerous from the standpoint of infection and warrants early medical care. It is not uncommon for the mentally deranged to swallow large numbers of bizzare objects, even silverware, or to insert objects into the rectum. One of the most important factors during such an emergency is to determine whether or not the foreign body has been swallowed into the stomach or has been aspirated into the respiratory tract. Usually it will not be difficult to differentiate the location of the foreign body. When it has lodged in the respiratory tract, difficulty in breathing, consisting of obstruction to respiration, will be the most prominent manifestation (see Chap. 14).

Most foreign bodies which are swallowed into the stomach are relatively harmless ones, such as stones, marbles or coins. Fortunately, these foreign bodies being round and smooth will pass readily through the intestinal tract without producing harmful effects. More serious foreign bodies are open safety pins. This is a remarkably frequent type of foreign body, particularly in infants. Although it might appear impossible for an infant to pass an open safety pin, experience has taught us that, in most instances, the pin will actually pass through the entire intestinal tract without producing serious harm. On some occasions, the pin may lodge at certain points and actually penetrate the wall of the intestine. When this happens, a local abscess will develop which may spread into a general peritonitis.

The *treatment* of patients who have swallowed foreign bodies is rarely an emergency. However, foreign bodies with sharp points may occasionally require operation to remove them to prevent perforation of the intestine. Large objects may cause partial or total intestinal obstruction. *Cathartics must not be administered* in the treatment of swallowed foreign bodies. The administration of cathartics may increase peristalsis so much that the sharp points of the foreign body may penetrate the wall of the intestine. If the foreign body is of such a nature that there are sharp points on it, a physician should naturally be consulted to determine whether it is permissible to drink fluids or eat a soft diet, or whether or not removal by operation is indicated. Naturally, the stool should be watched to determine when and if the object is passed.

THROMBOSED OR PROLAPSED HEMORRHOIDS. Hemorrhoids are extremely common, being present to a mild degree in perhaps 25 percent or more of adults past the age of 40. Complications, such as bleeding from hemorrhoids, thrombosis, or prolapse, are fairly common.

Thrombosis of a hemorrhoid usually occurs fairly rapidly and commonly without obvious cause. Severe pain develops and an indurated area represented by the thrombosed hemorrhoid may be palpated. The pain is usually so severe as to cause complete, or at least partial, disability. The recumbent position with applications of an ice bag to the affected area affords relief, but with conservative treatment of this type, it will usually require three or four days for the pain to subside. A much more effective method of eradicating the symptoms and the condition is to have a physician incise over the thrombosed hemorrhoid and express the blood clot. Invariably this affords complete relief. A small dressing consisting of cotton and gauze is applied and the patient allowed up as usual. Obviously, evacuation of the clot is done by the physician.

Prolapsed hemorrhoids usually occur only in the severe cases in which there is a redundancy of mucosa. This prolapse occurs during bowel movement, but usually is reduced spontaneously. At other times the patient obtains reduction by pressure with the padded finger. On certain occasions reduction by the patient may be unsuccessful. In this case the patient should be put to bed with the buttocks elevated and an ice bag applied to the perineum. The administration of sedatives, such as 10 grains of aspirin and one-half grain of phenobarbital, should be given in an attempt to obliterate spasm of the rectal sphincter which so commonly prevents reduction of the mass. Ordinarily it is advisable to have the mass reduced early by a physician before it becomes edematous and irreducible. In either event an operation will usually be necessary ultimately.

17 / Injuries of the Scalp, Skull, Spine, and Nervous System

ERIC OLDBERG

From the standpoint of first aid, injuries to the scalp, skull, spine, and nervous system form one of the largest groups of accident cases and are among the most important. Although statistics vary, it would probably be safe to say that one third of all important injuries during World War II involved these structures, that between one third and one half of the fatalities resulted from such injuries, and that close to 50 percent of the permanent disabilities resulting from injury were caused by damage in this area. Since these structures are of such importance to life and normal function, the principles of first aid for injuries to them are of paramount importance and of great assistance in cutting down the incidence of serious consequences.

Scalp

Although the scalp, anatomically, is not a part of the nervous system, injuries to it are considered here because of the possibility of a concomitant intracranial injury. The scalp is a very vascular integument and is rather loosely applied to the skull. Both of these features are of great importance, are different from the characteristics of tissues or integument elsewhere in the body, and are important with regard to treatment. Indeed, it may be said that because of them, the two chief complications of improper treatment are serious hemorrhage and infection.

With regard to *hemorrhage*, it is common knowledge that the scalp is richly supplied with blood vessels. Everyone who has had a laceration of the scalp or who has seen friends or relatives receive such injuries, is aware of the fact that a very small stab wound alone is sufficient to allow the escape of great quantities of blood. This is true even if a very small scalp laceration does not happen to cut an artery. If an artery of any size happens to be included in the laceration, the resultant bleeding may even be so severe as to be fatal. The areas of greatest predilection for such severe hemorrhage are in the temporal region, where the temporal artery has large branches; the occipital region, where the same situation exists with regard to the occipital arteries; and the forehead, where the supraorbital artery on each side supplies that region richly with arterial blood. Hemorrhage is least likely to be severe near the vertex of the skull, at which point vessels which are cut are of the smallest caliber.

Since the scalp is normally covered with hair, it is exceedingly difficult to control bleeding from it or to keep the area in a sanitary condition unless the hair is shaved. This should, therefore, always be done, and the usual rule is that the area to be shaved must leave a margin of at least two inches around the laceration. The removal of hair is often clumsily done, even by persons who should know better. Proper removal of hair requires two instruments, a hair clipper, either manually or electrically operated, both of which are easy to use and one or more old-fashioned straight-edged razors kept in good condition. Safety razors are anathemas to the experienced head surgeon, since they tend to pull hair out by the roots, cause pain to the patient, and open a large number of hair follicles which may serve as an ingress for infection. In shaving the head, as a matter of fact, except in dealing with female patients who in selected cases may have a valid reason for preserving hair, it is better to clip the entire head and then shave around the lacerated area for a distance of two inches as described above. Tincture of green soap should be properly lathered into the area to be shaved, beforehand, by means of an ordinary piece of gauze, preferably sterile. When the bleeding laceration has thus been properly exposed, it will usually be found to be rough and jagged. The chief function of the first aid worker is to stop hemorrhage by exerting pressure on a dressing in the wound; if this fails to control the bleeding, the artery should also be compressed (see also Chap. 8). *Repair of the wound* as described in the next paragraph is left to the physician.

If Novocain is available, it is very easy to inject several ml of a 1- or 2-percent solution into the tissues immediately surrounding the laceration. This is usually all the anesthetic that is necessary, and the laceration can then be spread apart by means of retractors or sterile dressings. If a general anesthetic is necessary, one of the many intravenous agents may be utilized. Pieces of dirt, cloth, hair, and the like, should be picked out as carefully as possible and the wound thoroughly irrigated with warm sterile water or saline solution. Ragged pieces of scalp may then be treated, and if the underlying tissues (galea and bone) seem to be intact, the wound may be closed if recent, i.e., less than 10 hours since injury. If there is active bleeding in the edges of the laceration, the novice will find it difficult to stop. The scalp is not adaptable to the clamping of individual blood vessels, and therefore hemostats are usually placed on the inner edge of the scalp and flopped over so as to inhibit bleeding by pressure. The wound is closed by applying numerous sutures, preferably silk, through the entire thickness of the scalp. If there is a considerable amount of soiling and contamination, it is advisable to administer antibiotics. A pressure bandage may then be applied, the best material being the elastic weave with which Ace Bandages are made. Tetanus antitoxin should be given in all cases in which contamination is significant.

The other possible complication from laceration of the scalp, as mentioned above, is *infection*. Infection in the scalp may occur for a number of reasons. In the first place, foreign material may be driven through a laceration into the loose tissues underneath the scalp. Second, the presence of hair, which has not been removed in time, and of seborrheic (dandrufflike) material means that there are organisms constantly in contact with the wound. Third, the loose application of the scalp to the skull allows pus to burrow rather freely underneath the scalp. Fourth, it may be impossible to attend a laceration within a reasonable period of time, in which case, the scalp, like any other tissue which is not cleaned properly, may become infected. The rule to prevent infection, if possible, is to debride all lacerations of the scalp as thoroughly as possible. Here again, shaving of the hair is of paramount importance. If the laceration of the scalp is old, i.e., inflicted more than 12 hours previously, and pus is already present along the edges or between the edges of the wound, then it is better to irrigate the wound, carefully remove any foreign bodies present, and leave it open so that it can drain; the gaping wound will then heal by granulation from the bottom. This is a tedious and time-consuming healing process, however, which carries with it some danger of infection of the underlying bone, and therefore it should be avoided, if at all possible, by prompt and early attention to all lacerations.

The above principles are, in general, utilized in denuding or scalping injuries; the denuded area should be washed off as promptly as possible and cleaned, the surrounding hair clipped and shaved, and petrolatum gauze laid in place over the raw area. The patient should then be sent to the hospital for further and more specialized treatment.

Skull

The skull itself is not inherently important except as a container for the brain (Fig. 1). By that is meant that ordinary fractures in it do not have the same importance as they do in weight-bearing bones, although they may be much more serious because of the damage sus-

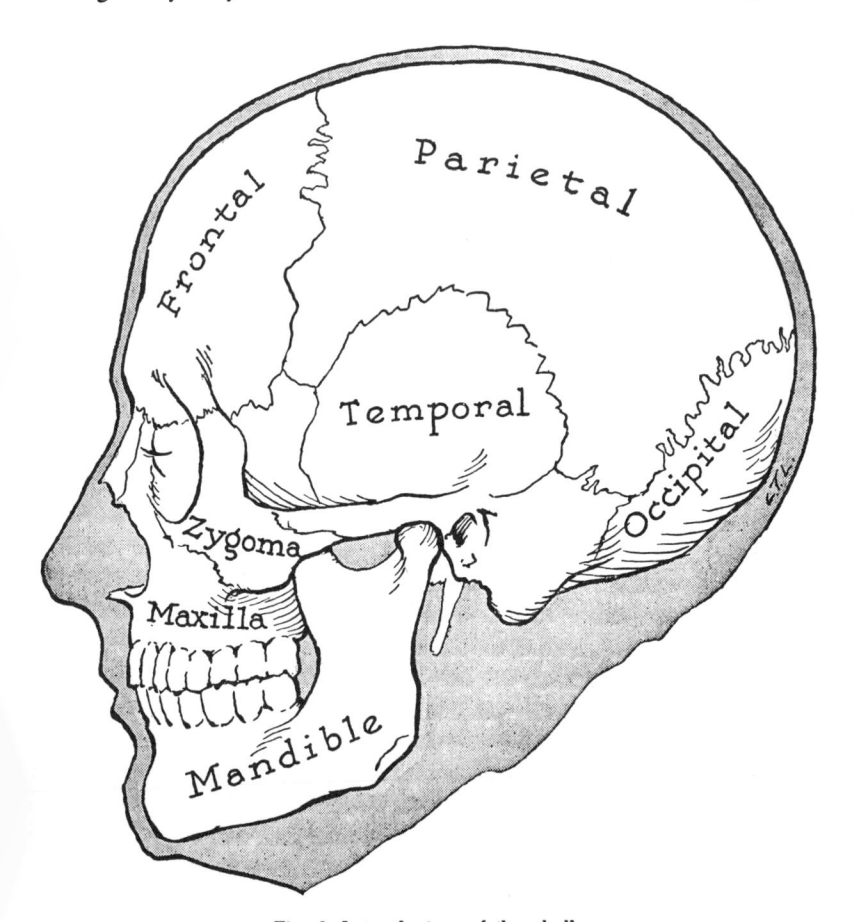

Fig. 1. Lateral view of the skull.

tained by the brain. Perhaps the most important pathologic manifestations of brain injury are *hemorrhage* and *laceration* of the brain itself. These injuries are, of course, the direct result of the blow inflicted on the head and not directly caused by the fracture, except in the occasional instance when loose bone fragments actually produce laceration of brain tissue. In addition to hemorrhage and laceration of brain tissue other pathologic conditions may be produced. For example, fractures of the skull may involve portions of it which allow the escape of cerebrospinal fluid from the spaces around the brain between the edges of the fracture and out through the soft tissues to the outside. The two more common places for this to occur are from the ear and from the nose. In wartime it may also happen, to a somewhat lesser degree, from compound fractures of the vault of the skull which tear the scalp, fracture the bone, and lacerate the dura underneath the bone.

In *leakage of watery cerebrospinal fluid* from the nose or ear, it will sometimes be surprising to the novice to see the large amount of fluid which may escape in this way—sometimes a quart or more per day. This causes loss of body fluids, which should, of course, be taken into consideration. A more serious aspect of the question, however, involves the fact that a route is open in such injuries for the ingress of infection into the brain or its membranes, causing abscess or meningitis. If a patient is leaking cerebrospinal fluid from his ear, this means that the eardrum has been torn in order to allow the fluid to escape, and there will be some blood and probably also some dirt in the ear canal. At first impulse it might appear desirable to syringe out this material in order to clean up the field of injury. Such a procedure, however, invites disaster, since syringing may wash organisms back through the laceration into the cranial cavity. For this reason, in patients with leakage of cerebrospinal fluid from the ear, merely swab out the ear canal gently with small pieces of cotton or applicators. The patient should then be gently placed on the side from which the leakage comes and the fluid allowed to drain onto towels, sterile gauze, cotton, or other appropriate absorptive material. Such drainage will usually continue copiously for two or three days and will then begin to lessen in amount, usually ceasing entirely in about 10 days. Manipulation and examination of the ear canal should be postponed until several days after the drainage has ceased. This, of course, does not mean that the canal should not be kept reasonably clean by means of sterile cotton applicators soaked in oil or glycerine.

When drainage of cerebrospinal fluid takes place through the nose, it is well to put the patient in a semireclining position to promote freer drainage. The patient should not attempt to blow his nose violently and should simply allow drainage to proceed. In these patients having leakage of cerebrospinal fluid from the nose, there is a greater probability that the drainage will persist indefinitely or will recur. This sometimes requires subsequent operative repair, which is a highly specialized procedure.

Drainage of the cerebrospinal fluid through the wound in a compound fracture of the skull is a separate problem which has to do with the care of compound fractures and will be discussed subsequently in this chapter. In all patients having cerebrospinal fistula, antibiotic therapy should be started as soon as possible as a prophylaxis against infection.

Occasionally *fractures of the skull may be depressed* and this may occur with or without laceration of the overlying scalp. Such depressions are rarely an emergency problem from the standpoint of surgical correction (Fig. 2). In the vast majority of cases, depressed fractures of the skull can be temporarily disregarded and the patient treated along the general principles advocated for the treatment of craniocerebral injuries, which will be described on page 277. It may be mentioned in passing here that the novice will sometimes be confused as to the presence or absence of a depressed skull fracture. In palpating the scalp he may feel a hematoma which has existed for a day or two, the center of which has become liquefied. This will sometimes give a cuplike impression and misleads the examiner into the fallacy of thinking that he is dealing with a depressed fracture. Since, as stated above, immediate operations for depressed skull fractures are almost never performed, such observation should be of little importance in first aid work, whether or not it is detected. However, subsequently most depressed fractures of the skull should be elevated, but this is not a first aid consideration.

Compound fractures of the skull are of the greatest importance from the standpoint of first aid, particularly in wartime when their incidence is multiplied many times. The term "compound fracture of the skull" implies that there has been a laceration of the scalp, fracture of the bone, very often a laceration of the membranes surrounding the brain, and a penetration of the brain itself (Fig. 3). Such fractures are produced by flying particles, by penetrating wounds, like those caused by bullets and other flying objects (shell fragments,

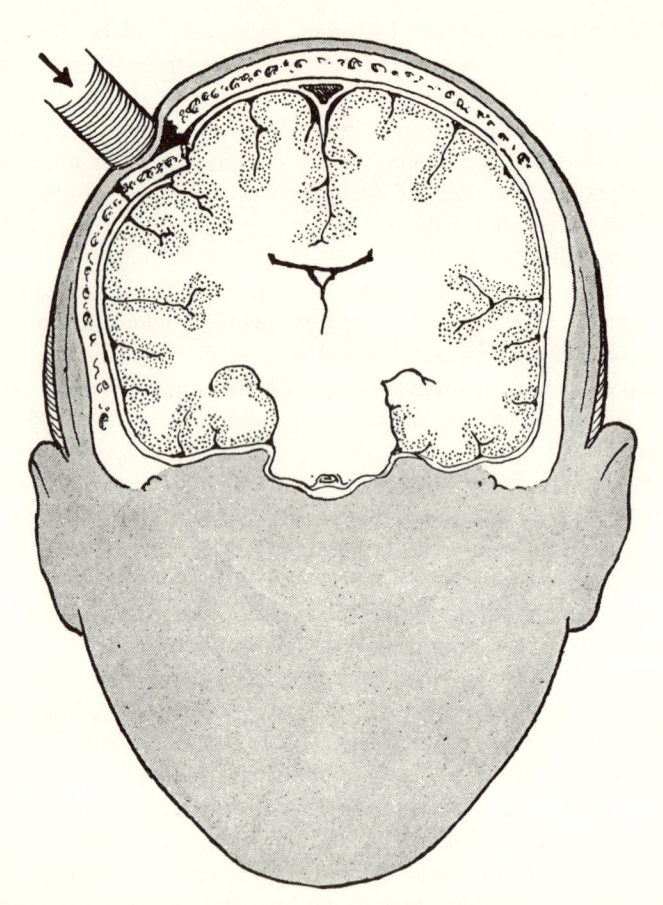

Fig. 2. Depressed fracture of the skull which requires subsequent, but not emergency, operative correction.

glass, and so on), or by severe falls. One usually finds that pieces of bone or metal accompanied by fragments of scalp, hair, and dirt have been driven into the brain. Of course, the immediate concern from the standpoint of first aid involves the possibility of such an injury producing an infection, which may take one or both of two forms, meningitis or brain abscess. The rule in first aid care, therefore, involves debridement of such injuries as well as is compatible with the existing conditions, but *only by the physician*. Gross particles of metal, bone, hair, dirt, cloth, head covering, and such should be removed as well as possible and the area irrigated with warm, sterile saline solution. If a good debridement is possible and the injury

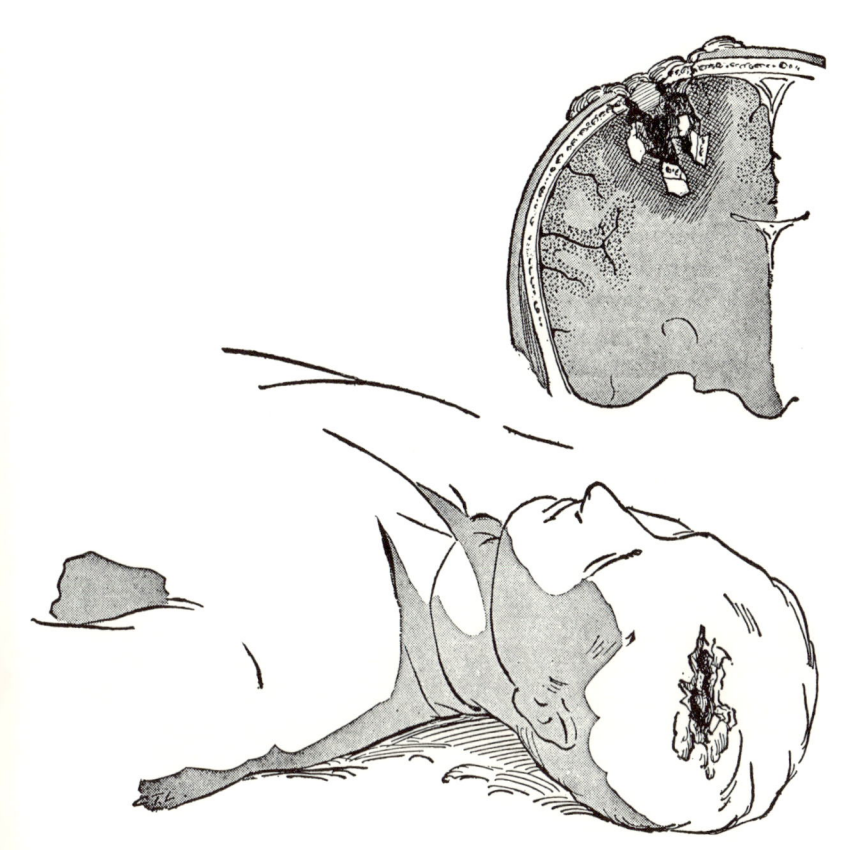

Fig. 3. Compound fracture of the skull. Note the pieces of bone and debris driven into the brain.

is fresh, the wound may be closed as described in the first portion of this chapter on page 267. If such is not the case and infection has already set in, the head should be shaved, chemotherapy started, and the patient taken to the hospital as quickly as possible. As has been emphasized in the discussion of wounds elsewhere in this text, cleanliness and debridement of the scalp and skull are of much greater importance than the use of antiseptic substances, such as iodine and Mercurochrome. Most head surgeons abjure the use of all such substances and rely entirely in their preoperative preparations on careful cleanliness, utilizing bland agents such as soap, water, and alcohol. If the wound is badly contaminated or infected, the patient should be treated with chemotherapeutic agents and antibiotics, such as penicillin.

Finally, other injuries to the skull may be mentioned for the sake of completeness which are more technical than the usual problem confronting the first aid worker. These involve fractures of the skull through nonsterile areas, such as sinuses, and fractures inducing hemorrhage of such extent that the patient's absorptive process cannot take care of it.

Brain

ANATOMY AND PHYSIOLOGY. By far the most important structure involved in head injuries is the brain. Injuries to it from the standpoint of immediate disability, death, and permanent disability are among the major items of the casualty list. A brief description of the anatomy of the brain should be borne in mind by the first aid worker. In the first place, it is a very soft, moist organ which is richly supplied with blood. It is enclosed in the cranial cavity, and except for the foramen magnum through which the spinal cord enters to its attachment to the base of the brain, it is so tightly enclosed that there is no room in the cavity for the swelling which occurs after injury. The cranial cavity is divided into compartments by two very tough and nonyielding membranes. One of them runs from front to back in the midline and separates the cerebral hemispheres. The other runs from side to side in the occipital region and separates the cerebrum from the cerebellum and medulla. Since these membranes are tough and inelastic, one mechanism by which head injuries affect the brain consists of laceration by them when the brain is shifted violently inside the cranial cavity by a gravitational or other force.

The brain is enclosed by membranes called the meninges. There are three of these. The innermost one, which is a thin membrane, is called the pia mater and is applied closely over the entire surface of the brain. Just outside of it lies the space in which the cerebrospinal fluid is enclosed. This space is about a millimeter or two in depth over the majority of the brain area, but over the crevices or sulci of the brain the depth of these lakes of fluid may be considerably greater. The fluid space is enclosed by a transparent, spiderweblike membrane called the arachnoid. The cerebrospinal fluid is therefore referred to as being enclosed in the subarachnoid space. Outside the arachnoid and intervening between it and the bone of the skull is a tough, thick protective membrane called the dura mater. The two inner membranes, pia mater and arachnoid, are referred to as the leptomeninges and the outer membrane, the dura mater, is referred to as the pachymeninx. All three layers together form the meninges of the brain. Infection usually involves the leptomeninges. This complication is serious, since the leptomeninges are in contact with the brain and since the cerebrospinal fluid circulates through them.

It should be stated at this point that the brain also contains cavities—one in each hemisphere, one in the midline between the hemispheres, and one underneath the cerebellum and lying between it and the pons and medulla. These cavities are called the ventricles of the brain and together contain about one ounce of fluid. They are connected by means of small openings with the fluid spaces surrounding the surface of the brain and spinal cord. They contain the organs which form the cerebrospinal fluid. As this fluid forms it passes out through the ventricular system, up around the surface of the brain, and down over the surface of the spinal cord, the latter structure having the same meninges as the brain. This cerebrospinal fluid, which is almost like water in its constituents, is being constantly formed at a high rate (perhaps 1 or more quarts per 24 hours) and is constantly being absorbed at the same rate by small clumps of veins which project into the fluid over the surface of the brain, particularly in the region of the vertex. Thus, it can be seen that with such an enormous free circulation, infection which gets in at one point is quickly carried by the fluid and spread to all other points over the brain and spinal cord. The ordinary forms of meningitis known to the lay person are such infections of the meninges which have been carried by the circulating fluid.

In order to do intelligent first aid work a minimal amount of knowledge regarding the localization of functions in the brain itself should be at hand. As is known to everyone, the brain contains comparatively large regions known as silent areas. They are under constant investigation, however, and it will probably be eventually found that there is no portion of the brain which does not have a function. The most important areas from the clinical standpoint are described in the following paragraphs.

Just in front of the ear and running up to the vertex of the brain there is a crevice or sulcus known as the Rolandic fissure, named after an early anatomist named Rolando. Immediately in front of this fissure lie the cells which control motor function. On the left side of the brain in the left hemisphere these cells control the motion of the right side of the body, including the right arm and leg, and vice versa. The cells nearest the top or vertex of the brain control the leg, and then as one comes down toward the ear over the surface of the brain, the cells in the lower region control the muscles of the trunk, the arm, the face, and so on. Just behind the Rolandic fissure the corresponding cells for sensation are located; they are distributed in approximately the same manner.

In all human beings, one side (hemisphere) of the brain is more important than the other; this hemisphere is called the predominant hemisphere. Since most persons are right-handed this means that in most brains the left hemisphere is predominant. Since it is predominant the right hand and the right leg are usually more powerful, more delicately coordinated, and more accurate. In addition, in such right-handed persons the areas governing expression, such as speech or writing, are located in the predominant hemisphere, namely, the left side. Therefore, a right-handed person who has received an injury to the left side of the brain, in the region of the Rolandic fissure, may be paralyzed on the right side of his body, including the arm and leg; in addition, if the injury has extended slightly frontward, he may also be unable to speak, although he may know what he wants to say. His ability to express himself verbally is gone because of injury to the speech center.

Just behind the Rolandic area there is an ill-defined area called the parietal region. This part of the brain is characterized by cells which give the individual the ability to integrate various common sensations into a complete conception. Thus, a person putting his hand in his pocket and taking hold of a match box is immediately aware of the article which he has grasped, even though he cannot see it and may not have known it was there. This implies that he could feel an object of a certain size, hardness, weight, temperature, roughness, configuration, and so on, and integrate all of the multiplicity of those impulses together in his parietal region and thereby instantly acquired the knowledge that his hand enclosed a match box. If the parietal area is damaged, however, the individual may still be able to tell sharp from dull, hot from cold, heavy from light, and so on, as separate sensations, but he is unable to integrate them, and if his hand were in his pocket, he therefore would be unable to distinguish, let us say, a match box from a coin. The parietal area of the predominant hemisphere also is the vicinity of centers for comprehension of expression by others; that is to say, the ability to understand what is said and to comprehend what is read. These functions are therefore impaired in injuries to the parietal region on the left side, in a right-handed person, and vice versa.

In the occipital region the centers for vision are located. Even though an individual may have no impairment of his eyes or of his optic nerves, the presence of the occipital lobes is necessary for him to comprehend what he sees. If both occipital lobes are injured or destroyed, the patient is blind as far as conscious vision is concerned. If the occipital lobe is destroyed on one side only, then the patient loses conscious vision for all objects which fall into his field of vision on the opposite side from the side of this injury. Thus, if the left occipital lobe is destroyed, the patient cannot see anything to his right with either eye.

The cerebellum is the organ having to do with coordination. If an individual has an injury or destruction of the cerebellum, his strength is not diminished, but he cannot coordinate his movements. Thus, he staggers like a drunken person in walking, cannot handle eating utensils with firm sure movements, and is generally clumsy and uncoordinated.

The stem of the brain and medulla oblongata contain the centers from which the cranial nerves spring, such as those which control rotating the eyeballs, moving the muscles of the face, protruding the tongue, swallowing, hearing, and equilibrium. In addition, this vital area contains the centers which are essential to life itself, such as those governing respiration, temperature, pulse rate, and possibly consciousness.

With the above brief summary of the gross and functional anatomy of the brain the first aid worker has a conception of the importance of the tissues with which he is dealing. The method of dealing with them from the first aid standpoint follows.

INJURY TO THE BRAIN. It should be the primary concern of all first aid workers to realize that a patient with a head injury, whether or not there is also an injury to the scalp or skull, or both, has first and foremost an injury to the brain; likewise, it is this injury which is probably going to mean life or death to him, or the possibility of a normal life later if death does not supervene. The brain, like any other organ, swells up when injured and there may be bleeding into it. Unlike other structures, however, this swelling is serious because there is no room for it to take place in the enclosure of the skull. The vital centers controlling respiration and so on are therefore placed under embarrassment, since their normal blood supply is squeezed out of normal function and since they may actually be injured by tears or hemorrhages. In addition, it should be borne in mind that the essential cells of the brain have no healing power whatever. If a bone is fractured, new bone is formed to heal the fracture. Not one single functioning brain cell, however, which is destroyed can ever be replaced. They are replaced instead by scar tissue, which not only has no function but acts as an irritating agent to remaining brain cells and sometimes stimulates them in later life to the point of setting off convulsions.

It should be the primary object, then, of all first aid workers to realize that the greatest service that they can do the injured person is to *treat him gently*. He should be subjected to the least possible handling. X-rays at the time of injury are rarely of value unless there has been a penetrating wound, and this question the operating surgeon himself should decide, not the first aid worker. The period of a patient's unconsciousness is of importance in evaluating the amount of damage done, and this should be carefully observed. A particular precaution regarding unconsciousness is that in cases of intracranial bleeding following head injuries, a patient may be conscious for a time and then lose consciousness. Such an occurrence is all the more reason for arranging for hospital care as soon as possible.

Other than the above admonishments, the first aid worker should attempt to evaluate the neurologic situation to the best of his ability. It is sometimes very important to know whether or not a patient was paralyzed on one side when first seen or whether this paralysis was a subsequent development. Other simple observations can be made which may be of importance, such as inspection of the pupils to see whether or not they are equal in size and which pupil is the larger. The larger of two unequal pupils will almost invariably demonstrate the side of greatest brain damage. Weakness or paralysis of the extremities on one side of the body is indicative of injury on the opposite side of the brain. If the first aid worker carries out these simple principles and observations in conjunction with the instructions and advice previously given in this chapter regarding wounds involving the brain, he will be fulfilling his obligations and will be sending back to the hospital an individual in whom proper treatment has been initiated. In summation, the watchwords in head injuries are 1, *cleanliness;* 2, *gentleness;* and 3, *quick hospitalization.*

Spinal Cord

Injuries to the spinal cord may result from direct or indirect trauma. Direct injury may be caused in war by bullets or shell fragments, but in civilian life most injuries are indirect and result from acute, forcible forward flexion of the spine, since the spongy bodies of the vertebrae are less resistant than the denser laminae (Figs. 4-9).

The thoracic vertebrae are somewhat splinted by the ribs, so that the vertebrae most often involved are in the cervical and lumbar regions. When acute pressure is brought to bear by forced flexion of the body of the vertebra, it collapses and is compressed, causing an angulation of the spinal cord. This angulation in itself is not enough to cause damage to the spinal cord, unless it presses on the anterior spinal artery, the chief nourishing artery to the cord. But bony fragments may be broken off and project into the canal, or the softer cartilaginous disc between the vertebral bodies may be forced backward so as to compress the spinal cord. Also, the vertebrae may be

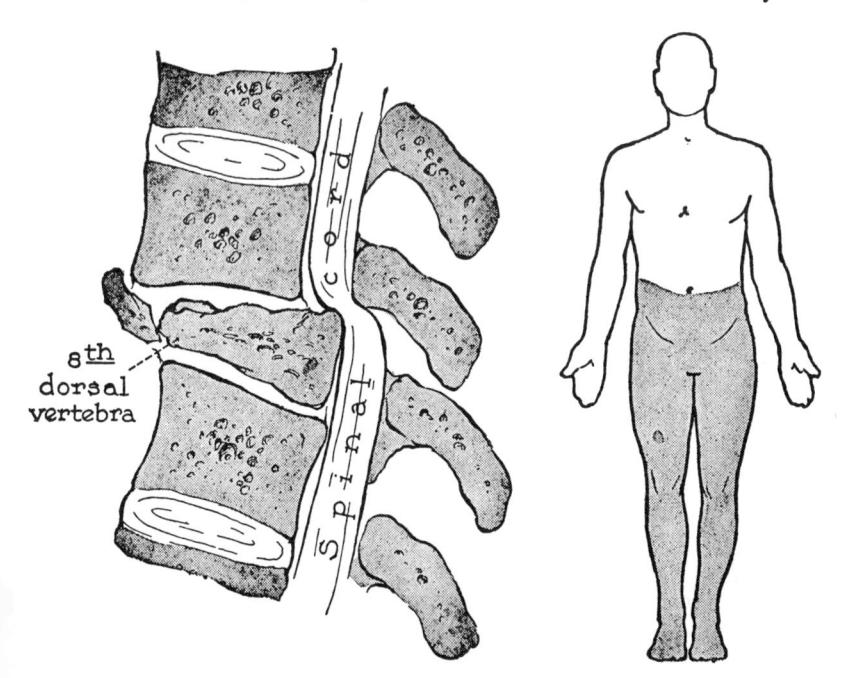

Fig. 4. Injury of the spinal cord sustained by fracture of a vertebra.

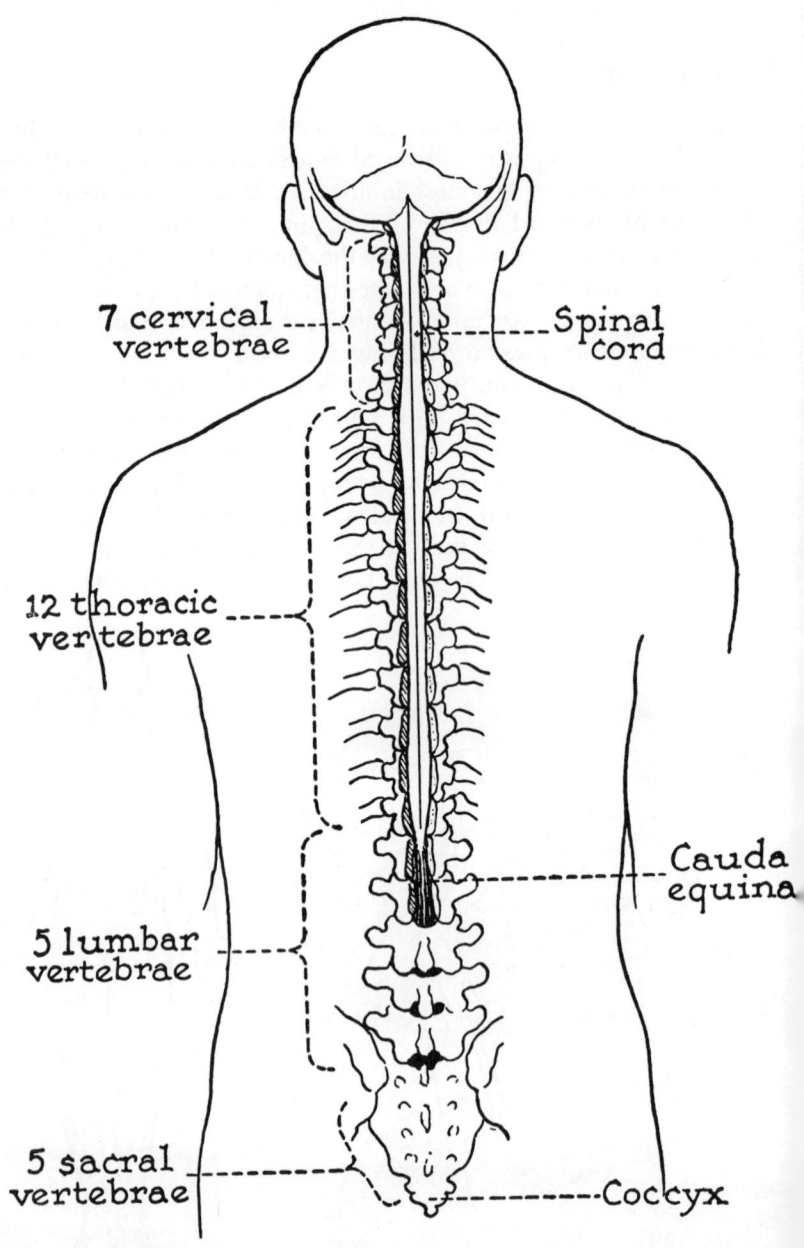

Fig. 5. The vertebral column. The vertebral column is divided into segments corresponding to the vertebrae; however, the spinal cord segments are two spaces higher than the corresponding vertebrae.

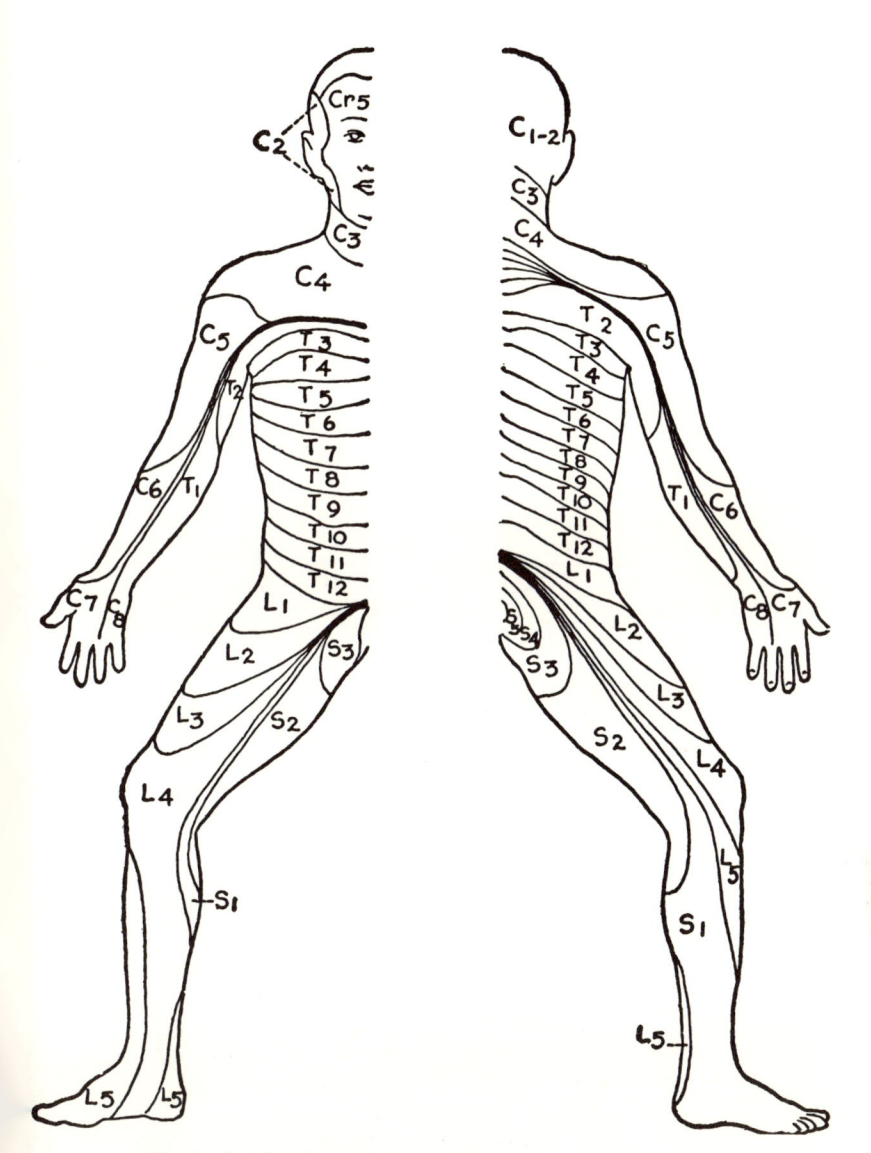

Fig. 6. Peripheral distribution of the various spinal nerves.

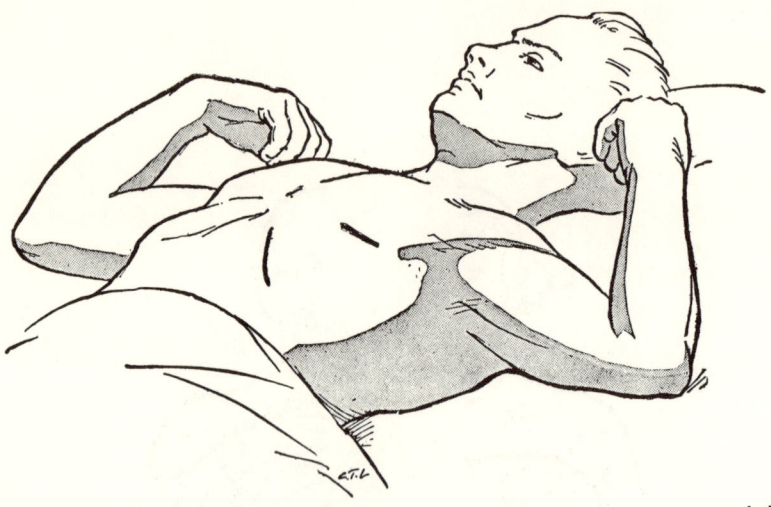

Fig. 7. Position and attitude of the arms in a fracture located in the region of the sixth cervical vertebra with injury to the spinal cord.

Dislocated disc

Spinal cord

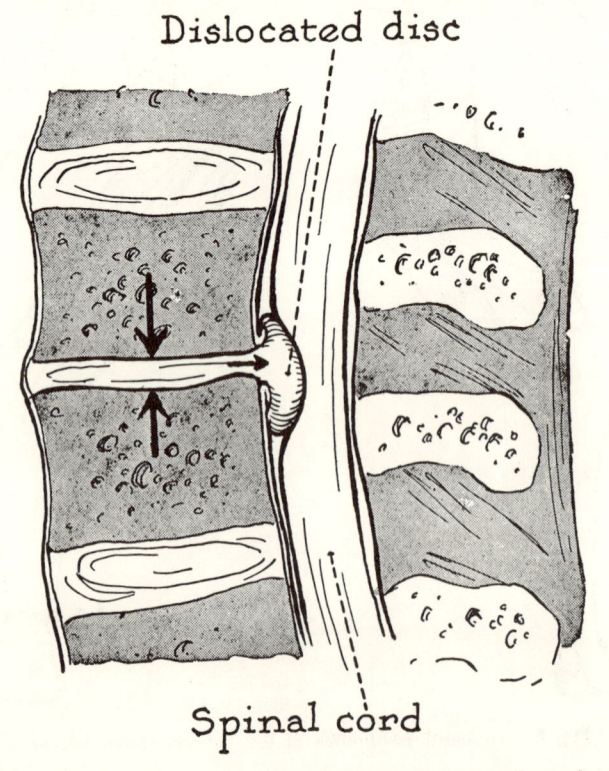

Fig. 8. Dislocation of intervertebral disc backward into the spinal canal compressing the spinal cord.

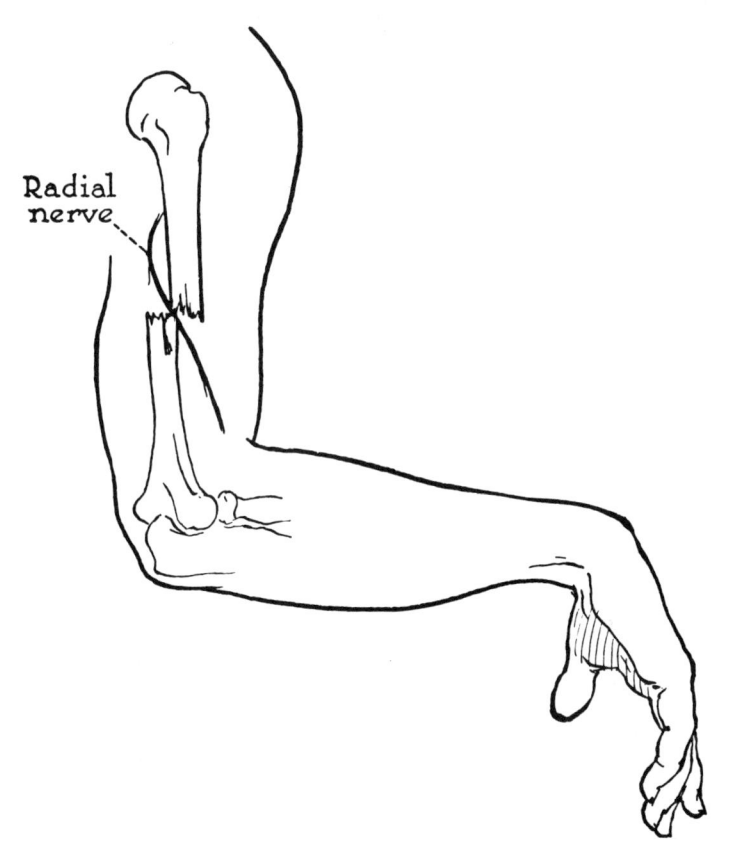

Fig. 9. Wristdrop resulting from paralysis of radial nerve afflicted by fracture of the humerus.

dislocated from their normal alignment and so impinge upon the spinal cord.

If the *spinal cord itself is injured* the results are grave. The resulting symptoms tell the neurologist at what level the spine is involved, since the relationship of the spinal segments to the vertebrae is known in great detail. Let us suppose first that there is a complete transverse lesion of the spinal cord. This may result either from severance of the cord or from local shock which prevents impulses passing the level involved. The primary result of such a lesion would be to suppress all motion and all sensation below the level of the lesion. By determining the level at which sensation is possible, for example by pricking the skin with a pin, the examiner determines the level of the lesion, since the region innervated by each segment of the spinal cord has been accurately determined. Moreover, one can get some idea by simply watching the patient. If he does not move any of his extremities, and cannot do so on command, the lesion must lie in the upper cervical (neck) region, since the upper limbs are innervated from the lower cervical cord. If, on the other hand, the arms are moved freely but the legs are not, then the lesion must lie below the lower cervical cord and above the lumbar cord, from which the lower limbs are innervated. Any serious lesion of the cord will cause retention of urine.

In addition to the neurologic signs, other means exist to determine the location of the lesion. By pressure on the spinous processes one may find that the spine of the involved vertebra is much more sensitive. But by all means the most important adjunct to our examination is the roentgen ray. X-rays are to be made by directing the rays both anteroposteriorly and laterally. The lateral plate is very important, since the compression of the vertebral body may not be visible on the anteroposterior photograph.

The *treatment of spinal cord injuries* is very important because such injuries are so serious. The fact that the vertebral body is usually collapsed and the angulation of the spinal canal is forward, is very important in the handling of a patient with an injury to the spine, since an attempt to move or carry the patient in the usual way, or on the usual stretcher, will tend to increase the anterior curvature of the spine and may cause further damage to the spinal cord.

When called to see a patient who is suspected of having an injury to the spine, a very careful inspection should be made before attempting to move him. If the patient cannot move either arms or legs or cannot move the legs and only imperfectly the arms, the injury is to the cervical region and the problem of moving him becomes very grave. The important feature in the treatment of fractures of the spine with suspected or proved injury to the spinal cord is to insure safe transportation to a hospital and *avoidance* of further injury which might be inflicted during transportation. Carelessness in transporting patients with a fracture of the cervical vertebrae is particularly liable to result in damage to the spinal cord. Three or more strong people are necessary to move a patient with a cervical fracture. The head must not be rotated but must be held rigidly in perfect alignment with the thoracic spine and extended. The body must be lifted by two strong men, while another pulls the head and holds it straight and a fourth pulls in the opposite direction at the feet. The patient is then laid flat on his back on a rigid floor or plank (if necessary take a door off its hinges and use it as a stretcher) with a sandbag or other solid object on either side of the head to keep the neck in alignment. When the patient reaches the hospital the same care must be exercised, especially in taking x-rays.

If the patient, when first seen, moves the upper extremities freely, the lesion must be below the cervical region, and it suffices to roll the patient over on his face and transport him in that position. To place a person with a fractured spine on his back in the usual stretcher is only to invite trouble for reasons already given.

The important matter in the treatment of fractures of the spine is, therefore, to prevent injury to the spinal cord which may be irreparable and leave the patient permanently paralyzed. The person who first sees such a patient should remember that any attempt to move him may cause irreparable damage and should go at once for a physician. The first aid attendant should not even lift the patient's head to try to shift him into a more comfortable position.

The Peripheral Nerves

Any of the peripheral nerves may be injured in one way or another, especially those of the extremities because of their long and exposed course. The problem of first aid in these cases does not differ from that of fractures and lacerations in general. One must stop the hemorrhage and place a clean bandage over any external wound and get the patient to a physician as soon as possible. It is very important to prevent infection, since this complicates and delays suture of the nerves involved. Success in nerve suture depends on clean end-to-end anastomosis.

18 / Eye Injuries

WILLIAM A. MANN

While the medical and surgical management of most ocular diseases and injuries is strictly in the province of the trained ophthalmologist, there are frequently occasions when the prompt rendering of first aid treatment by the nonophthalmologist may be the means of saving an eye and preserving vision.

Anatomy and Physiology

There are certain anatomic and physiologic characteristics peculiar to the eye which need to be understood for the application of anything but the most superficial first aid. We can think of the eye as an approximately spherical end-organ of vision connected to the brain through the optic nerve and consisting of three layers. The *outer* (protective) *layer* comprises the opaque white sclera and anteriorly the transparent cornea. The smooth surface of the cornea (producing the "highlight" seen in Fig. 1) together with the transparency must be maintained if a clear image is to be obtained. The normal cornea is supplied with nerves so that any loss of the corneal surface (epithelium) causes severe pain in the eye. The epithelium when damaged is quickly repaired but damage to the deeper layers (stroma) may result in permanent scarring and thus cause visual impairment. The *middle* (vascular) *layer* comprises the iris, ciliary body, and choroid. The iris is the diaphragm regulating the size of the pupil and controlling the amount of light entering the eye; the amount of pigment determines the "color" of the eye. Behind the iris lies the ciliary body which supports the lens through the zonular fibers and thereby controls accommodation. Posteriorly lies the choroid, lining the sclera and supplying through its rich vasculature the *inner* (ner-

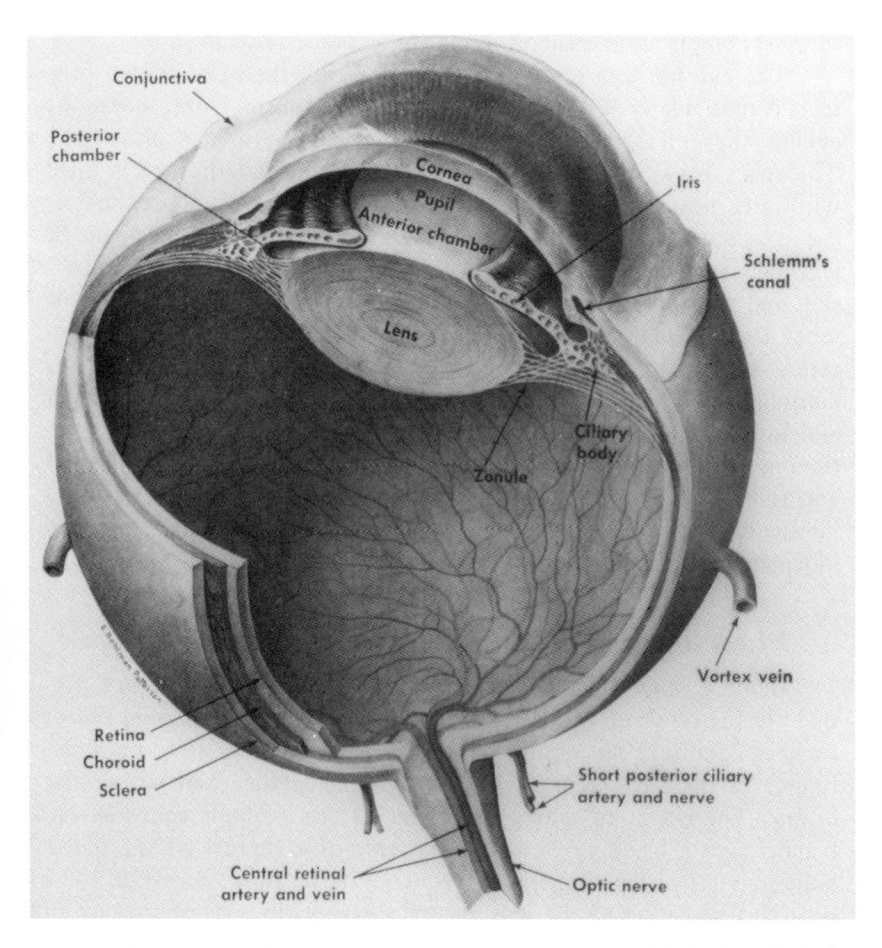

Fig. 1. "The human eye". (Frontispiece illustration. **In** Newell. **Ophthalmology** 2nd ed. 1969. Courtesy of C. V. Mosby Co.)

vous) *layer* which is the retina. On the retina are formed the images for transmission to the higher centers in the brain.

The interior of the eye is filled with aqueous humor in front of the lens (and ciliary body) and vitreous humor behind the lens. The aqueous is a water-like fluid formed continually by the processes of the ciliary body and draining away through the Canal of Schlemm lying in the cornea in the angle of the anterior chamber. If aqueous is lost through injury or surgery, it is replaced in a few minutes. This is not true of vitreous, a complex gelatinous structure occupying the space between the lens and retina. Loss of vitreous through injury or surgical complication is therefore not to be desired usually.

The eye lies in a bony cavity in the skull, the *orbit*, which protects it particularly well from injury except from the front, where the eyelids through the blinking reflex offer some further protection. The space between the bony walls of the orbit and the eye is filled with fatty tissue and tendinous sheaths which serve to support the eye, the extraocular muscles, nerves, and blood vessels. The eyelids may be considered to consist of two layers. The outer layer comprises the skin and subcutaneous tissue with the eyelashes at the lid margin; the inner layer is composed of a dense tarsal plate covered on the posterior surface by conjunctiva. This mucous membrane lining, the conjunctiva, is reflected onto the surface of the eyeball at the upper and lower fornix and at the inner and outer canthus becoming continuous with the corneal epithelium at the limbus (junction of cornea and sclera). The two layers play an important part in the repair of lid lacerations since they can readily be split and each layer repaired independently.

Blunt Injuries

Blunt trauma to the eye (concussion, contusion) is most frequently the result of an impact from a fist, a ball, or other solid object such as occurs in an automobile accident or running into a protrubrance in the dark. Blunt trauma may also be the result of a blast injury. The extent of damage may vary from a simple subcutaneous hemorrhage ("black eye") to the extreme of a rupture of the globe. Subconjunctival hemorrhage is frequent. If the blow is severe, there may be dislocation of the lens, cataract, traumatic iritis or rupture of the sphincter, hemorrhage in the interior of the eye, disturbance of the retina (commotio retinae), rupture of the choroid or sclera, or detachment of the retina. In severe injuries there may be a fracture of the floor of the orbit with the eye lying at a lower level that its fellow (blow-out fracture of the orbit).

While all cases of blunt injury should be referred to an ophthalmologist to determine the extent of intraocular damage the immediate treatment consists primarily in rest and sedation after cleansing the lids and removing any dirt or foreign particles in the skin. X-rays for orbital fracture should be taken in suspicious cases. Rest is important because, following such trauma, there may be a secondary hemorrhage in the eye even several days after the injury. For this reason *heat is to be avoided* and atropine is contraindicated. If there is considerable swelling of the eyelids cold applications during the first 24 hours may help reduce the edema and make the patient more comfortable. If there is no damage except subcutaneous and subconjunctival hemorrhages, no local treatment is indicated as these hemorrhages absorb spontaneously in one to two weeks. Hemorrhages in the anterior chamber (behind the cornea) clear spontaneously in a few days but sometimes cause a secondary rise in pressure (glaucoma) requiring treatment with diamox or evacuation of the clot if permanent bloodstaining of the cornea is to be avoided.

Incised Wounds (Lacerations)

This type of injury is frequently encountered and may arise from a tremendous variety of objects, such as a knife, scissors, broken spectacle lenses, claws of animals, fingernails, teeth, the edge of a paper, and even contact lenses. There may be involvement of the eye itself, the eyelids, or both. In all cases, there must be thorough inspection to determine the retention of any foreign material, the removal of which will be subsequently discussed.

Incised wounds involving the *margin* of the eyelids require special suturing to avoid the development of a notch. This calls for very meticulous aseptic suturing, usually by splitting the lid margin along the "gray line" on each side of the incised wound and repairing the defect in two layers so that the healing of the two layers is in slightly different zones. To accomplish this, a small strip of skin to one side of the laceration may have to be removed and the skin of the other side slightly undermined. If the canaliculus has been severed, an attempt should be made to find the two ends and place a suture or plastic material through the punctum and severed canaliculus to be retained while healing occurs. This type of surgery should only be done by an ophthalmic surgeon if at all possible.

Much more common are injuries to the globe, especially the cornea. These may be of a penetrating nature or more frequently nonpenetrating in character. *Penetrating* injuries, usually from some sharp instrument as a knife or a needle, may result in prolapse of the iris, cataract, or even complete destruction of the eye. Especially where there is injury to the ciliary body the possibility of sympathetic ophthalmia (with loss of the fellow eye) must be born in mind.

The possibility of a retained foreign body in the eye should also be considered. These penetrating injuries must be referred to an ophthalmic surgeon for definitive care; first aid treatment should be limited to instillation of an antibiotic and a patch on the eye; sedatives may be given as required.

Nonperforating injuries are of daily occurrence, frequently resulting from contact with finger nails, paper, twigs, contact lenses, or a foreign body which has become dislodged. If the cornea is involved, the patient complains of severe pain, tearing, and blepharospasm. It may be necessary to instill a drop of local anesthetic (½ percent tetracaine or ½ percent ophthaine) in order to open the lids and examine the eye. Since a small abrasion may be difficult to see, it is well to instill one drop of two-percent fluorescein solution into the lower cul-de-sac, have the patient blink the eye several times, and irrigate the excess dye out of the eye with normal saline solution. This will cause any defect in the corneal epithelium to stain a brilliant green. If available papers impregnated with fluorescein should be substituted for the solution since the latter may not always be sterile. Abrasions which are not infected heal very promptly (24 to 48 hours). They may be treated with instillation of antibiotic drops or ointment (such as chloramphenicol, neosporin, or aureomycin) and application of a pressure dressing. Local anesthetics should *not* be prescribed. While they relieve pain, they retard healing. If the patient has not been seen shortly after the abrasion has occurred and infection is present, the abraded cornea will appear gray due to the infiltrate. The corneal *ulcer* then present may need to be treated by cauterization with application of a caustic such as trichloracetic acid exactly applied to the ulcer and frequent instillation of an antibiotic. Some corneal injuries, especially those due to fingernails, may heal in a few days but subsequently break down on numerous occasions over a period of years, a condition known as recurrent erosion. If in any corneal abrasion or ulcer there is iris irritation as evidenced by a small pupil, congested iris, and photophobia, a weak cycloplegic drug such as two percent homatropine should be instilled; atropine should ordinarily not be used for minor conditions as its effect lasts for 7 to 10 days.

Foreign Bodies

Foreign bodies may become lodged in the superficial layers of the eye or if propelled with sufficient force may pass into the deeper layers or the interior of the globe. If there is suspicion of a retained foreign body within the eye, prompt x-ray examination and referral is indicated. Most foreign bodies however are found either under the upper lid or on the cornea and can be removed without much difficulty. The upper lid can be everted readily by grasping the lashes between the thumb and index finger of one hand and using an applicator or thumb of the other hand as a fulcrum; by pulling slightly outward and upward the lid is everted and the conjunctiva on its posterior surface exposed (Fig. 2). Any foreign body, such as a cinder may then be gently wiped off with the tip of a clean handkerchief or applicator moistened with sterile saline solution.

Foreign bodies imbedded in the cornea require instillation of several drops of an anesthetic solution such as ½ percent tetracaine. If the foreign body cannot be dislodged by directing a stream of normal saline solution against it, a spud or small sharp sterile knife is then placed tangentially just under the foreign body, which is lifted out. It is not advisable to wipe the foreign body off with an applicator as this removes considerable surrounding corneal epithelium; on

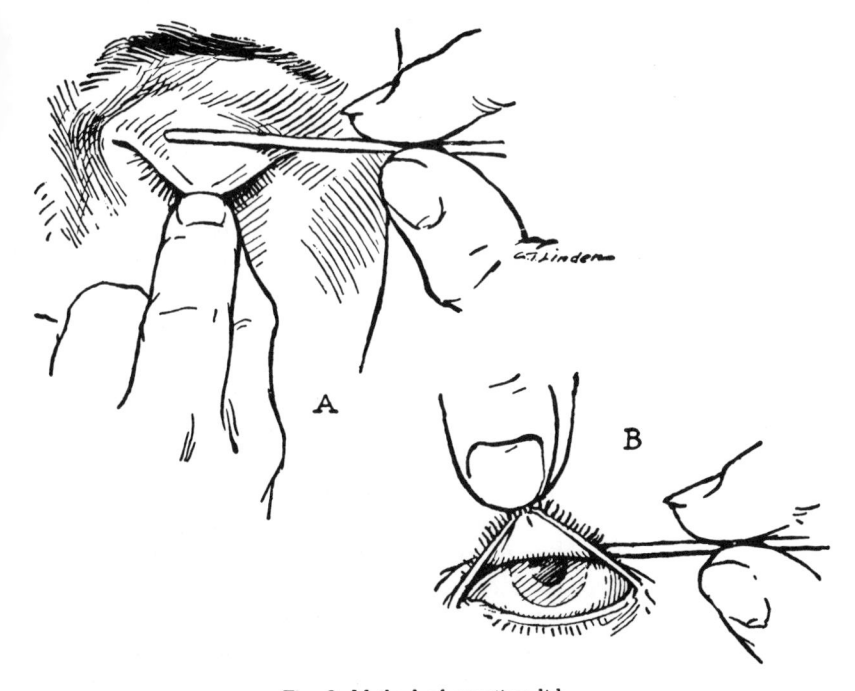

Fig. 2. Method of everting lid.

the other hand, the instrument must not be placed too deeply as damage to the corneal stroma results in eventual scarring with possible visual impairment. It is important that all the foreign body including metallic staining, be removed. An antibiotic ointment should then be instilled. If the foreign body was not quite superficial, it is well to patch the eye for 24 hours. The patient should be advised to return for inspection the following day. Barring secondary infection, the cornea will usually be healed in that length of time.

There is sometimes a complaint of foreign body sensation when no foreign body can be visualized with the naked eye. A hand magnifying lens and illumination with a flashlight should then be used to detect the presence of a microscopic particle. If this reveals nothing, fluorescein should then be instilled as described under "lacerated wounds" as there may be an abrasion (from a dislodged foreign body or an ulcer. Dendritic (herpetic) ulcers may be recognized with the magnifier after use of fluorescein as a branching linear "dendritic" figure. The ordinary bacterial ulcer appears as a small gray infiltrated area which stains with fluorescein. One should not overlook the presence of an inverted cilium of the eyelid which may be causing the foreign body sensation.

Burns

Nonmechanical injuries or burns may be the result of tissue damage from thermal, electric, radiation, or chemical origin. The principles of treatment of burns due to excessive *heat* or *cold* are elucidated elsewhere in this book (Chap. 10). In nearly all cases, a large area of the face and lids is affected and this must be treated according to the principles outlined for burns of the skin. In most cases, the eye is sufficiently protected by the lids so that damage may be limited to a hyperemia of the conjunctiva. In more severe burns, such as from phosphorus and magnesium, there may be corneal damage and even destruction of the globe. Emergency treatment is usually limited to instillation of an antibiotic ointment, sedatives, and supportive treatment with subsequent skin and conjunctival grafting where necessary. Freezing of the cornea is extremely rare even in severe frostbite. When it does occur, the cornea appears edematous (gray) but unless the entire cornea is involved, it will usually clear in a few days. Use of cryosurgery in cataract extraction has shown that the cornea can clear in a few days from a mild freezing without permanent loss in transparency. Treatment of thermal burns of the eye is largely limited to asepsis and the local use of antibiotics.

Electric injuries from lightning or high voltage electric contact may cause a conjunctival hyperemia, opacities in the deeper layers of the cornea or even destruction of the eye. Lenticular opacities (cataract) usually appear days to months later and will not be noted at the time of the initial examination. Emergency treatment is the same as for thermal burns.

Radiation burns seen as emergencies are most frequently due to *ultraviolet* and are most apt to occur following exposure to a welding arc or ultraviolet lamp when the eyes have not been protected by proper goggles. "Snowblindness" and overexposure at the beach may also be the cause. Since the ultraviolet rays do not penetrate far into the eye, they involve especially the corneal epithelium. There is usually excruciating pain in the eyes occurring some four to six hours after exposure. Instillation of fluorescein reveals the presence of innumerable small staining dots in the corneal epithelium, both eyes usually being involved. There is marked blepharospasm; instillation of a drop of local anesthetic (tetracaine or ophthaine) may be necessary to examine the eyes. The condition is self-limited with recovery in 24 to 36 hours. During this period, the use of an anesthetic ointment (tetracaine, ophthaine, or butyn) may be justified, together with cold compresses and sedatives.

Infrared causes very little effect on the anterior segment of the eye except occasionally in the so-called "flash burn" in which there is instantaneous release of infrared, visible light, and ultraviolet. The net effect is a thermal burn. Prolonged exposure to infrared may result in "glass blower's cataract" since these rays are absorbed by the lens but this condition will not be encountered as an emergency. Eclipse blindness, caused by gazing at the sun, may, however, be seen since there is a sudden loss of central vision due to a focusing of the infrared rays on the retina in the macular area. There is no definitive treatment; milder cases recover in days or weeks but more severe cases have permanent loss of central vision due to the chorioretinal scar.

Other types of radiation burns from x-ray and short-wave diathermy are not usually in the province of first aid therapy; their treatment is basically prophylactic and belongs in the realm of the specialist.

Chemical burns are exceedingly common in industry, in the

laboratory, as a result of household accidents, and occasionally from intentional injury. A wide range of chemical substances may be involved. For most of these there are no specific antidotes but certain general principles of therapy will apply to all chemical injuries. The first principle is immediate and copious irrigation to remove any excess of chemicals which may not have already damaged the tissues. While theoretically the use of a nontoxic neutralizing chemical would be ideal this is usually not practical and a stream of water or normal saline solution should be utilized as promptly as possible. Workers in industry and the laboratory should be instructed to hold the lids open and let water from the tap (lukewarm if possible) wash out the chemical as soon as they can reach the running water. Many eyes have been saved by this immediate self-treatment. When seen by the physician, the damage will usually have been done. If there is marked blepharospasm, it may be necessary to instill a drop of local anesthetic (never cocaine) in order to examine the eye. The latter should then be irrigated, preferably with isotonic saline solution and if any particles of a chemical substance are seen, these should be removed. An antibiotic ointment should be instilled; if the burn is extensive, one drop of 1 percent atropine should be instilled. If the reaction is severe, local corticosteroids may be helpful. It is usually better *not* to bandage the eye. One of the chief late complications is the formation of adhesions between the burned conjunctiva of the lid and the globe (symblepharon) which in some cases can be prevented by use of the ointment and daily separation of the bulbar and tarsal conjunctiva with an applicator. In severe cases, it may be necessary to remove the burned conjunctiva and place a mucous membrane graft.

Acid and *alkali burns* are particularly common. Of these, the alkali burns are the more serious since the chemical can penetrate through the outer coats of the eye and cause severe damage to the interior of the globe. Thorough, prompt irrigation is therefore particularly important as some free alkali may remain in the conjunctival sac for a period of time. Corneas burned by strong alkalis tend to perforate at a later date. Recent investigation suggests that this is due to the enzyme collagenase rather than the chemical itself. Favorable results have been reported in use of the collagenase inhibitor cystein used several times a day as an irrigant (0.15 M). Acids do not penetrate the eye as do alkalis but cause a local tissue destruction at the point of contact; their ultimate prognosis is therefore better. A frequent source of alkali burns is household *lye*, not infrequently used on an erring husband or suitor. *Calcium*, especially in the form of unslaked lime, is a frequent offender in industry and may give rise to a prolonged reaction in the eye. It is here important that in addition to irrigation any particles of calcium should be removed from the conjunctival sac. This can be done, after instillation of a local anesthetic, with a moistened applicator, or camel-hair brush dipped in equal parts of soft and liquid paraffin. The use of the neutral sodium salt of ethylene-diamine tetra-acetic acid in .01M solution as an irrigant has been advocated. This is said to produce a soluble calcium salt.

Of the metallic salts, *silver* preparations are perhaps the most common as they are used not only in certain preparations for dyeing of eyelashes, but especially in the form of the nitrate for therapeutic purposes. Even the use of 2 percent silver nitrate in the eyes of the newborn, according to the Crede method, has in a few cases resulted in corneal damage. Long continued use of silver protein preparations may result in silver staining of the tissue (argyrosis). After accidental instillation of strong silver solutions, immediate irrigation with saline solution will neutralize the effect by producing soluble silver chloride. This will, however, not act on tissues which have already suffered corrosive action.

Of the vesicant gasses, *mustard gas*, used primarily in World War I has been extensively studied but no effective antidote has been found. It is unlikely to be encountered in civilian life; the treatment is largely symptomatic: extensive irrigation, antibiotics to combat secondary infection, atropine, and a minimum of local anesthesia. The eyes should not be bandaged. Late mustard gas keratitis is usually best treated with contact lenses or keratoplasty. Of the arsenical gaseous compounds, *lewisite* is perhaps the best known example; its effect is neutralized immediately if 20 percent BAL (British Anti-Lewisite) is immediately instilled. BAL is also effective in neutralizing other arsenicals, as well as gold, cadmium, and mercury. Treatment must be instituted within a few minutes of contact.

Tear gas injuries to the eyes, most recently in the form of Mace, are becoming increasingly frequent. As ordinarily used in police action or riot control, the effect is only irritation, tearing, and blepharospasm which is resolved with recovery in a short span of time. If the concentration is large, however, as when a tear gas pistol is (usually accidentally) discharged into the eyes at short range, extensive permanent damage may be done to the lids and eyeball. There may be complete desquamation of the superficial layers of the cornea and conjunctiva, formation of symblepharon, iritis, and eventually a vascularized corneal scar which may necessitate keratoplasty. Treatment consists in irrigation to remove any remaining chemical on the skin or in the eye, removal of any necrotic tissue, an antibiotic to prevent infection, sedatives for pain, atropine if there is iritis, and subsequent treatment to prevent symblepharon.

Medical Emergencies

Medical emergencies, without any history of injury, will usually be encountered because there is *severe pain* or *sudden loss in vision*.
THE PAINFUL EYE. When there is severe pain in one or both eyes, one should suspect an attack of acute narrow-angle *glaucoma*. The pain usually radiates towards the back of the head and may be accompanied by nausea and vomiting. Vision is blurred due to the steamy cornea; the pupil is dilated; and the eye inflamed. Because of the redness of the eye, the condition must be differentiated from *conjunctivitis* (which is not extremely painful and usually produces a purulent discharge) and *acute iritis* (with a contracted pupil, muddy iris, precipitates on the back of the cornea, and frequently photophobia and tenderness on palpation.) In acute glaucoma, the intraocular pressure is extremely high and on palpation between the two index fingers the eye may feel stony hard. Measurement with a tonometer may give a reading of 60 to 100 mm Hg instead of the normal 10 to 24 mm range.

If one is certain of the diagnosis of acute glaucoma, an immediate effort should be made to reduce the pressure if ophthalmologic aid is not available. A carbonic anhydrase inhibitor such as diamox 500 mg should be given orally or by intravenous injection (in 5 cc normal saline) if the patient is nauseated. Oral glycerin, best tolerated as osmoglyn 3 to 6 ounces or glyrol 2½ to 4 ounces, is frequently very effective if the patient is able to retain it. Miotics in the form of 4 percent pilocarpine or ¼ percent eserine should be instilled in the eye at frequent intervals (every 15 to 30 minutes at first). These patients should usually have surgery (most frequently a peripheral iridectomy) to prevent further attacks, preferably after the attack has subsided.

Other causes of a painful eye include: styes and acute meibomitis, corneal ulcer, orbital cellulitis, and acute dacrycystitis.

SUDDEN LOSS IN VISION. A sudden loss in vision, partial or complete, is most commonly due to an occlusion of the central retinal artery or vein, a hemorrhage into the vitreous, a retinal detachment, or an optic neuritis. All of these require examination with the ophthalmoscope. Occlusion of the central retinal *artery*, recognized by narrow or empty retinal arterioles and edema (graying) in the retina is the only one of these conditions requiring immediate treatment. A paracentesis of the cornea near the limbus, performed with a sharp knife under local anesthesia, will reduce the intraocular pressure and may help any embolus in the vessel to pass on to smaller branches. A vasodilator, such as priscoline, may be injected retrobulbarly. This treatment is more of theoretical than practical value since it must be performed within half an hour after the occlusion to be successful. Occlusion of the *vein* may be helped with anticoagulant therapy if instituted within the first week. Vitreous hemorrhage requires no treatment except rest. If should be born in mind that in the absence of trauma, hypertension, or diabetes, the hemorrhage may be due to retinal detachment which may be visible only after the hemorrhage has cleared. Retinal detachment and optic neuritis usually require hospitalization and treatment by a specialist.

Do's and Don't's in Emergency Eye Care

The observance of certain basic principles in the treatment of eye injuries is important to the preservation of vision. It is assumed that in a hospital emergency room there will be available a visual acuity chart, pocket flashlight, magnifying lens, tonometer, ophthalmoscope, sterile spuds or knives, and a minimum of drugs to include local anesthetics, fluorescein, antibiotic and corticosteroid eye preperations, 1 percent atropine and 2 percent homatropine with other drugs readily available when indicated. It will be assumed that special examinations such as slit-lamp microscopy and gonioscopy are not included in emergency treatment as performed by the non-ophthalmologist.

The following suggestions should be born in mind:
1. Take a brief history, finding out what happened and when.
2. Estimate the visual acuity if possible, as this may have subsequent medicolegal significance.

3. Examine the eye with focal illumination or pocket flashlight and magnifying lens, using an ophthalmoscope when indicated.
4. Be gentle in all manipulations so that no damage is done by examination or treatment.
5. Use a local anesthetic such as ½ percent tetracaine or ½ percent ophthaine (*never* cocaine) only to enable examination and treatment but not to be prescribed for subsequent treatment.
6. Examine the cornea carefully under magnification, using fluorescein when necessary.
7. Remove all foreign substances promptly and completely whether chemical (by irrigation) or solid (by mechanical removal).
8. Avoid any irritating substance or strong medication except in the few instances where a specific antidote is available.
9. Instill and prescribe antibiotic or chemotherapeutic agents where secondary infection is a possibility. Chloramphenicol, polysporin, neomycin, tetracycline, or sulfacetamide may be used. Avoid penicillin because of its frequent allergic incidence.
10. Use corticosteroids only when an undue inflammatory reaction is present. The possibility of damage in herpes simplex and in the production of glaucoma must be remembered.
11. Use atropine only in the presence of an iritis and never after simple foreign body removal. If iris irritation is present (small pupil, muddy iris) it is better to instill a short-acting mydriatic such as 2 percent homatropine.
12. Do not patch the eye after chemical injuries or in the presence of suppurative discharge.
13. Have x-ray examination in all cases of suspected intraocular foreign body or orbital fracture.
14. Refer all but the most simple cases to an ophthalmologist for subsequent care.

19 / Head and Neck

*CHRISTOPHER H. SOUTHWICK AND
HARRY W. SOUTHWICK*

Wounds of the head and neck can be the most distressing that the average individual experiences. The change in the patient's physical appearance as well as the functional impairment from residual disability may have far-reaching psychologic and financial consequences. Early and proper first aid treatment is necessary not only from a lifesaving standpoint but also for successful rehabilitation. With the constant emphasis on increased speed of travel in our modern society, accidents with injuries particularly to the head and neck area continue to rise.

In the isolated accident first aid is exactly what the term implies: emergency care until the patient can be transported to an area where definitive treatment can be performed. However, in a mass disaster it must be remembered that first aid may be the only treatment available, especially for the minor injuries. A thorough understanding of the procedures involved thus assumes an even greater significance under these circumstances.

General Considerations

There are some general principles which apply to all wounds in this area. A fatality can occur quickly from either respiratory obstruction or massive hemorrhage, and the first evaluation should ascertain if either of these problems exist. Fortunately, simple first aid promptly applied can usually contain either situation.

RESPIRATORY OBSTRUCTION. Maintenance of an adequate airway is essential to any successful treatment. As was pointed out in Chapter 14, four minutes is probably the critical period of time for reestab-

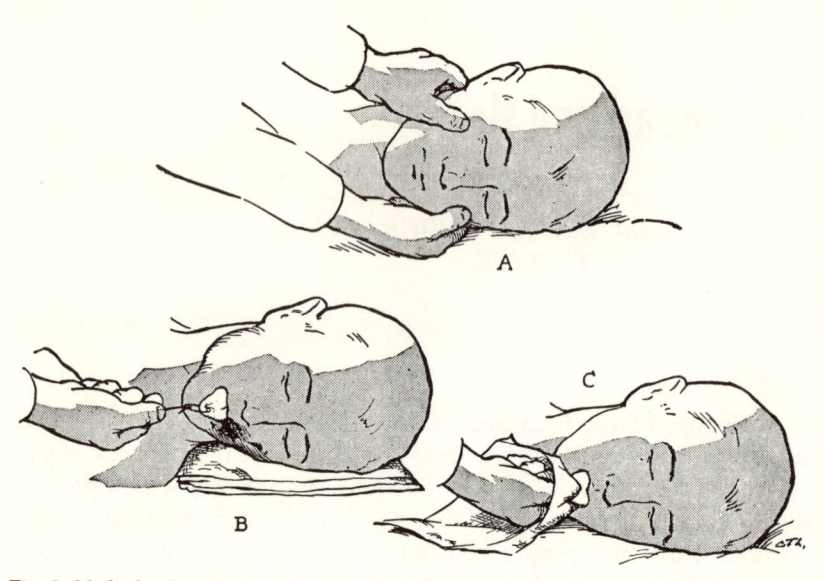

Fig. 1. Methods of correcting pharyngeal obstruction due to the jaw falling backward in unconscious or seriously injured patients. A, the jaw is held forward by pressing anteriorly against the rami. B, if the patient must be transported some distance and obstruction is serious, the tongue may be transfixed with a safety pin and pulled forward. C, grasping the tongue with fingers covered with a handkerchief is effective temporarily in relieving obstruction.

lishing an airway. First the oropharynx should be checked for any foreign bodies present such as broken dental plates, bridges, or fractured or avulsed teeth. In the unconscious patient, the tongue may fall backward and this should be grasped usually holding the tip between pieces of gauze or a handkerchief for traction and pulled forward (Fig. 1). Bilateral mandibular fracture can also interfere with the patient's holding his tongue and jaw in a position to prevent respiratory obstruction and he may have to be manually assisted. The color of the patient, audible air exchange through the oropharynx, and adequate respiratory movements of the chest are the best indications of an adequate airway. There is a simple plastic tube, a double oropharyngeal airway, which is becoming increasingly available in major first aid equipment. While originally designed as a means of giving mouth to mouth artifical respiration, it also provides a reasonable and efficient oral airway. Indications for a tracheostomy outside of a hospital are present only if it is not possible to secure or maintain an airway by any of the above conservative methods. The technique of tracheostomy has been outlined in Chapter 14. With very few exceptions it will be performed only by physicians.

HEMORRHAGE. Major hemorrhage in wounds of the head and neck can be of either arterial or venous origin. Because of the large size of the veins and the proximity to the heart, the two types sometimes may be confused in the head and neck area. Venous bleeding will generally present itself as a continuous though possibly massive flow, dark red in color, and should be controlled by direct pressure with a sterile gauze pad if available; a clean handkerchief may be a useful substitute.

Pressure points to control arterial bleeding are noted in Figure 2. Some caution should be exercised in carotid artery compression (Fig. 2A) in an elderly patient as the patency of the circle of Willis may be compromised, and the circulation to the brain may be impaired by common carotid artery pressure. If a patient loses consciousness following carotid artery pressure and other signs of profound shock are not present, the circulation should be restored immediately and other methods used to control the bleeding. Because of the rich collateral circulation in this area, proximal pressure points may not be effective since blood can flow in both directions. If the usual pressure point does not control bleeding direct pressure over the wound should be applied. Care should be taken to avoid incidental direct pressure on the airway and thus produce secondary respiratory obstruction.

SHOCK. Chapter 8 covers this subject in considerable detail. It must be remembered that injury to any area including the head and neck is a potential cause of shock. General measures such as loosening of

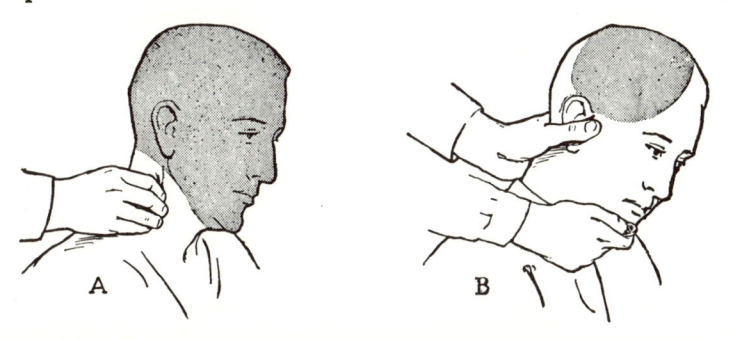

Fig. 2. Pressure as illustrated in A can compress the carotid artery, and theoretically controls the blood supply of the shaded area. B. Similar pressure in front of the ear will control the blood supply to a portion of the scalp. Collateral circulation from the opposite side is extensive in most individuals, and bleeding by pressure point in the head and neck is generally slowed at best. Pressure directly over the wound with some type of pad is generally superior in the control of bleeding and should be tried first.

restrictive clothing, external warmth, and elevation of the body and lower extremities above the level of the chest and head are indicated in all seriously injured patients until the severity of the injury has been evaluated.

INFECTION. In the modern age of broad-spectrum antibiotics there is a great tendency to rely on them to compensate for careless first aid. As near sterile technique as possible should be followed with any open wound with prompt covering to prevent further external contamination. Any wound with potential soil contamination should be considered as exposed to tetanus infection and appropriate measures taken (see Chap. 7).

Blunt Trauma

MOUTH. Contusions in this area are usually of minor consequence. Superficial breaks in the mucosal lining usually caused by compression against the teeth require no treatment except primary cleansing and subsequent good oral hygiene during the period of healing especially after meals. If the mucosal wound gapes widely, it should be evaluated by a physician for possible loose approximation with sutures to shorten the time of healing.

Teeth should be checked when time permits. Any teeth completely unseated should be removed from the mouth to prevent aspiration. When they are whole, especially in the younger patient, they should be saved and brought in with the patient as it is now possible to reimplant them under favorable circumstances. A loose tooth in the unconscious patient should be removed to prevent aspiration during transportation to a medical facility. If the patient is conscious, it should be left in place as there will be a better result if the nerve root is kept intact. Hemorrhage from a tooth socket can be controlled by local pressure of a small pledget of cotton.

Dislocation of the mandible is generally bilateral and characterized by pain just below the ear as well as inability to occlude the teeth properly. The lower jaw will protrude forward and if the dislocation is unilateral to the normal side, reduction can usually be delayed until the patient can be seen by a physician. In circumstances where this is difficult or impossible an effort may be made to reduce the dislocation immediately. Both thumbs are wrapped with a protective towel and then placed over the lower molars. By pressing down and backward a definite click is noted when the reduction has been accomplished. The

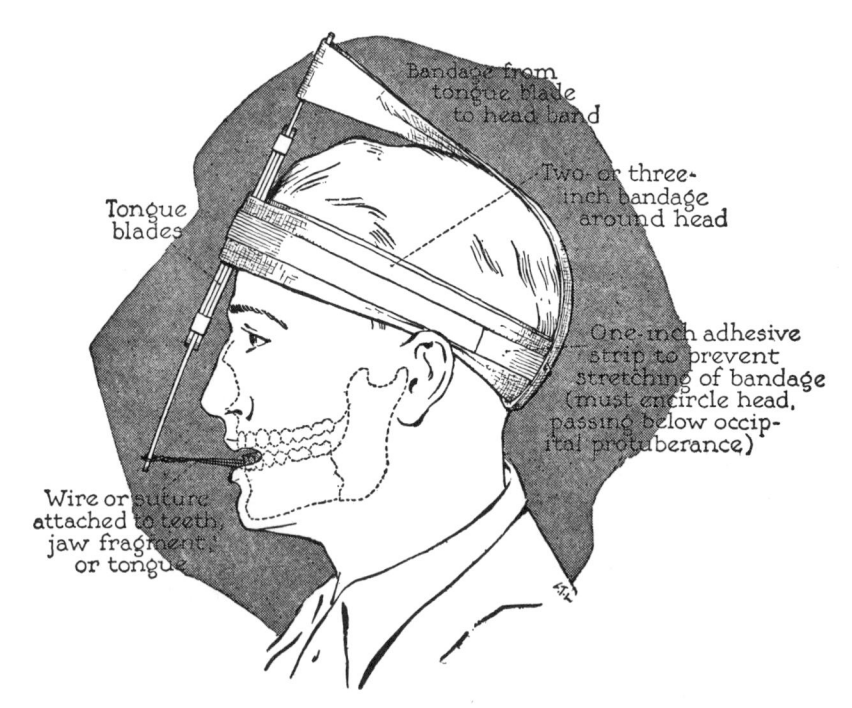

Fig. 3. Apparatus for transport of patient requiring traction of the jaw and tongue for maintenance of airway. The tongue may be pierced with a safety pin or suture, or wires may be anchored to the teeth or jaw. If teeth are used, at least three should be included in the wiring, since use of only one would put excessive strain upon it. Bending the head well back will also straighten the airway and facilitate breathing.

patient will then be able to open and close the mouth and the teeth will occlude properly.

Fracture of the mandible can take place in any area and is usually caused by a direct blow. Except for treatment of secondary airway obstruction or the overlying wound, no first aid is necessary. Reduction and immobilization involves x-rays and wiring and should be done only in the hospital by trained personnel (Fig. 3).

FACE. The most common blunt wound of the face is the superficial abrasion. If the loss of skin is not full thickness, the problem is not serious as long as early and proper cleansing is carried out. People thrown from automobiles or children falling off bicycles will grind dirt into the superficial layers of the skin. If this is left in place a permanent tattoo may develop that can be removed later only by abrasion surgery. If the area is small and the patient cooperative, gentle persistent cleansing with a piece of gauze and warm soap and water until the dirt is no longer present will suffice. It is not necessary to use harsh pressure to remove most dirt. If the area is extensive or the patient is a small child, it may be necessary to defer anything but superficial cleaning until some type of anesthesia can be obtained.

Fracture of the nose is relatively common secondary to a direct blow. Before swelling has taken place it is usually obvious that the symmetry of the face has been altered. An effort can be made early to mould the nose back to a more normal position. Permanent reduction and immobilization with an external splint should be performed by trained physicians and can be done anytime during the first few days after the injury. It is not a true emergency.

Fracture of the maxilla is characterized by mal-occlusion of the upper teeth or mobility of the roof of the mouth. This can be checked quickly by grasping the upper teeth between the thumb and index finger and testing for motion. Fracture can also occur in the infraorbital ridge formed by the maxilla and zygomatic bones (Fig. 4). If there is any degree of displacement present, the support of the orbit will change and secondary diplopia may result. These are complicated fractures usually requiring wiring for fixation and should be repaired as soon as possible by a specialist in this field.

Nosebleed associated with a nasal injury is probably secondary to rupture or tear of one of the submucosal vessels along the anterior portion of the septum. If there is no other injury present, nosebleed is best treated by mild elevation of the head, application of cold to the bridge of the nose, and direct pressure to the bleeding point if it can be visualized. The patient should be cautioned not to blow his nose after the bleeding has stopped as this may remove the obstructing clot and hemorrhage will recur. If nosebleed persists, the local bleeding point will probably have to be cauterized by a physician. Occasionally, in a severe injury, there will be a watery discharge from the nose which may be cerebrospinal fluid. No effort should be made to stop this flow as increased intracranial pressure can result. The patient should be taken into the hospital as soon as possible for complete evaluation.

EYE. Blunt trauma to the eye is best evaluated by the degree of visual acuity. Hemorrhage in the sclera or lid will not change the vision and can be treated by cold applications to minimize the swelling. If the injury is severe enough to cause hemorrhage within the eye, a hazing or total loss of vision will occur and the patient should be treated promptly by an ophthalmologist (see Chap. 18).

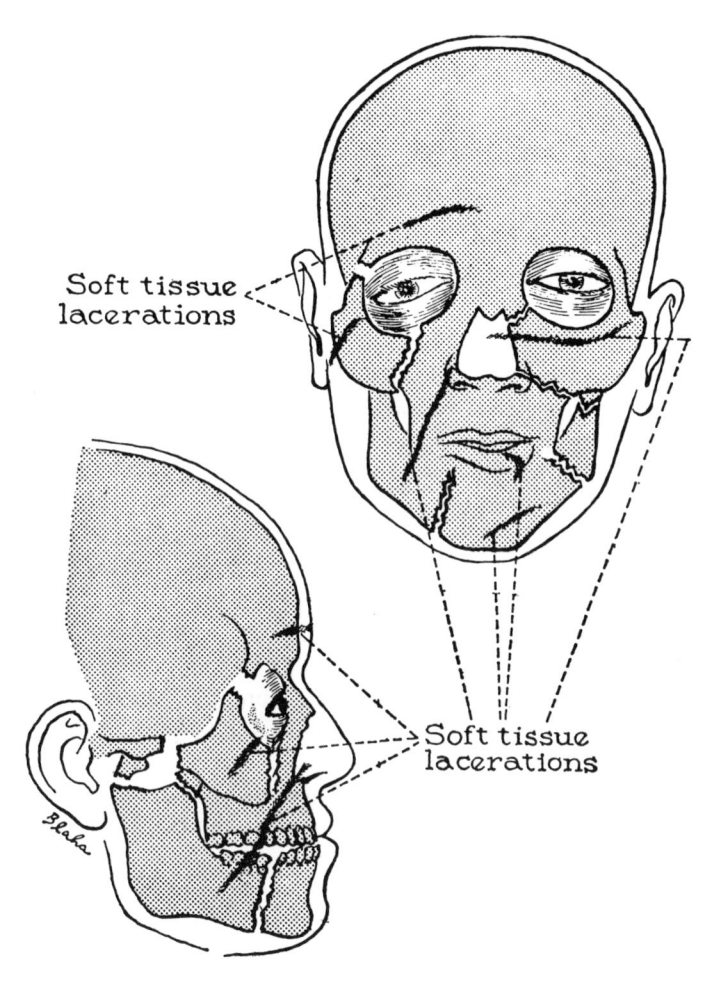

Fig. 4. Clinical manifestation of acute trauma in soft tissue lacerations. Thorough evaluation of clinical findings will often reveal multiple fractures of the facial bones.

NECK. Compromise of the airway due to collapse of the trachea or larynx can result from a blunt injury to the neck by compression of these structures against the bodies of the cervical vertebrae. If hyperextension of the neck does not produce adequate air exchange, this type of injury is an indication for an emergency tracheostomy for the relief of respiratory obstruction. Subcutaneous hemorrhage can occur with blunt trauma but usually will be venous and can be controlled with application of cold and pressure.

Sharp Trauma

LACERATIONS. In contrast to blunt trauma, injuries sustained from a sharp instrument are much more likely to sever structures deep to the skin. Careful attention should be directed not only to the surface wound but to the potentially damaged underlying structures as well. A thorough knowledge of the nature of these structures is essential.

MOUTH. Small lacerations in the oral cavity can be treated as mentioned previously by good cleansing and oral hygiene. If the wound is bleeding severely and cannot be controlled by pressure, then exploration of the wound in a hospital with direct ligation of the bleeding vessel will be necessary. If the mucosal wound gapes, it should be approximated well enough to facilitate early healing. Lacerations of the tongue are similar to lacerations of the scalp. Specific ligation of individual vessels is impossible and control of bleeding is best accomplished temporarily by pressure followed by suture in the hospital.

FACE. Because of the severe bleeding that can result from a facial laceration, many times the first impression will be that the cut is more extensive than it actually is. After bleeding has been controlled by pressure, careful cleansing of the surrounding area can be done to determine the severity of the wound. In general, because of the importance of the final cosmetic appearance of the scar, any cut which goes through the full thickness of the skin and exposes the underlying fat or other tissues should have surgical attention. A butterfly dressing or band-aid is no substitute for careful debridement and reapproximation of the edges of the wound with fine sutures. While secondary plastic repair of facial wounds can usually improve the final appearance of the scar, every effort should be made in the initial treatment to make this further surgery unnecessary.

Before the patient is taken to the hospital care should be taken to check for any full thickness loss of vital tissues such as the tip of the nose or a portion of the ear. If noted, this tissue should be found if possible, wrapped in as sterile a carrier as can be located, and sent to the hospital with the patient. There is no completely satisfactory substitute for facial skin and usually the missing part can be cleansed in the hospital and used in the repair.

EYE. Lacerations of the eye most commonly involve the cornea. The symptoms of some pain, burning, and watering of the eye following injury when a branch of a tree or some similar object brushes across the eye warrant further examination. Corneal lacerations, while not readily visible to the naked eye, will continue to give increasingly severe pain. If left untreated, the cornea can become infected and ulcerate, greatly complicating the treatment and possibly giving permanent decrease in vision secondary to corneal scarring. In the case of the obvious laceration of the orbit, the eye should be covered with a sterile patch and an ophthalmologist consulted as soon as possible (see Chap. 18).

NECK. Lacerations of the neck are particularly significant because of the size of the superficial vessels, especially the jugular veins. This bleeding should be controlled by pressure until the bleeding points can be isolated and ligated. In the case of very large veins, even though bleeding is controlled, a pressure seal should be maintained to prevent the sucking of air into the vascular system. This could result in an air embolus which can be a fatal complication. Under no circumstances should a circular bandage be placed around the neck to hold the dressing in place. Even if placed loosely at first, with motion and wetting with blood, it will tighten and can function as an inadvertent tourniquet with actual increase in the venous bleeding and possibly secondary respiratory obstruction.

PUNCTURE WOUNDS. An adequate history is essential in evaluating any puncture wound. With a basic knowledge of the underlying anatomy, the instrument with which the wound was made, and the direction and depth of penetration of this instrument, some evaluation of the potential seriousness can be made. It must be remembered that the neck not only contains the vascular and nerve supply to the head, but that injuries here can also injure these same structures to the arms. In addition, the apex of the lung can be cut with the potential hazard of pneumothorax. In general, any patient with a puncture wound which penetrates beyond the thickness of the skin should be taken to a hospital as soon as possible to determine the full extent of the injury.

Burns

While the general subject of burns has been discussed in Chapter 10, there are some specific points in reference to the head and neck which should be reiterated. The most important of these from the lifesaving standpoint is the laryngeal burn. It must be realized that with a flash fire there may be very little external evidence of burn while the larynx can still be exposed to sufficient heat and chemical irritants to cause laryngeal edema. The development of this complication can be quite rapid, but it may be delayed for 24 to 36 hours. Any person exposed to a burn of this nature should be taken to a hospital for observation. The signs of huskiness of the voice, mild respiratory distress or minimal cyanosis should alert the person at the scene to this potential problem. In some cases it may be necessary to perform an emergency tracheostomy. When sufficient laryngeal edema develops, nothing short of this procedure will supply the necessary relief.

Burns of the eye present specific problems. Thermal burns are not a frequent injury because of the protective mechanism of the eyelids. However, chemical burns secondary to a solution spattering into the eye are frequent. With tissues as delicate as those of the eye, it is better not to look for a specific neutralizing solution but rather to wash the eye out with copious amounts of water immediately. Following this, the patient should be taken to the hospital where a complete examination can be made.

As with injuries of the mouth, face, and neck particular attention in the management of burns of this area should be directed toward the conservation of as much normal tissue as possible. Control of infection is especially important as this can convert a deep second degree burn to a full thickness tissue loss which may result in further damage to the surrounding previously unaffected tissues.

Foreign Bodies

ORAL. Most ingested foreign bodies are seen in small children who eventually will attempt to put anything they are playing with in their mouths. If the object is lodged above the larynx, it usually can be removed by inverting the child, gently tapping him on the back, and sweeping the oral cavity with the finger. As mentioned previously, all posttraumatic cases with injury to the mouth should be checked for loose or free objects which may be present. In the case of a small sharp foreign body, such as a fishbone in the posterior pharynx, the patient should be reassured and taken to an emergency room where adequate lighting and material are available for its removal rather than to attempt extraction under unfavorable circumstances.

LARYNGEAL. Treatment should be directed to relief of the respiratory obstruction as stated earlier. This may require the performance of a tracheostomy before the foreign body can be removed.

ESOPHAGEAL. If it can be determined that the foreign body has passed beyond the larynx, no true emergency exists. As long as no respiratory distress is present, the patient can be reassured and taken to a hospital for x-rays and further examination.

EYE. Foreign bodies in the eye are potentially serious especially if they involve the central portion of the cornea. If the material is embedded in the cornea, as is frequently the case with small pieces of metal, only direct lifting with a sharp instrument under local anesthesia can dislodge the foreign body. This obviously should be done by a trained physician in a hospital. While no true emergency exists with a superficial foreign body, its removal should not be delayed unnecessarily. If it is metal, a secondary rust ring can develop in the matter of hours which requires more extensive damage to the cornea in its removal (see also Chap. 18).

Injuries of the head and neck, more than any other anatomic area, may present both an immediate lifesaving and future rehabilitation challenge to one called upon to administer first aid. Life or death from hemorrhage or respiratory obstruction may be decided in a matter of a very few minutes. Improper treatment may result in the loss of vision or in a grotesque physical appearance that can ruin an otherwise promising career. Judicious handling of these injuries requires previous training and forethought; they cannot be managed well by intuition.

20 / Genitourinary Trauma

ORMOND S. CULP

Injuries of the genitourinary tract usually are serious or inconsequential. Most of the system is so deep-seated and protected by other structures that there are few opportunities for first aid per se. But familiarity with these organs and some of their peculiarities should spare one ignominious and tragic pitfalls.

Delayed recognition of damage to the urinary tract, initial mismanagement, and inadequate treatment have resulted in an inordinate number of "urologic cripples" who have died prematurely of renal insufficiency. Prompt, expert care usually can prevent such catastrophes.

Increased speed in all modes of transportation and continued mechanization of home, farm, and industry have produced a higher incidence of grave complex injuries involving multiple anatomic systems. Growing rates of mass violence, stabbings, gunshot wounds, vicious beatings, and perfection of more efficient weapons of destruction have added to the toll on the genitourinary tract. But it also can be traumatized seriously by commonplace incidents of everyday life.

Anatomy

Customary arrangement of the urinary system is shown diagrammatically in Figure 1. Usually both kidneys are situated just below the diaphragm, which separates the abdomen and the chest. They lie on each side of the spinal column, against the heavy muscles of the back, at the level of the lowermost ribs. However, one or both kidneys may be located much lower behind the abdominal contents. Kidneys also can be fused or one may be missing. If only one kidney is present it is considerably larger than average.

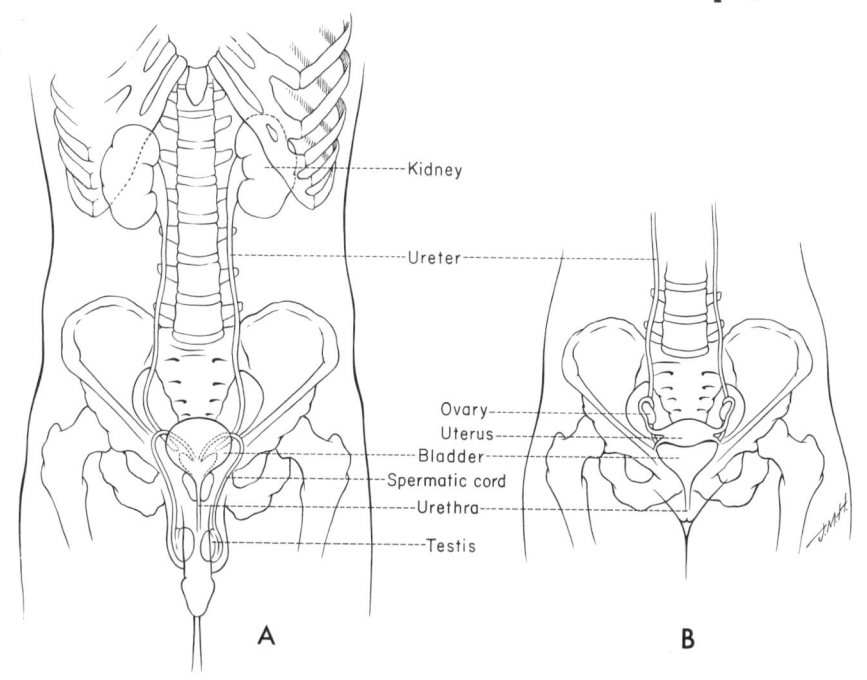

Fig. 1. Distribution of genitourinary structures. A, male. B, female.

Some individuals are born with partial blockage of the outlet of a kidney. In such instances the organ may be tremendously distended, thin, and much more susceptible to rupture.

Normally the kidney consists of a thick meaty portion that produces urine (parenchyma) and a funnel-like device (pelvis) which collects the urine. Since all of the circulating blood passes through the renal parenchyma every few minutes, that portion of the kidney is especially capable of bleeding profusely.

A relatively thin, muscular, elastic tube (ureter) connects the pelvis of the kidney to the base of the bladder and drains the urine. It descends near the spinal column, is not fixed rigidly, and is able to undulate throughout its course.

The urinary bladder is a muscular sac deep in the cavity of the trunk and shielded by the pelvic bones. Normally it holds up to a pint of urine comfortably but may undergo amazing overdistention if the individual has certain systemic diseases, obstruction to the outlet, injury to its nerve supply, or deep sedation. Once normal capacity is exceeded the bladder protrudes above the sheltering pelvis and becomes more vulnerable to lower abdominal trauma.

A "beer binge" produces not only excessive quantity of urine but also a bladder that may simulate late pregnancy as the degree of intoxication and analgesia (even anesthesia) increases. Unconsciousness (from any cause) may be accompanied by spontaneous involuntary urination or by progressive retention of urine and overdistention of the bladder.

Urine is expelled from the bladder through a tubular channel (urethra) which includes a most important control valve (sphincter). The female urethra is only about an inch in length and opens into the vagina. Fortunately, urethral injuries in females are extremely rare. But the male urethra is especially vulnerable to devastating damage.

The male urethra has three significantly different segments: 1) *prostatic*, which is the deepest portion, adjacent to the bladder, surrounded and protected by the prostate, a substantial, accessory-sexual, glandular structure after puberty but one that is attenuated and provides unreliable urethral protection during childhood; 2) *membranous*, which is an unprotected quarter of an inch beyond the prostate that is subjected frequently to trauma in this region; and 3) *anterior*, which is the remainder of the passageway to the opening at the tip of the penis.

Other male genital organs include the scrotal contents, spermatic cords, seminal vesicles, and ejaculatory ducts which open in the prostatic urethra.

Female genital structures (ovaries, tubes, uterus) communicate with the external aperture (vagina) deep within the recess and are not within the scope of this review because they are exceedingly well-protected and are not accessible for first aid measures.

Basic Principles

Blood at the urethral opening or in the urine is indicative of injury to some part of the urinary tract. Presence of a mass or discoloration in the flank or lower part of the abdomen is always suggestive of damage to the kidney or lower urinary tract.

Appearance of the male external genitalia is more meaningful and provides the chief opportunity for conventional first aid.

Injuries to the concealed segments of this system can be so elusive that they tax the ingenuity of experts and frequently require sophisticated diagnostic procedures. These in turn must be timed properly to avoid jeopardizing the victim's general physical status.

Basic Principles / 313

In most instances, therefore, initial efforts should be confined to control of obvious external bleeding, general support of the patient, and prompt transfer to an appropriate facility for additional study.

KIDNEY. Although the normally situated kidney is well-protected and cushioned further by an envelope of fat, it does not withstand trauma well. Even tiny wounds permit massive hemorrhage because of the rich blood supply.

External forces may damage the kidney by varied routes (Fig.

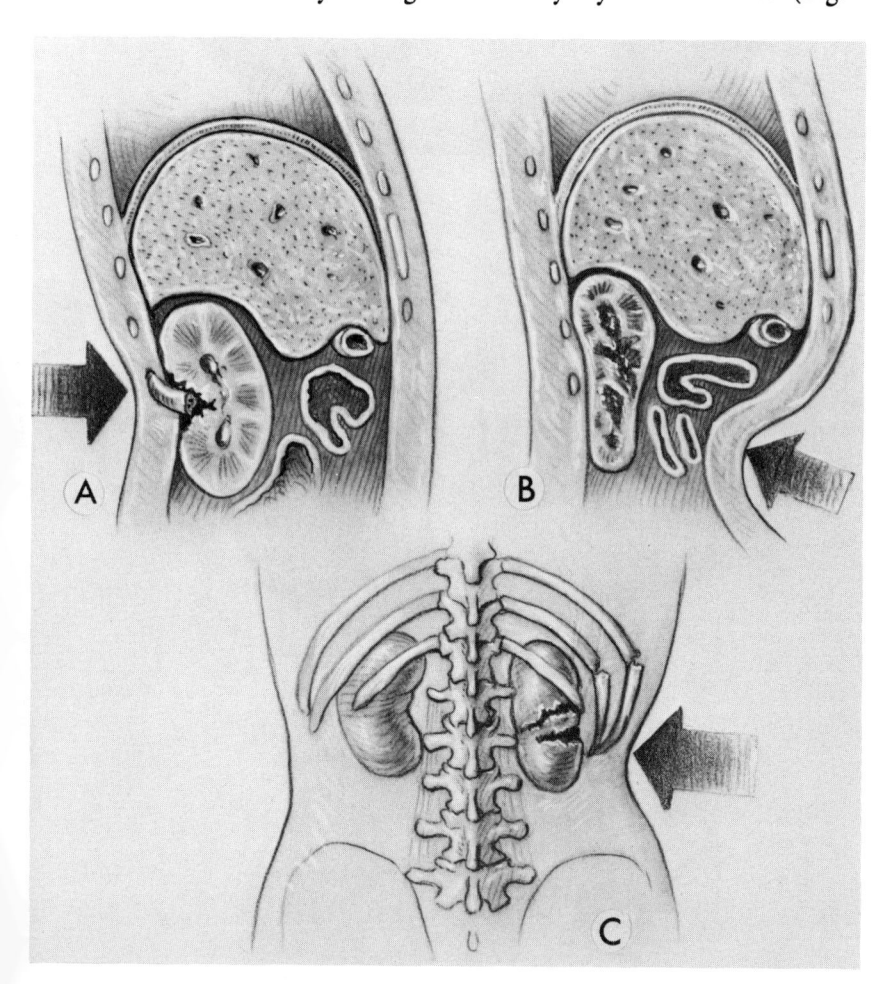

Fig. 2. Forces that may injure the kidney. A, fracture of part of a vertebra. B, blunt force transmitted through the abdomen. C, fracture of a nearby rib. (From DeWeerd. **J. Int. Coll. Surg.**, 29:567-572, May, 1958.)

A, contusion. B, laceration. C, fragmentation. (From DeWeerd. J. Int. Coll. Surg., 29:567-572, May,

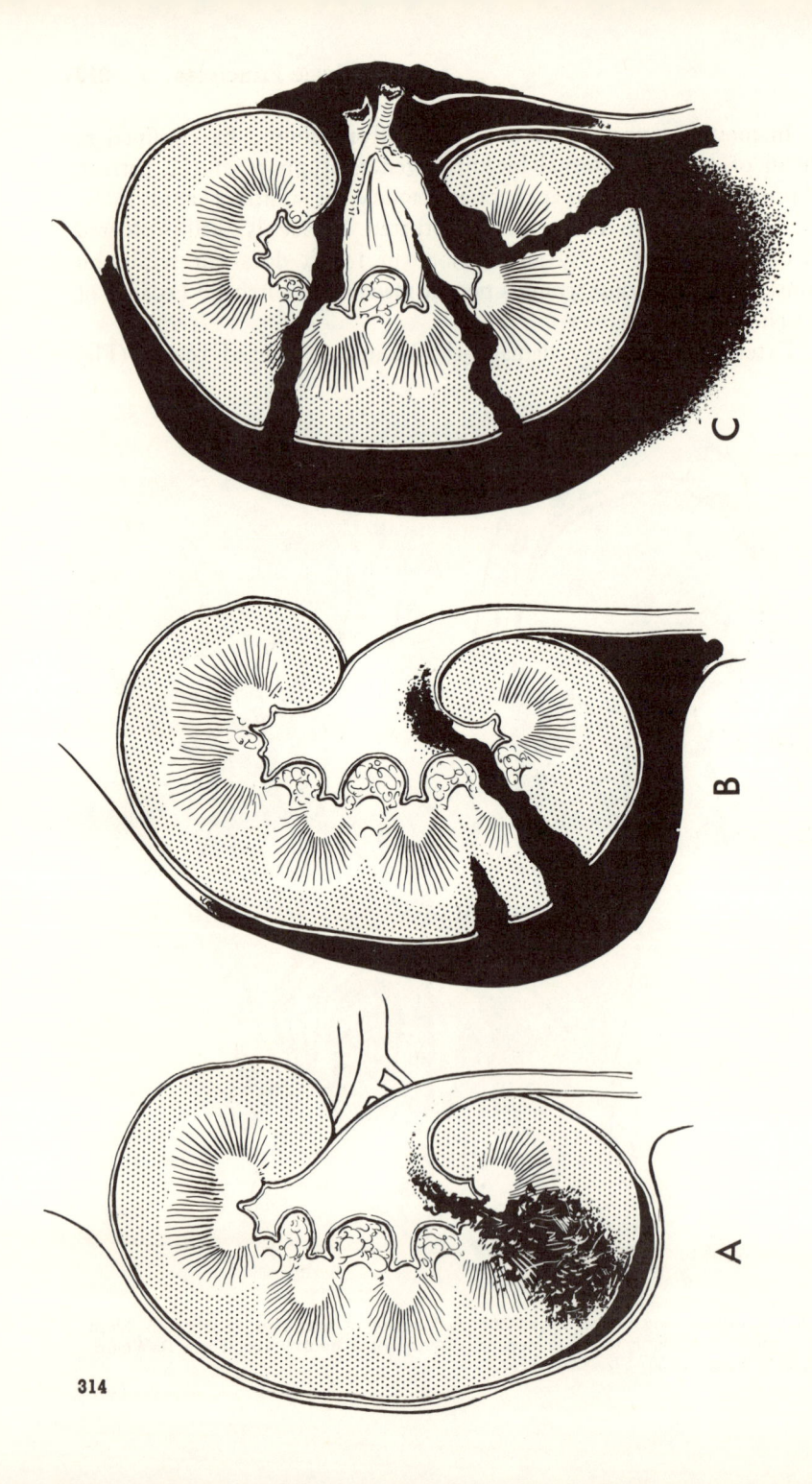

2). The result may be contusion, laceration, or extensive destruction (Fig. 3).

Frequently injuries in the region of the kidneys involve other organs as well, notably the spleen on the left and the liver on the right.

Profound shock is common and demands early correction (see Chap. 8). If the collecting system of the kidney also has been disrupted, the extravasating fluid will contain urine as well as blood. This increases the toxic condition of the patient and usually dictates some type of surgical intervention.

So much progress has been made in precise preoperative identification and evaluation of renal injuries that all victims are entitled to thorough study. This permits salvage of increasing numbers of damaged kidneys which were removed in the past.

URETER. This worm-like tube is injured almost exclusively by missiles and errant surgeons. Defects are not likely to be suspected at the time of the accident. Not infrequently they are missed during exploratory operations. Fortunately, they are rare.

BLADDER. As noted previously, the bladder is sheltered within the bony pelvis except when overdistended. A thin layer of tissue (peritoneum) separates the bladder from the abdominal cavity. If the bladder is ruptured, dissemination of its contents and associated blood depends on the integrity of the peritoneum (Fig. 4).

Perforation of the bladder below the peritoneal reflection permits

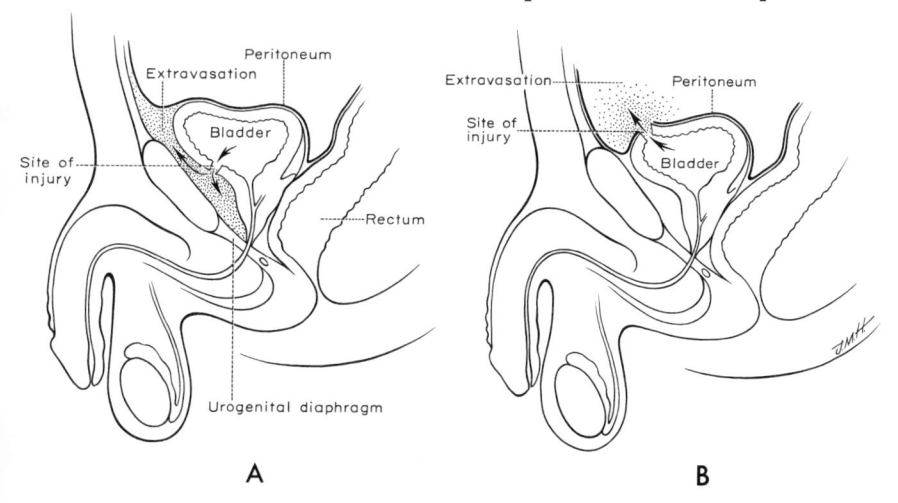

Fig. 4. Types of leakage after rupture of the bladder. A, extraperitoneal. B, intraperitoneal.

leakage only around the bladder, even though this may involve most of the deep pelvic cavity. A dense fibrous barrier near the tip of the prostate prevents spread into the genital region.

Pain, tenderness, and swelling will be confined to the pelvic and lower abdominal regions if other systems are intact. Indwelling urethral catheter drainage with suction may suffice, if instituted promptly. Late pelvic abscesses are not uncommon.

If the defect in the wall of the bladder includes the thin layer of peritoneum, urine and blood promptly pour into the spacious abdomen. Diffuse pain, tenderness, and muscle spasm ensue as with any form of generalized peritonitis. Early operation is of paramount importance.

Both intraperitoneal and extraperitoneal extravasations are possible in the same individual if damage is extensive or if the perforation is located at one of the peritoneal reflections.

URETHRA.

PROSTATIC AND MEMBRANOUS, OR POSTERIOR/DEEP SEGMENT. Fractures of the bony pelvis usually spare the female urethra and are more likely to rupture the bladder. But the short, unprotected, membranous urethra of the male is a common target.

Force of the impact and displacement of the bone fragment tend to sever the membranous urethra just beyond the lower limit of the prostate (Fig. 5).

An experienced examiner usually can detect the malposition of the prostate by rectal palpation (Fig. 6). Indeed, it is possible to displace the gland further and leave no doubt regarding the diagnosis.

Since the partition between pelvis and external genitalia usually remains intact, this type of injury simulates extraperitoneal rupture of the bladder clinically. Inability to catheterize is a notable difference.

Reestablishment of urethral continuity is vitally important. Simple drainage of the bladder alone results in obliteration of the separated ends of the urethra, formation of diffuse intervening scar tissue, and creation of an especially refractive clinical problem that often requires many years of vigorous and complicated treatment.

ANTERIOR (OUTER SEGMENT). Below the deep pelvic barrier, well-developed fibrous investments (fascias) control the course of extravasation if they remain intact (unlikely with gunshot wounds and stabbings). Straddle falls over a rigid object are the most common cause of injury to the deep anterior part of the urethra.

Swelling, distortion, and purplish discoloration of tissues vary with the severity of the trauma and the elapsed time after the accident (Fig. 7). There may be only a small tender bulge behind the

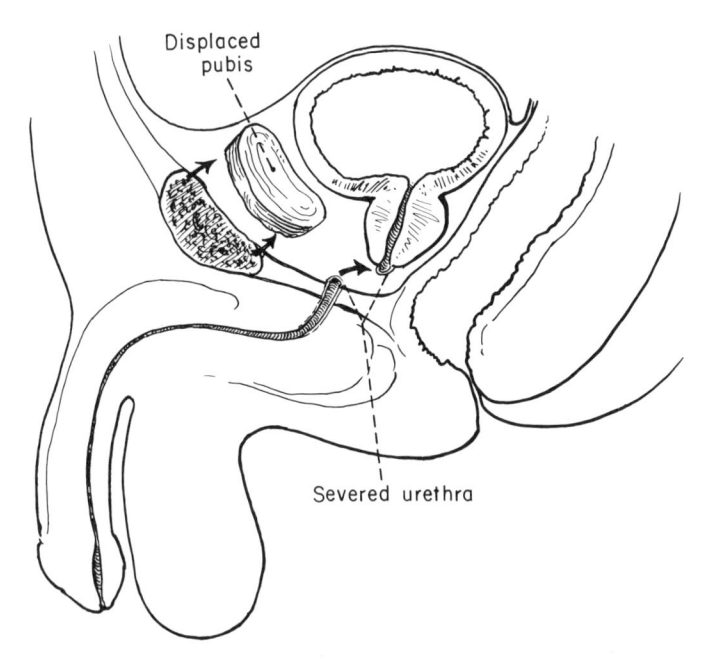

Fig. 5. Mechanism of complete division of the urethra by fracture of the pelvis.

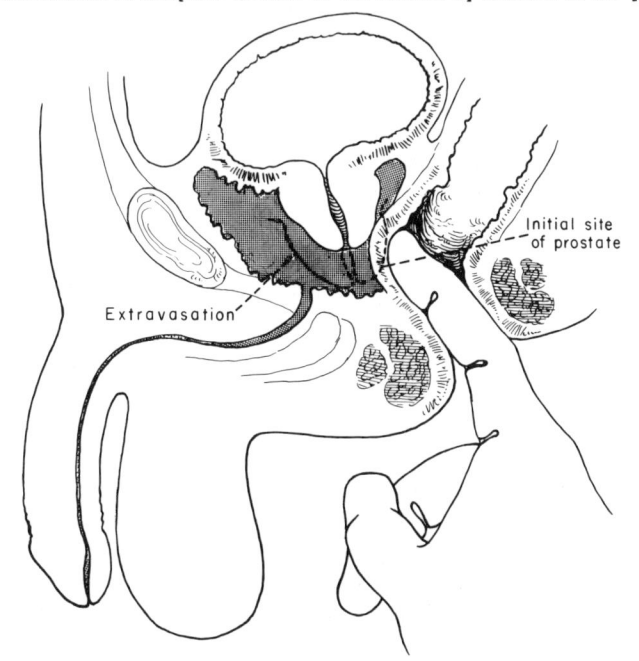

Fig. 6. Palpable displacement and abnormal mobility of the prostate after complete division of the urethra. Note extraperitoneal extravasation confined to the pelvis.

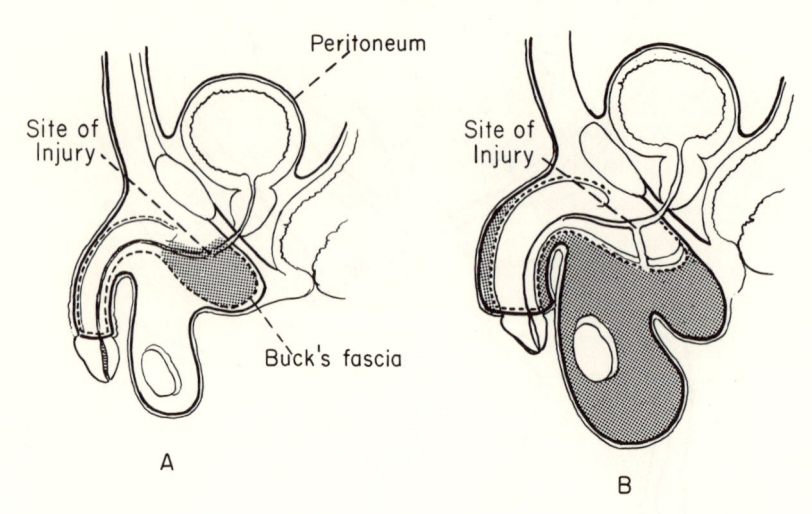

Fig. 7. Injury to the anterior urethra with extravasation. A, localized. B, diffuse.

scrotum; or the extravasation may involve the entire external genital region. It may extend onto the lower abdominal wall.

The defect in the urethra may vary from a small laceration to complete division. The same general external appearance can prevail regardless of the site of the urethral perforation.

Individuals with significant urethral injuries are unable to urinate and are in severe pain. They go into shock quickly and classically have some blood at the urethral meatus. Catheters customarily deviate into the soft tissues and do not drain urine.

Prompt repair of the urethra and appropriate drainage of all involved soft tissues are essential for prevention of serious sepsis, extensive necrosis, and intractable strictures.

GENITALIA.

FEMALE. There are no first aid measures adaptable to the female reproductive tract because of its concealed nature, as postulated previously.

PENIS. Simple contusion of the penis is accompanied by swelling and discoloration but does not interfere with urination. Bed rest and ice packs usually suffice if the process does not continue to spread.

Blunt trauma to an erect penis may rupture one or more of the turgid vascular bodies. Hemorrhage produces marked swelling, pain, and discoloration, and prevents urination. Surgical repair is inevitable.

Superficial lacerations (for example, foreskin caught in zipper) are amenable to customary techniques of cleansing and dressing.

Stab wounds, gunshot wounds, and deep lacerations require investigation regarding the integrity of the urethra. Pressure dressings usually will control bleeding at the time of injury.

Psychotics and sexual deviates occasionally attempt to amputate the penis and sometimes succeed. This also is an established form of retaliation by other individuals. A tourniquet may be required to arrest massive hemorrhage. Victims invariably are in shock and in urgent need of emergency care. The penis should not be discarded. Successful reattachment has been accomplished.

A special type of trauma is endemic to rural areas. Clothing caught in the unguarded power take-off of farm equipment can avulse virtually all penile and scrotal skin. Special care must be taken to preserve the testicles and any remnants of the scrotum. Bleeding is seldom a major problem. Avoidance of unnecessary contamination and prompt hospitalization are important.

SCROTUM. Severe blows to the scrotum and penetrating or perforating wounds often pose a problem in control of bleeding because of the elasticity of the scrotal wall. Since it has no intrinsic tamponading ability, the scrotum can attain tremendous size. Early application of a pressure dressing and ice packs often help to minimize enlargement.

Testicles are sufficiently mobile to escape injury in most situations. Even damaged ones have remarkable recuperative power and should be preserved.

Trauma to the cord that is attached to the testicle may produce excessive bleeding from its artery. This can be controlled by pressure against the nearby pelvic bone.

Other Emergencies

Not all urgent problems concerning the genitourinary tract are related to injuries. Some untraumatic situations can be just as challenging.

RENAL COLIC. Extreme pain in the flank or back radiating into the groin and, at times, into the scrotum or vagina is usually caused by movement of a stone in the kidney or ureter. It may occur at any time or place. The urine may be bloody. Heat administered by hot tub, water bottle, or electric pad may afford some relief but the patient generally requires prompt attention by a physician.

ACUTE URINARY RETENTION. Sudden inability to urinate may be precipitated by a variety of factors but prostatic enlargement in elderly men is the most common cause. Sitting in a tub of hot water may initiate urination but, more often, catheterization is required. If relief is delayed unduly, the bladder may become flabby and decompensated. Only properly trained personnel should insert catheters and must do so with strictest aseptic precautions.

FOREIGN BODIES. Strange personalities have been known to insert bizzare objects into the urethra. Frequently, they escape the grasp of that individual and move quickly into the deeper recesses of the channel. No attempt should be made to remove them because they require special instruments and expert manipulation.

Occasionally the penis has been inserted into or through a rigid circular structure. Metal rings have been especially popular. The end of the penis soon swells because the circulation becomes impaired and the object cannot be removed. Copious lubrication is effective only during the incipient stage. Most of these items must be removed with high-speed cutting equipment such as dental drills.

PARAPHIMOSIS. When a tight foreskin is left retracted, it often swells and produces a tight ring behind the head of the penis. The head of the penis becomes congested and enlarged and the foreskin cannot be replaced.

Frequently the paraphimosis can be reduced by placing both thumbs on the head of the penis and the index and middle fingers over the constriction. Pushing with the thumbs and pulling with the fingers may force the head through the tight ring. If this maneuver fails, prompt professional attention is needed to avoid possible gangrene.

TORSION. Some testicles are abnormally attached to adjacent structures and the cord that provides the blood supply may become twisted. To many urologists, this is the one bona fide emergency in the specialty. Since the circulation of the testicle may be shut off completely, time is vitally important. Only a few hours of strangulation can result in irreversible destruction. The patient has severe pain, moderate swelling, and exquisite tenderness. The condition may be indistinguishable clinically from local trauma and certain infections.

Professional advice should be sought immediately. A prophylactic operation on the contralateral side is mandatory.

Summary

With only isolated exceptions, most of the acute problems arising in the genitourinary tract are not amenable to conventional first aid.

Immediate hospitalization and timely surgical efforts are required in numerous situations. The patients need early supportive measures because of the gravity of their injuries.

Some of the anatomic, physiologic, and clinical peculiarities of this system have been reviewed in hope that this knowledge will increase the proficiency of paramedical personnel.

21 / Care of the Injured Hand

JOHN H. SCHNEEWIND

General Principles

The hand is a highly specialized organ that is expected to perform very delicate tasks as well as those requiring power grip and strength. Because of the presence of many complex and delicate structures as well as the bony architecture, it is important that first aid be rendered skillfully in order to avoid infection and additional tissue damage which may lead to stiffening and loss of function.

In the case of patients with several injuries, it must be ascertained that the life of the injured patient is not being threatened by an obstruction to his airway or by severe hemorrhage. Such injuries must be given priority despite the presence of serious hand damage.

Types of Injuries to the Hand

The constant use of the hands in all walks of life exposes them to injury as much or more than any other part of the body.
LACERATIONS. Cuts on the hand may be very simple with only the skin itself injured or may be extremely serious, covering a large area and injuring the blood vessels, tendons and nerves. One cannot assume that any of these structures are intact as even very small lacerations or puncture wounds may damage vital structures and require prompt and highly specialized care.
CRUSHING AND ROLLER INJURIES. This type of injury may cause a great deal of damage to the hand because of the compressive forces involved. If the rollers are hot, burns may be superimposed on the crushing injury to the hand. Washing machine *wringer* injuries sustained by children are still common and may be very deceptive. The hand and arm may appear to be only slightly damaged but the com-

pressive force of the rollers may cause hemorrhage and subsequent swelling with severe injury to the nerves, blood vessels, muscles, and other structures.

AMPUTATIONS. Amputations of the digits and hand may be partial or complete. With complete amputations, if the parts can be found they should be brought with the patient as it may be possible to utilize them. However, this must be done immediately because such amputated tissue will not survive if more than a few hours intervene between injury and repair. If the amputated part is kept at low temperature (slightly above freezing) the chance of its survival following replacement is improved. A fingertip amputation, for instance, is far from a trivial matter since, without good padding, the amputation stump becomes very sensitive or stiff resulting in significant loss of function.

Care of the Injured Hand

Proper first aid treatment of injuries of the hand include the basic principles of protection against infection and immobilization in a "position of function" (Fig. 1).

PROTECTION AGAINST INFECTION. If the patient is to be taken promptly to the hospital, it is better not to wash the hand and arm for fear of contamination if an open wound is present. If a significant delay is anticipated then the parts around the wound may be washed with soap and water but it is better not to wash the wound itself. The best protection for the wound is coverage with *sterile gauze squares*. If these are not available, freshly laundered towels may be used. The purpose is to create a resilient compression dressing (Fig. 2), as this serves to minimize bleeding and swelling, and tends to keep the in-

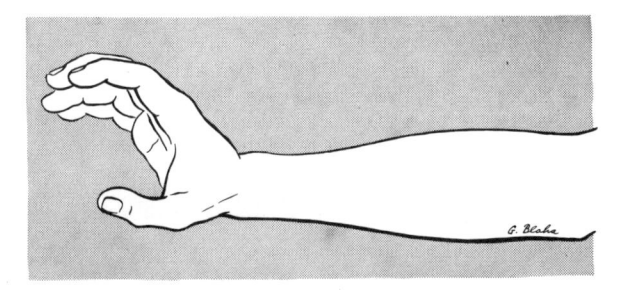

Fig. 1. Position of function.

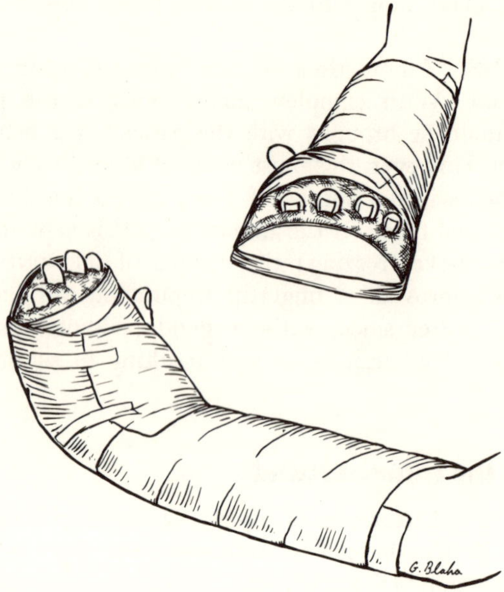

Fig. 2. Resiliant compression dressing.

jured parts at rest. After application of the clean dressings, they should be held in place with some type of roller dressing. The fingers should be kept separated from each other and in a natural, curved position.

IMMOBILIZATION IN THE POSITION OF FUNCTION. The purpose of immobilizing the hand and upper extremity is to minimize further damage in the case of injury to soft tissues and bones. The position of function generally maintains the most favorable relation of fractured bones and lacerated soft tissues. If an undue delay occurs between the time of injury and definitive care, muscle contractures and joint stiffness may be minimized.

Almost any material can be helpful in immobilization including wooden splints, rolled-up newspapers or magazines.

It should be emphasized that it is important to avoid putting anything into a deep or large wound such as antiseptics, instruments, or gauze. Rapid, specialized care includes a most careful cleansing of the tissues and this is done with adequate instruments and other equipment.

Infections

Any break in the skin, however small, may allow bacteria to enter and result in an infection. If infections are allowed to progress without the proper treatment they may cause complete loss of function of a digit or even an entire hand by destroying tendons or causing a great deal of scar formation.

Any small cut or pin prick should be treated immediately by washing the affected part in soap and warm water for ten minutes, drying with a freshly laundered towel and applying an adequate dressing. The affected part should be kept out of water when covered and, if the dressing becomes wet, it must be changed.

The symptoms of an infection which is becoming more severe include swelling, redness, pain and tenderness, and if more severe, the formation of pus. It is most important that infections be seen by a physician as early as possible, because when the first signs of pain and swelling appear it may be possible to treat the infection with antibiotics and rest and cure it.

For severe infections the basic principles of treatment are as follows: immobilization, elevation to reduce swelling, antibiotics, and drainage of abcesses by properly placed incisions.

Bites

Human bite wounds are most dangerous and difficult to treat. They frequently are sustained by striking the knuckle against an adversary's tooth. There are many dangerous germs in the mouth and if these cause an infection in the knucklejoint a patient may lose his ability to bend or straighten the affected digit.

Animal bites, such as inflicted by teeth, as well as human bites are potentially dangerous and should not be irrigated or closed.

The best treatment of human and animal bites is applying a protective dressing and seeking medical care.

Burns

There are several types of burns, the most common of which is flame burns. Burns of the skin may be caused by chemicals and other agents.

The best treatment of a significant burn is the careful washing of the affected area with soap and water. If the burn is extremely painful, the hand may be put in cold water which helps temporarily to relieve the pain.

A common error in the treatment of burns is to apply a thick coating of some ointment. With a significant burn it is much better to simply cover it with a dressing and seek medical care.

Frostbite

Frozen fingers and hands are quite common in the wintertime and, if severe, can lead to gangrene and loss of part of a finger. If it is possible to get medical care immediately, some physicians advocate immersing the frostbitten part in warm water at a carefully regulated temperature. If medical care is going to be delayed, it is better to wash the affected part with soap and warm water and protect it with a clean dressing. Rubbing snow or applying additional cold to a frostbite is not recommended.

The Tourniquet

The use of a tourniquet to prevent bleeding is most dangerous. It is not possible to tell how much pressure a tourniquet, such as a belt or rubber hose, exerts and there is great danger that the tourniquet will be put on and forgotten. This can easily result in complete lack of circulation to an injured extremity with resultant gangrene and necessity for amputation.

It is rare that bleeding from hand injuries cannot be controlled by the use of a resilient compression dressing. In case of a very severe injury, such as complete amputation of the hand or forearm, it may be necessary to use the tourniquet. If so, it *must* be loosened every 15 minutes for a short period to allow some circulation even though the extremity continues to bleed. In summary, although the use of a tourniquet is highly dangerous, if used with extreme care, it may be helpful.

Immediate Hospital Treatment

It is important for all who may be called upon to render first aid for the injured hand to understand the principles of early definitive treatment. After the patient has arrived at the hospital he must receive a general physical examination in order that correct priority of treatment be established. This is especially true for patients with multiple injuries or for elderly patients. It will be necessary also to summon sufficient personnel and have the proper facilities prepared.

PERSONNEL. In addition to a surgeon experienced in the treatment of hand injuries there must be an available operating room, nurses, an anesthesiologist, and assistants for the operating surgeon.

FACILITIES. Full operating room facilities are required. Operations on the hand are major ones requiring strict aseptic technique, including masks, gowns, drapes, and other material. A full supply of instruments, good lighting, and a pressure cuff to insure a bloodless operating field must be available. General anesthesia often will be required.

PRELIMINARY EXAMINATION. A preliminary examination is necessary to evaluate the hand injury before taking the patient to the operating room, but this examination must never be careless with respect to asepsis, or cursory with respect to the extent of injury. The preliminary examination should be done in a clean area, personnel should wear gowns, caps, and masks. A few sterile instruments and bandages should be ready to protect the wound against further contamination. After determining the details of when and where the injury occurred, and the extent of first aid treatment rendered, the wound itself must be evaluated as to the type, i.e., incised, contused, crushed, and so on, and the degree of damage and contamination present. Assay of the structural damage includes:

Extent of skin loss.
Major bleeding.
Evidence of tendon laceration, (by testing motion).
Assay of nerve damage, (by sensory and motor tests).
X-ray for bone and joint injury.

OPERATIVE TREATMENT. Principles of proper operative technique include:

Thorough soap and water preparation of the entire hand and forearm with the wound protected.
Meticulous draping and a bloodless field.
Thorough wound cleansing and removal of foreign material and any devitalized tissue.
Ligation or repair of severed blood vessels.
Repair of damaged nerves.

Repair of divided tendons if not contraindicated by long duration since initial injury or location.
Adequate skin coverage with skin grafts, if necessary.
Reduction of fractures and immobilization in the proper position.
A carefully applied resilient, protective dressing with moderate, even pressure.
Administration of tetanus toxoid and antibiotics as indicated.

22 / The Feet

CHARLES B. PUESTOW AND ROBERT J. JOPLIN

On first thought it might appear that devotion of an entire chapter to lesions of the feet requiring first aid treatment is allocating too much space to such a subject. However, there are no more minor ailments that can be so incapacitating as those of the feet. This fact is always reemphasized among military personnel, although the problem is always present among civilians but not concentrated sufficiently to be impressive. Therefore, it does not appear inappropriate to devote considerable discussion to various aspects of this subject, particularly since so many of the lesions are acute ones requiring first aid treatment and not complicated surgical therapy. As long as military training of at least a fair number of our people seems to be with us indefinitely, it appears to be more than justifiable to devote considerable attention to the numerous conditions discussed in this chapter.

Commercialization and indiscriminate use of so-called arch supports, bunion pads, corn plasters, solutions for "dissolving" corns, and various powders and ointments have tended to create in the public mind the impression that the use of these sundry products is the answer to all foot ailments. As a result of this, many individuals come to see the orthopedic surgeon with disabilities of the foot far more severe than would have been the case if proper treatment had been instituted early.

Anatomy of the Foot

Perhaps more so than in any other part of the body, a knowledge of structure of the foot is necessary in order to understand the methods of treatment employed.

The 26 bones of the foot (Figs. 1 and 2) are considered in

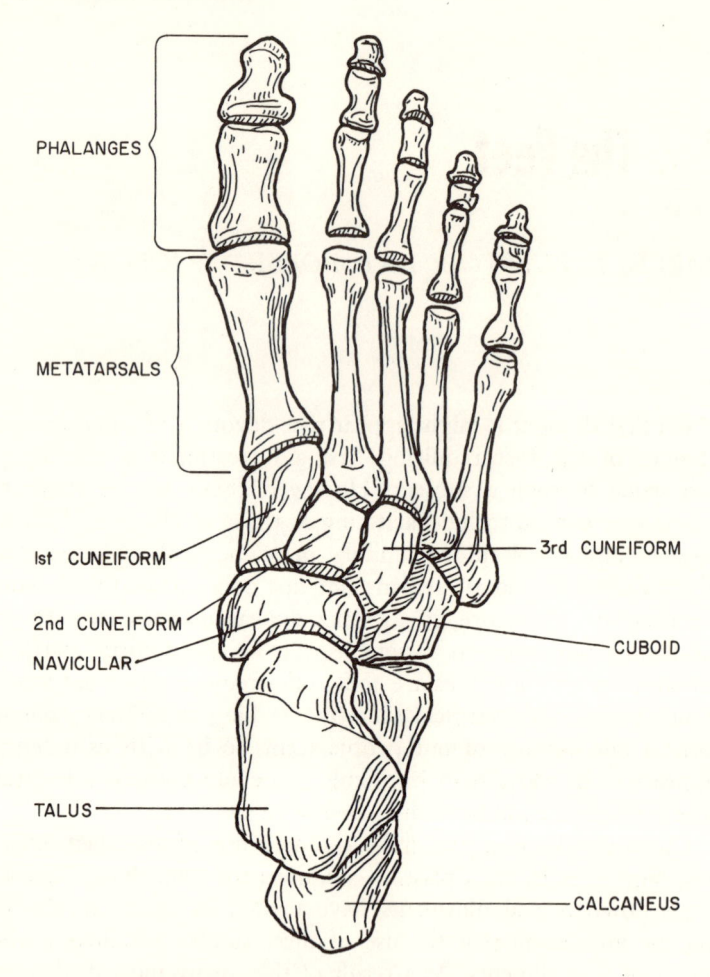

Fig. 1. Bones of the foot, dorsal view.

three groups: hindfoot of 7 *tarsal* bones, forefoot of 5 *metatarsals* and the five toes with 14 phalanges. Functionally, the foot provides:
1. A *support* for the body weight (primarily through the massive calcaneus and astragalus lying directly under the tibia)
2. A *shock absorber* action for the body by resilience, spring, and elasticity through the multiplicity of joints
3. A *lever arm* to raise and propel the body into motion

The *arches* (Fig. 3) of the foot are formed by the tarsal and metatarsal bones, fastened together by ligaments, tendons, and mus-

Anatomy of the Foot / 331

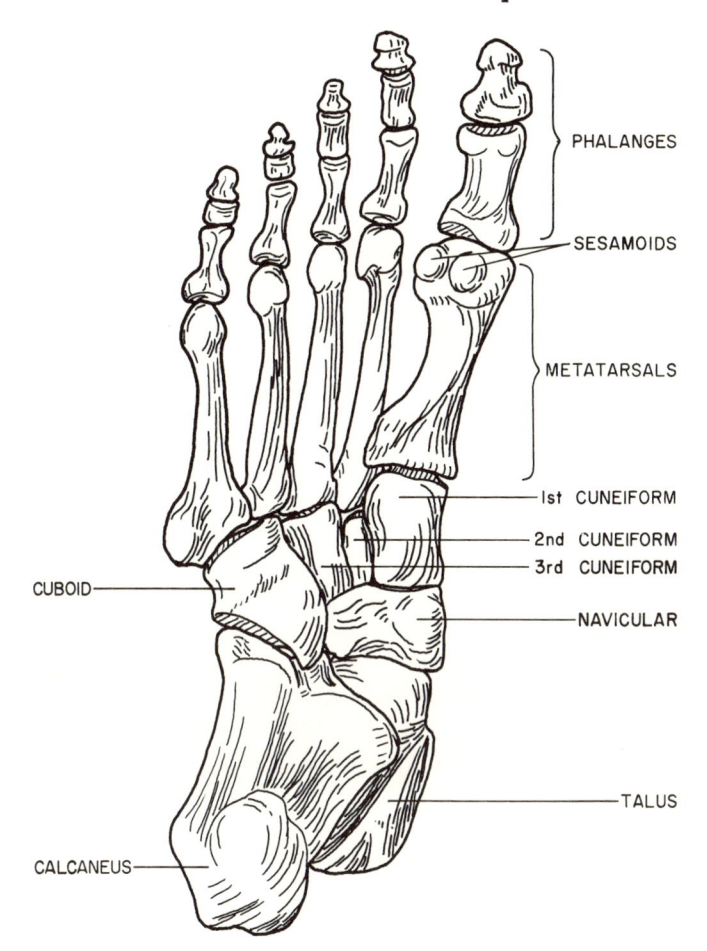

Fig. 2. Bones of the foot, plantar view.

cles. It is generally accepted that the arches are maintained by the ligaments, while the muscles through their tendons intermittently raise and lower the arches maintaining balance.

For first aid purposes there are two major arches: the *longitudinal arch* in the long axis and *the metatarsal or anterior arch* in the transverse axis across the heads of the metatarsals. The longitudinal arch consists of an inner or *medial* and an outer or *lateral* pillar. Posteriorly, both pillars rest on the os calcis. Anteriorly, the medial pillar rests on the head of the first metatarsal and to a lesser extent the second and third metatarsal heads. The lateral pillar rests on the heads of the

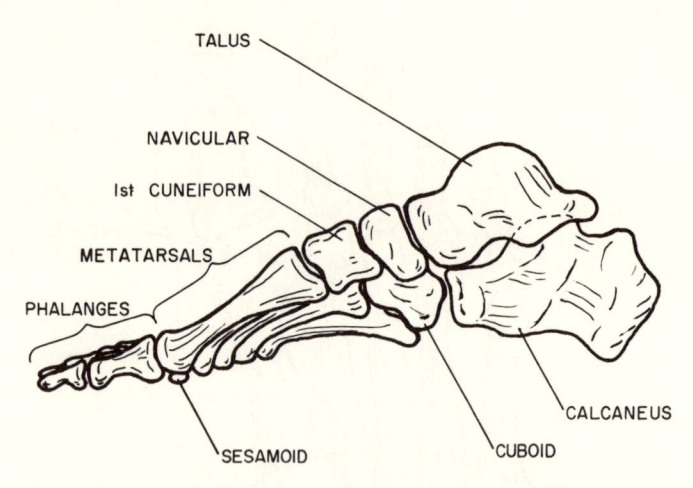

Fig. 3. Bones of the foot, lateral view, showing longitudinal arch.

fourth and fifth metatarsals. The high medial pillar consists of the astragalus, tarsal navicular, the three cuneiform and the medial three metatarsal bones. The low lateral pillar, almost flat, consists of the cuboid and the lateral two metatarsals. The longitudinal arch is maintained by the plantar ligaments and fascia. Within this arch are housed the blood vessels, nerves, and muscles. That there is sufficient room for these structures to be free and unrestricted is all important.

The anterior arch is formed by the heads of the five metatarsal bones and is rather shallow. It becomes flattened and disappears upon weight bearing but resumes an arched form when the weight is removed. Because of this, many do not consider this to be a true arch.

Movements of the foot occur through the various joints. By a combination of movements through the use of two or more joints, various positions of the foot may be assumed.

The *ankle joint* is formed by mortising an irregularly shaped bone, the ankle bone (astragalus), into a groove formed medially by a downward projection from the medial side of the tibia (medial malleolus) and laterally by the distal end of the fibula (lateral malleolus). This joint is hingelike in character and allows the foot to bend upward (dorsiflexion) or to be dropped (plantar flexion). It is the astragalus which receives the body weight and transmits it to the rest of the tarsus.

The subastragaloid joint lies between the lower portion of the astragalus and the upper border of the os calcis. This joint, in connection with others, permits side-to-side motion (inversion and eversion) of the foot on the leg.

The *midtarsal joint* lies immediately in front of these two bones and permits a limited amount of movement and also adds elasticity to the foot.

The *metatarsophalangeal joints* and the *interphalangeal joints* of the toes provide motion in a manner similar to the corresponding joints in the hands and fingers. The toes, particularly the great toe, when functioning normally add power and smoothness to the gait.

Affection of the Arches

By far the greatest proportion of painful feet is due to a change in the arch structure with a resulting abnormal distribution of pressure upon the foot.

The direct cause for painful feet may be that of strain or trauma by: A, excess weight as in obesity; B, excess exercise as in long walks or marches on the untrained foot; C, excess standing; D, abnormal positioning of the foot; E, poor posture and gait; F, poor shoes and support; and G, actual injury to the foot. However, these are often superimposed upon some deep-seated condition as: 1, hereditary errors in muscular, neurotrophic, or osseous structures (such as spina bifida, accessory bones, fusions, and shortening of the first metatarsal); 2, infections producing fibrosis locally and toxic relaxations of supporting structures at a distance; 3, arthritis, metabolic or traumatic; 4, toxic states; and 5, relaxing of ligaments after prolonged illness.

Flatfoot has been generally considered as the most common cause of painful feet. This is not true as very young children normally have *hypermobile flaccid (flexible) flatfeet*, which may persist with growth so that this is the normal relationship for the bones of the arches.

Such a foot is asymptomatic unless there has been some superimposed stress or injury. In flatfoot the longitudinal arch is flattened, the forefoot is turned out (abducted), the heel rolled outward (everted). In the early stages this happens only on weight bearing, while at rest the arch may be normal, and all movements of the foot may be carried out. As the condition becomes chronic, with continued foot strain and stretching of capsules and ligaments on one side and contractures of opposing structures occurring on the other, the deformity becomes more and more fixed, even at rest (*rigid flatfoot*). At this stage the foot is again asymptomatic, but with very limited motion.

The *peroneal spastic flatfoot* is considered to be the result of congenital anomalies of the tarsal bones on the basis of studies of recruits in the Canadian Army by Harris and Beath. They found an astragalocalcaneal bridge (fusion of the accessory os sustentaculi to the astragalus). Previously, a calcaneonavicular bar (fusion of the anterior process of the calcaneus to the navicular) had been observed and associated with severe rigid flatfoot. In these conditions the peroneii become shortened and spastic, placing the plantar fascia under strain. If the fascia maintains its integrity, the whole foot is everted and the strain directed to the gastrocnemius and soleus muscles. If the fascia is weak and stretched, the forefoot first abducts, and later with progression, the heel is pulled out and the heel cord shortens. When the foot becomes fixed in this position it is called a rigid flatfoot. It may or may not be painful but neither does it function well.

Acute foot strain may have its inception in any one of the several ways mentioned. It is manifested by pain, swelling, and inability to bear weight. With *chronic foot strain* the lower extremity is fatigued, tiring easily after standing or walking a short time. Discomfort, aching, and a burning sensation of the arches of the feet are among the first symptoms of foot strain. The strain may be felt on the medial side of the ankle. The aching may extend upward to involve the calves of the legs as the result of strain on the stretched and bowed gastrocnemius and soleus muscles. Cramps occur in the leg, especially at night, and the feet often swell as noted by the patient when the shoes become tight. On examination, the foot is seen to turn outward and the weight rests on the medial side of the heel. If the condition is allowed to progress, the feet will feel cold and numb as a result of impairment of the circulation (due to loss of the protection of the neurovascular structures by the longitudinal arch). There is marked tenderness under the arch over the plantar fascia with trigger points under and in front of the lateral malleolus. Callosities form at the new pressure sites under the metatarsal heads in direct proportion to the strength of the plantar fascia. The weaker the fascia the greater the abduction, with increasing callosity formation under the head of the first metatarsal to a point where the pressure site moves back under the tarsal navicular. As this occurs, the gait assumes a slouching, shuffling character.

An apparent flatfoot may be perfectly painless due to fixed contractures and bony development in this position, whereas a foot with normal anatomic appearance may be very painful because of strain on ligaments, which may eventually result in the development of flatfoot. The *cavus* high-arched foot is prone to have complaints of any or all of the affections involving the feet.

Treatment objectives are the reestablishment and maintenance of normal mechanical relationships in the foot. This is done by restoring the strength and tone of the muscles. It must be remembered that the only indication for treatment of flatfoot is pain. However, prophylactically, proper foot function (including weight reduction and correct posture) is the goal to be sought rather than correction after symptoms appear.

In the acutely painful flatfoot, *bed rest* with as complete relief from weight bearing as possible should be insisted upon. Application of *local heat* in the form of hot soaks and baking, or alternate hot and cold baths (*contrast baths*) and *massage* may be used to relieve pain. If prompt relief of pain is not secured by these measures, the injection of Novocain and hydrocortone into the tender areas or trigger points may give relief. When the tenderness and swelling have disappeared, the foot should be strapped, holding the foot in inversion and supporting the longitudinal arch for walking.

The patient may then be allowed up with progressively increased weight bearing and activity. The subsequent treatment is the same as that for a chronically painful flatfoot. Here, bed rest is usually not necessary. A *correctly fitting shoe*, (Figs. 4 and 5) is essential: The shoe should have a straight last, the counter holding the heel snugly

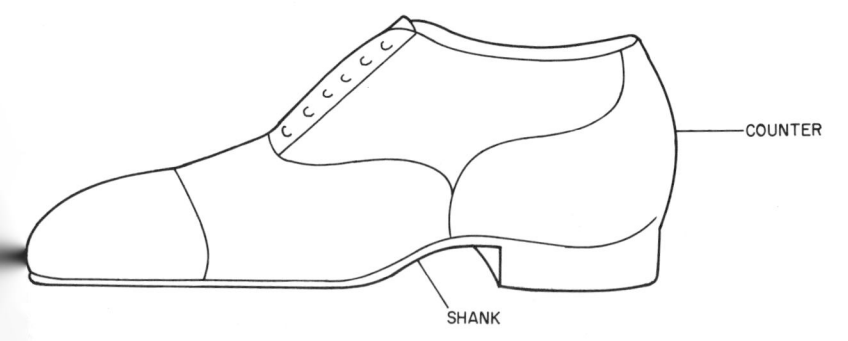

Fig. 4. Lateral view of the shoe to show the counter, which should be stiff to support the correctly aligned foot, and the shank, which should be stiff to support the longitudinal arch.

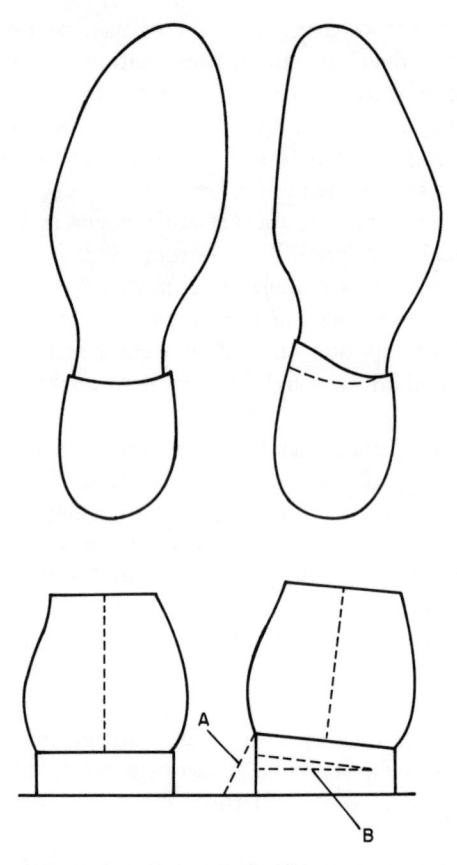

Fig. 5. Sole of straight last shoe (on right) compared with sole of conventional shoe. Thomas heel (on right) compared with conventional heel. Note: Flare "A" and wedge "B" which may, or may not, be indicated in maintaining correction of pronation in some children's feet.

and extending forward past the medial pillar of the longitudinal arch to the head of the first metatarsal, the medial border of the heel prolonged forward (Thomas heel) with slight medial elevation of one sixteenth to one fourth inch. Enough room should be allowed in the front portion so that the toes are not constricted. The arches should be supported by firm felt or other suitable padding material (Fig. 6) (not rigid or too resilient) fitted to the individual foot, depending upon the specific requirements. Experience has indicated that this should be done by a physician or by the intelligent patient under his doctor's guidance.

It is occasionally necessary to resort to forcible overcorrection

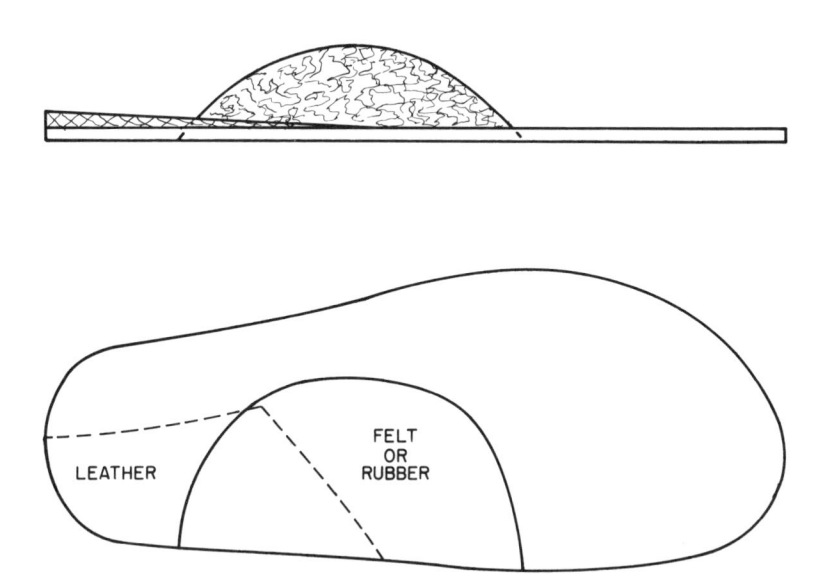

Fig. 6. Child's foot pad: If made of felt, it should have the consistency of piano felt; if of rubber, the consistency of sponge rubber. A little tilt of the heel may be had by inserting a slip of leather if pronation is a factor.

of the foot under anesthesia and immobilization in a plaster cast. The same treatment as in a flexible flatfoot is then prescribed. In extreme cases it may be necessary to utilize various soft tissue and bony operations.

Metatarsalgia

The term metatarsalgia has been used to denote pain in the region of the anterior arch. Many orthopedic surgeons and anatomists maintain that there is no arch in this area, since on pressure the heads of all the metatarsals touch the ground and bear weight, but there is some question as to how much weight each metatarsal head bears. In the presumed normal foot it has been theorized that the weight distribution carried by the first metatarsal head is twice that carried by each of the other four metatarsal heads (or two sixths under the first metatarsal and one sixth under each of the lateral four metatarsals). The causes of disturbances in this part of the foot are the same as those of the longitudinal arch. Anything which will throw unusual

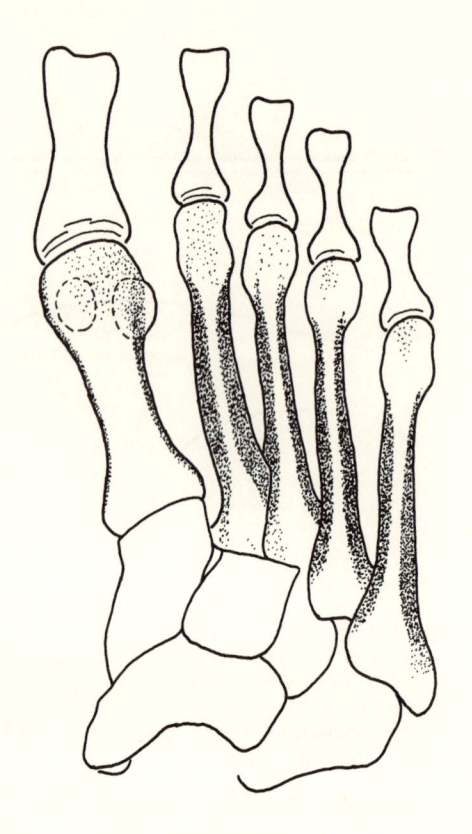

Fig. 7. Disturbances of structural relationships lead to unequal stress as shown in increased thickening of the metatarsal shafts in so-called atavistic first metatarsal syndrome. Note: Cortex of first metatarsal appears thinner than that of each of the four lesser metatarsals. Normally, the first should bear twice the weight of each of the others—when shorter than the others, it cannot carry its share even if heels of only moderate height are worn.

stress on the forefoot can produce pain. Therefore it is frequently found in:

1. Women wearing narrow, high-heeled shoes where there is constant strain and the weight is concentrated on weight bearing, well forward on the ball of the foot, without adequate support of the arches and heel. This position forces the toes into continuous hyperdorsiflexion, and on full weight bearing the toes are jammed forward

into the narrow point of the shoe. This with the limited stretch of the flexor tendons frequently produces marked hammer toe deformity.

2. The foot with high longitudinal arch (as a *clawfoot*) may have similar problems.

3. Shortening of the Achilles tendon with an intact strong plantar fascia, throwing an excessive proportion of the weight on the head of the first metatarsal.

4. Shortening of the first metatarsal with undue pressure carried by the second metatarsal head.

All of these are frequent causes of disturbances of structural relationships (Fig. 7) leading to unequal stress with ensuing distressing symptoms. These are static changes in which the metatarsal heads are allowed to spread, called *relaxation metatarsalgia*, or are crowded, called *compression metatarsalgia*. In the latter, the plantar digital nerve (Fig. 8) is frequently irritated, or actually pinched, pro-

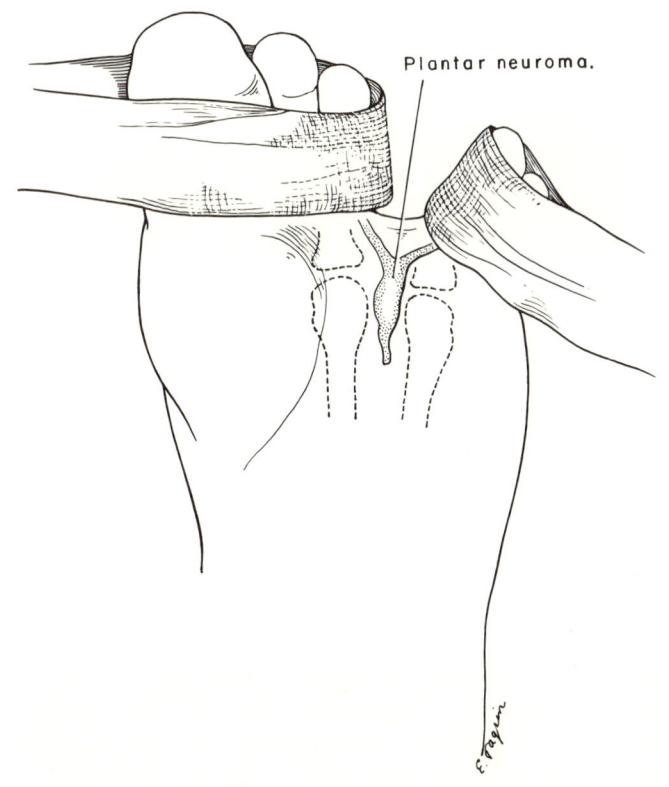

Fig. 8. Morton's Toe Syndrome (perineural fibrosis) of the plantar digital nerve between the 3rd and 4th metatarsals.

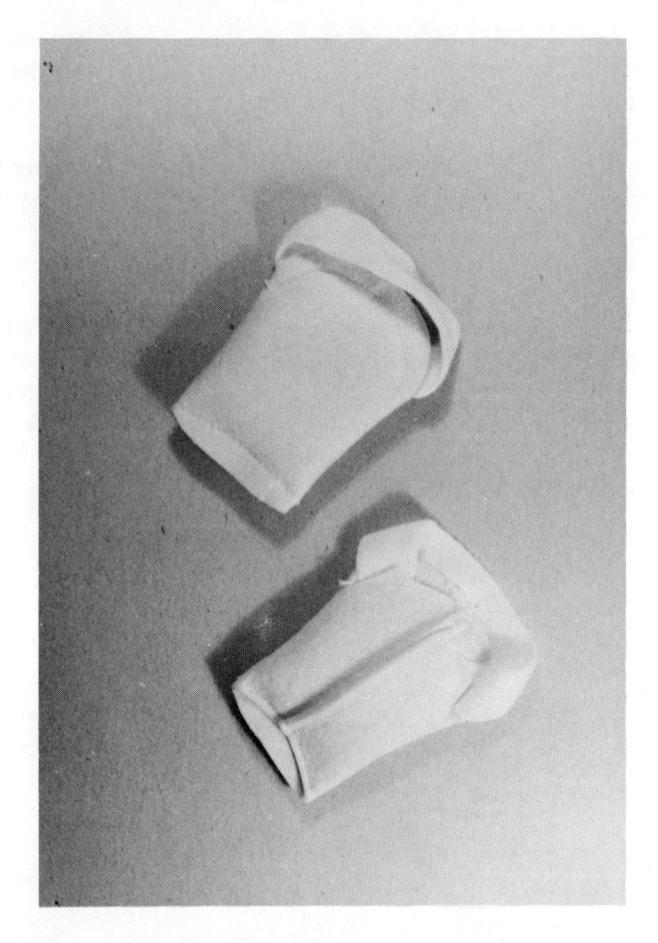

Fig. 9. A felt and foam rubber pad may be used effectively as a first aid measure to relieve acute symptoms. Footnote: This pad is made of felt sewn into the shape of a pocket into which a piece of foam rubber is placed. A thin, soft, woven cotton tape is attached. This tape is looped around the second and third toes; it is long enough to permit the pad to rest just proximal to the metatarsal heads.

ducing a painful neuroma as it passes between the heads of the metatarsals, usually the third and fourth. It is known as *plantar digital neuroma (Morton's toe)*. The symptoms may appear acutely with a step which twists the forefoot. Early distress may be spasmodic but soon becomes constant, if treatment fails. The burning pain begins under the metatarsal heads (Fig. 9) radiating into the toes supplied by the nerve. Weight bearing aggravates the pain so that the patient must stop, remove the shoe, and massage the toes and foot to relieve the pain. Metatarsalgia may also result from trauma and inflammation of this area whether of bacterial or metabolic (arthritic) origin. Symptoms of the relaxation metatarsalgia are those of strain in the ball of the foot with a constant burning toothachelike pain under the metatarsal heads. Callosities appear under the heads of the metatarsals that carry more than their proportionate share of the weight.

Relief of pain is of primary importance. Rest and freedom from weight bearing should be followed by physiotherapy and corrective exercises. Shoes redistributing the weight so that each portion of the foot bears its proportionate part are necessary. A straight last, rounded box-toed, with a firm well-fitting shank and a heel of moderate height should be worn (one and one half to two inches for women, one inch for men). The rigidity of the shank depends on the degree of involvement of the longitudinal arch. Pressure on the metatarsal heads is relieved by felt or other carefully fitted resilient padding placed in the shoe just behind the metatarsal heads, or occasionally by a metatarsal bar in the same relative location on the sole of the shoe. Manipulation and sometimes the application of a plaster cast may be required. A check on the general medical status of the patient should be made, and any problems found should be corrected before further treatment of the foot is carried out.

March Foot (Marching Fracture of the Metatarsal Bones)

Infrequently in civilian life, and with much greater frequency in military service, there occurs a fracture of a metatarsal bone, usually the second or third, with no history of a single severe injury, but following long and repeated foot strain under the stress of unusual exertion, as in marching and the trauma (injury) occasioned by weight bearing.

Various theories have been advanced as to the cause, but the pathogenesis is still not clearly defined. Continuous minimal mechanical insult (*microtrauma*), piling up beyond the ability of the bone to bear this strain, is the immediate cause. In the majority of cases, however, the metatarsal strength has been reduced by several factors, such as inflammation of the bone (*periostitis*) or of the muscle (*myositis*), disturbances in circulation (*ischemic changes*), relaxation of the muscular and tendinous support of the foot as in a flatfoot, relative shortening of the first metatarsal throwing added body weight on the adjacent metatarsals, and following certain infections.

The onset may be abrupt, with a sudden, severe pain at the site of the fracture, or there may be a complete absence of symptoms at the time the fracture occurs. As a rule, the course is insidious, the individual becoming conscious of a discomfort and burning pain on the plantar surface of the forefoot, gradually increasing in severity. This is present when the body weight is borne, and absent in most instances while at rest, although it may be constant. To lessen the amount of weight on the affected foot, the individual begins to limp. There is

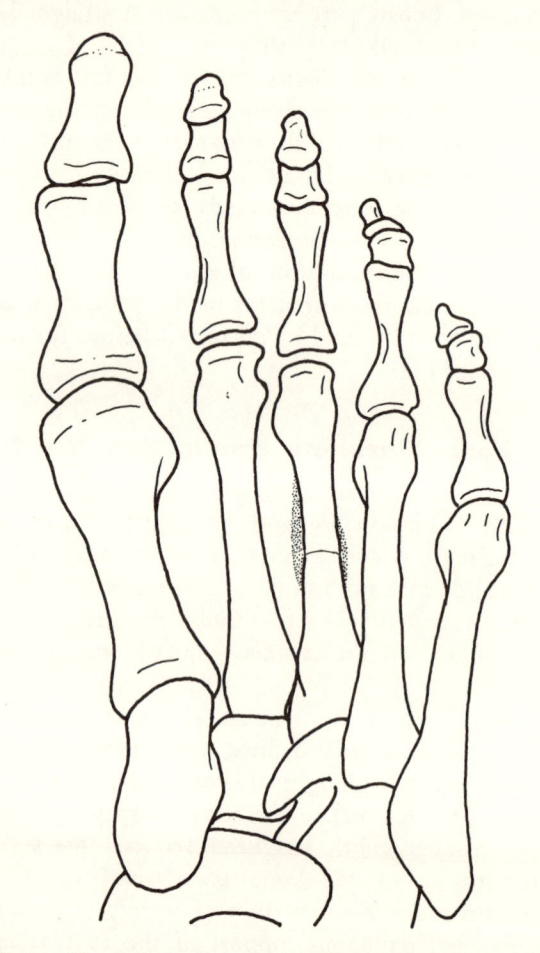

Fig. 10. March foot. The fracture line without displacement is now visible with the surrounding callus, four weeks after injury.

an exquisite tenderness localized to the fracture site. In very mild cases a swelling over the dorsum of the foot is present, while in more severe cases the plantar surface also becomes involved. This disappears when the foot is elevated and put at rest. Unlike most fractures, crepitus cannot be elicited.

The diagnosis is confirmed by an x-ray (Fig. 10), but in the early stages this may be difficult, since the fracture line is poorly defined and often is incomplete. After two or three weeks, however, a profuse amount of callus is formed, and the fracture line is usually more pronounced. This is especially true if the foot has not been immobilized.

In most cases rest and the application of a fitted arch support in a stiff shanked shoe may be all that is necessary in treatment. If the first metatarsal bone is shorter than the second, the arch support should be fitted slightly high behind the head of the first metatarsal.

In severe cases, the foot must be immobilized at right angles or above in a walking plaster cast extending from the toes to the knee and kept in the cast for three to six weeks. This should be followed by physiotherapy, graduated weight bearing, an arch support and metatarsal bar as the need is indicated.

Painful Heels

Pain in the region of the heel may be due to involvement of either the soft tissues or the bone, or both. The etiologic factors are *trauma* caused by actual injury or poorly fitting shoes, *infection* which may be either local or general, *static defects* such as a flatfoot, *metabolic*

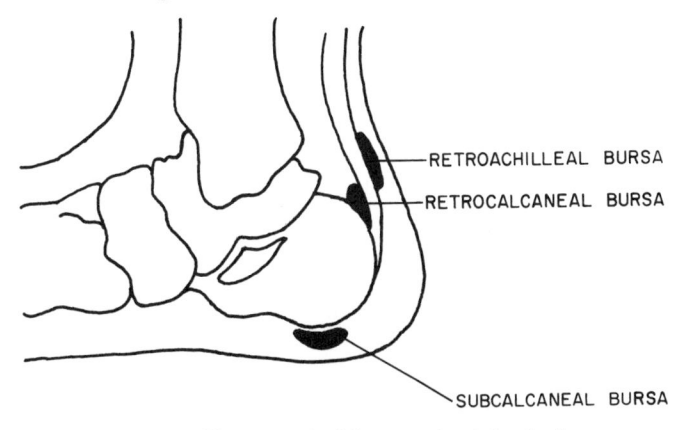

Fig. 11. Three principal bursas about the heel.

disturbances such as various arthritides, and *anomalies* in the structure of the foot with strain and secondary periostitis at the origin of the plantar fascia.

BURSITIS. There are three principal bursas (Fig. 11) about the heel. The *retrocalcaneal bursa* lies between the Achilles tendon and the posterior surface of the os calcis, immediately above the insertion of the tendon. Inflammation of this bursa is usually caused by trauma due to pressure from the shoe, or by infection, and manifests itself by pain on motion and localized tenderness. A superficial bursa between the Achilles tendon and the skin (*retroachilleal bursa*) is sometimes present, and bursitis here is most often due to irritation from a tight-fitting shoe. The treatment consists of rest, the application of moist heat, and the usual measures in the treatment of inflammation. If the bursa is fluctuant, aspiration and the injection of one-fourth to one-half milliliter of hydrocortone into the sac, followed by a tight dressing, may be indicated. Elevation of the heel, using a felt pad, and sometimes the removal or splitting of the back of the shoe to relieve the pressure follow the emergency treatment. If the inflammation does not subside, incision or resection of the bursa should be done only as a last resort after intensive prolonged conservative measures have failed. Scars in this area are easily irritated, causing considerable disability in themselves.

A bursa may form on the inferior surface of the heel (*subcalcaneal bursa*), most frequently centrally, and it may be over a bony spur in the origin of the plantar fascia. Bursitis or fasciitis is often responsible for the pain attributed to the exostosis. A felt pad, hollowed out in the center, placed under the heel removes the pressure on the bursa and relieves the pain. Correction of the strain on the plantar fascia is also indicated. Injection of the tender point in the fascia with Novocain and a cortisone is often curative. Excision of the bursa in addition to the spur is essential for cure when surgery is resorted to.

TENOSYNOVITIS. Inflammation of the Achilles tendon and its sheath may be caused by injury, infection, or a strain, such as produced in walking uphill, in which case the foot is dorsiflexed, stretching the tendon. It is symptomized by acute local pain, considerable disability, crepitus (grating) of the tendon on movement, and swelling behind the malleoli. It is treated by rest, elevation of the extremity, the application of heat in the form of moist dressings to the tender area, and the injection of hydrocortone into the tendon sheath. When the pain is gone, the heel of the shoe should be elevated by means of a pad.

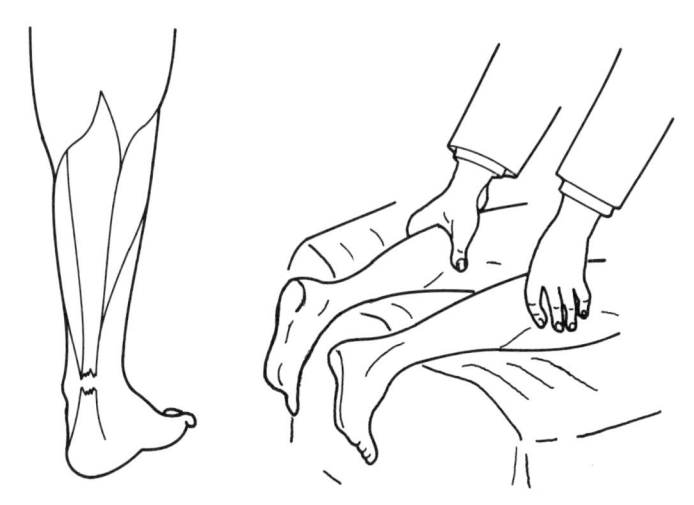

Fig. 12. Rupture of Achilles tendon on right—demonstration to show absence of foot movement on affected side and the presence of plantar flexion on normal (left) side by squeezing each calf muscle.

In this way, the tendon is relaxed by not allowing it to stretch its full length. Strapping of the ankle for a short while is also beneficial. It may be necessary to remove the counter of the shoe to relieve pressure on the tendon. This condition seldom occurs in the other tendons of the foot.

RUPTURE OF THE ACHILLES TENDON. The Achilles tendon may be completely ruptured (Fig. 12) in a number of ways—by a projectile, cutting instrument, or a fall from a height and landing upon the strongly extended foot. The victim has a sudden severe pain, the foot is dorsiflexed and cannot be extended (plantar flexed), or at most only partially. A gap in the tendon can be seen or felt at the site of the rupture, and the disability is at once apparent. Tenderness and swelling increase with time; in a matter of hours the defect in the tendon may be hard to detect, and the pain may become so severe that the patient can make no effort to extend the foot. Suture of the tendon ends should be done immediately and the tendon protected in a plaster cast for six to eight weeks.

Incomplete lacerations and partial ruptures of the Achilles tendon amazingly enough may very easily be overlooked due to the extreme range of motion carrying the point of injury of the tendon a considerable distance from the site of the bruise or laceration in the skin. Also the examiner may not recognize the severity of the injury, even complete rupture of the Achilles tendon, due to the power of plantar flexion of the posterior tibial and peroneal muscles. However, they are not strong enough alone for the patient to stand on his toes, and there is great danger of completing the rupture of a partially torn tendon. In the absence of treatment a partial rupture may be secondarily ruptured by very slight trauma, even walking, as a result of the ensuing degeneration in the tendon. Varying degrees of trauma may completely or partially rupture the tendon in which degeneration has occurred as the result of frequently repeated fairly mild injury or if involved by some disease process. Treatment of the partially lacerated Achilles tendon is best treated acutely by full exploration and repair when repairing the skin wound. The partial rupture if relatively asymptomatic or if seen late may be treated by rest, elevation of the heel by a pad, supportive strapping of the ankle or application of a cast for six to eight weeks.

CALCANEAL SPURS. These bony outgrowths usually appear on the inferior-medial aspects of the os calcis (Fig. 13). Their production has been attributed to both focal and general infections, trauma, static defects, metabolic disturbances, and a short plantar fascia. Large spurs are frequently present but may not produce symptoms. The onset is usually gradual, with increasing pain along the medial border of the os calcis, or at the attachment of the plantar fascia. The pain may be acute if a periostitis is present. Walking on the ball of the foot relieves the pain.

Treatment includes finding and removing foci of infection, rest,

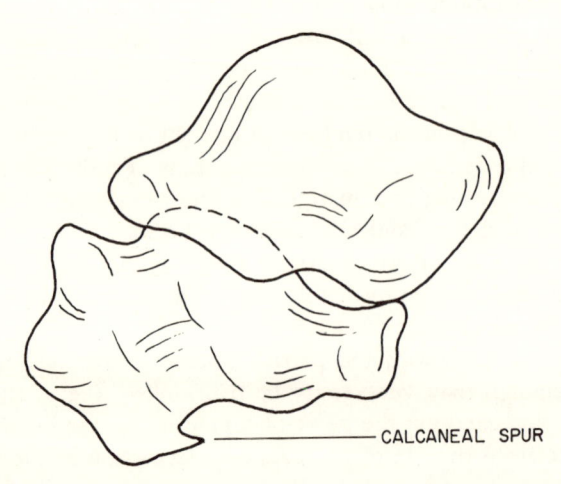

Fig. 13. Calcaneal spur at the attachment of the plantar fascia.

keeping off the feet, and heat. After the pain and tenderness subside, proper shoes should be prescribed. A rigid shank, supporting the longitudinal arch, is better than a flexible one. A felt or rubber heel pad with hollow center will relieve pressure on the involved area. Rubber heels are better than solid leather. If there is associated arthritis, diathermy may be of some value. Injecting the tender area with saline solution, Novocain, or hydrocortone often helps, x-radiation therapy in small doses may be of value in acute cases. Operative procedures, to be resorted to only as a last measure, include resection of the spur and the bursa usually associated with it. Removal of the spur without the bursa will not be curative. If the plantar fascia is tight it should be stripped loose from the os calcis.

PERIOSTITIS. Inflammation of the bony covering (the *periosteum*) of the os calcis may occur at the attachment of the Achilles tendon, the lateral or the inferior surfaces. Irritation from the shoe, infection, or trauma may be the cause. Localized pain and tenderness, and swelling over the involved area are the principal symptoms. The treatment is essentially the same as that for a bursitis, with rest, heat, and relief of pressure being indicated.

APOPHYSITIS CALCANEAL. The *apophysis* (*epiphysis* of a growth center that contributes to size, not length) contributes the posterior portion of the body of the calcaneus (heel bone). *Apophysitis* (*osteochondrosis*) (Fig. 14) is an inflammation of the epiphysis. It occurs most often in boys 10 to 15 years of age.

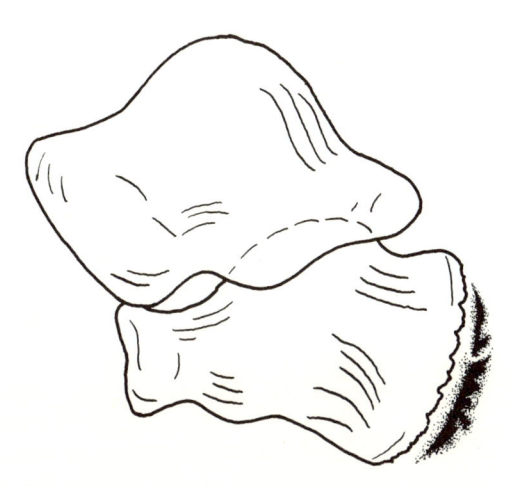

Fig. 14. Apophysitis calcaneal (osteochondrosis, or Sever's Disease).

Direct trauma or strain is most frequently the factor while systemic infections, circulatory and endocrine (hypopituitorism), are occasionally the cause. Symptoms start with an insidious slight limp and increasing pain. Lateral palpation of the heel between thumb and forefinger will generally serve to distinguish this condition from those of the adjacent bursae. Treatment is complete rest with a plaster cast for two or three weeks, followed by an adhesive strapping and elevation of the heel on a pad.

Affection of the Skin and Toenails

ATHLETE'S FOOT (EPIDERMOPHYTOSIS). This disease (Fig. 15), which is caused by fungous types of bacteria, is extremely common. The fungi are now considered to be more or less common inhabitants of the skin, invading it whenever the resistance is lowered. Fungi are known to infest and to propagate best in warm, alkaline, moist areas. Thus, the foot in a shoe provides a rather ideal environment for trycophytotic infections, and occasionally the fingers and other parts of the body are infected.

The primary lesions are tiny blisters (vesicles) which itch and burn. This causes the victim to rub and scratch the area breaking the vesicles, spreading the infection by means of the serum infested with numerous fungi to adjoining and distant areas. The small ulcers left by the blisters soon become secondarily infected. Maceration of the skin is a frequent complication, particularly between the toes if open ulcerations and fissures are present. Secondary infection occasionally is severe enough to develop a lymphangitis with red streaks extending up the leg. The disease may occur at any time but is most common in the summer (hot and humid), especially in people who are active on their feet. Soldiers are particularly subject to this condition as they live under ideal conditions for contracting and developing the disease.

Prophylaxis should be practiced and foot hygiene is extremely important as is the care of shoes and stockings (see Care of the Feet).

Treatment starts with redoubling the hygienic measures for the care of the feet. Direct treatment includes staying off of the feet as much as possible or entirely if the ulcerative stage spreads much beyond the webs of the toes. Application of a heavy metal antiseptic or gentian violet to the blisters or the resulting ulcers will usually stop their spread. Among the many remedial agents are potassium per-

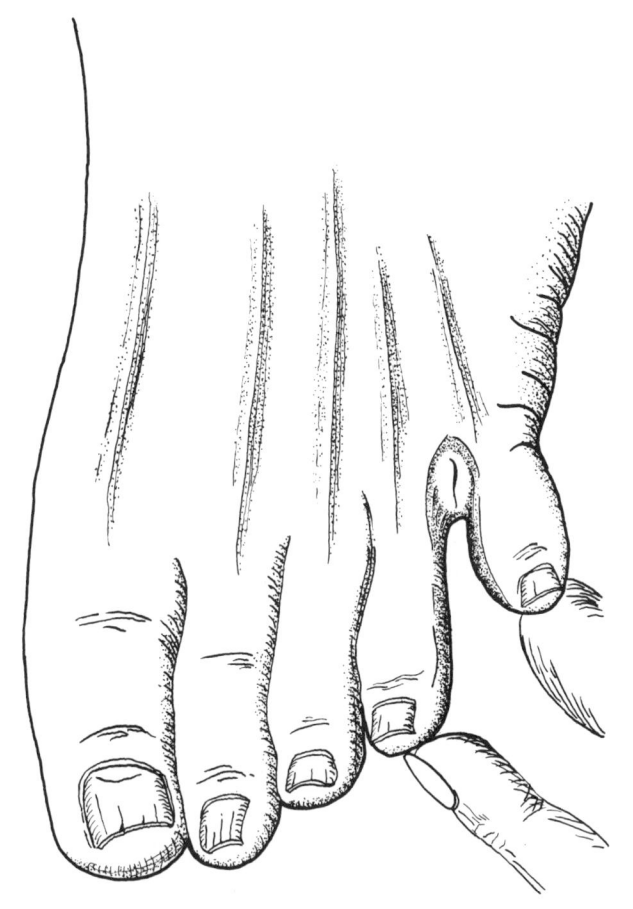

Fig. 15. Athlete's foot (epidermophytosis, acute dermatophytosis). Note the characteristic crack or fissure in web space between the toes affected and the blanched base within which the fissure appears.

manganate (1 to 9,000 solution) soaks daily and local application of half strength Whitfield's ointment. Some of the antibiotics may be helpful.

BUNIONS. This is thought by many laymen to be an involvement of the skin similar to a corn. It is the term used to describe a bursitis on the medial aspect of the great toe at the metatarsophalangeal joint. It is rather uncommon for simple bursitis to cause distress for long. Generally, after a number of years of recurrence of symptoms, there is lateral deviation of the great toe (*hallux valgus*) with either, or both, arthritis of the first metatarsophalangeal joint and/or exostosis of the medial aspect of the head of the first metatarsal under the bursa. The principal etiologic factor is short, pointed shoes. Prophylaxis and treatment call for the wearing of shoes large enough to prevent pressure. During the acute stage, the side of the shoe over the bunion may be cut out, and conservative measures for treatment of the bursitis carried out. Frequently a wedge of felt or lamb's wool placed between the first and second toes will straighten out the great toe, relieving the medial pressure of the first metatarsophalangeal joint. Surgical removal of the exostosis may be indicated in advanced bunions. The bursa should be resected only if it is calcified and thickened. Special procedures are required if an arthritis or hallux rigidus fails to respond to conservative measures.

BLISTERS. There are two schools of thought on the treatment of blisters. One is to keep them closed, the other is to open them and treat them as an open wound immediately. The first method, if successful, will require the patient to be off his feet for a much shorter period of time. Treatment of all blisters requires surgical cleansing and preparation of the entire area. If the blister is tense and thin-walled, drainage through a small border puncture is indicated in the closed method. The application of tincture of benzoin to the blistered epithelial cover whether drained or not will, with a thin petrolatum pressure dressing, often lead to resorption of the serum and reattachment of the epithelium to the underlying bed as a skin graft.

If the blister is accidentally broken or is so large that it is very likely to be broken and the epithelial bleb cover displaced, the open method of treatment is indicated. After surgical preparation of the area, the raised skin is completely removed and a thin petrolatum pressure dressing applied. No matter which method of treatment is used, signs of infection must be watched for.

INGROWN TOENAILS. Short, pointed shoes, tight stockings, and improper trimming of the nails cause the margin of the nail to turn down and to become embedded in the flesh of the nail groove. The soft tissues are soon penetrated by the nail being pinched against the side or sole of the shoe with ensuing infection. Proper shoes and hosiery, cutting of the nail straight across, and thinning the center of the nail longitudinally will prevent this condition. Insertion of cotton under the nail edge will assist the nail to grow above the skin margin. If diffuse infection occurs, all or part of the nail should be removed.

MISCELLANEOUS AFFECTIONS. A *corn* is an abnormal increase in the horny layers of the skin, compressed to form a thickened cone-shaped mass, which when pressed upon from the outside, impinges upon the small nerves in the body of the skin producing pain and disability in the foot. It is caused by pressure and the friction of the shoe against the skin; it occurs at the sites of greatest pressure, as on the dorsal aspect of the toes or on the lateral side of the fifth toe. Frequently there is an associated deformity of the foot, such as a hammer-toe, in conjunction with a high-arched foot. Both prophylaxis and treatment call for proper shoes and hosiery, and gait correction for prevention and cure alike. Removal of the pressure and correction of the deformity will often cause spontaneous separation of the corn. Removal of the corn is accomplished by softening it with daily hot soaks or plain petrolatum, followed by scraping of the softened layers of skin and keeping it level with the skin. The use of a scalpel or razor blade is best restricted to the hands of a surgeon. For scraping, however, an emery board or pumice stone is relatively safe in the hands of the patient. Covering with adhesive will reduce rubbing. Various preparations containing salicylic acid are used, but these should be prescribed by a physician and used cautiously on the corn alone.

Soft corns are formed in the same manner, but since they occur between the toes, usually between the fourth and fifth where there is greater perspiration, the corn is macerated and softer than the hard corn. They are due to the pressure of the toes against each other, especially when a narrow, pointed shoe is worn. Usually there is a spur on one of the phalanges, increasing the pressure. They may prove resistant to treatment unless shoe and foot hygiene are completely corrected. The skin should be kept dry and clean. A pad may be used between the toes to separate them. Raising of the anterior arch accomplishes the same purpose. Resection of the exostosis and its overlying bursa may be necessary. A shoe with a wide anterior compartment should be worn.

Calluses. Plantar corns and warts are produced by intermittent pressure and rubbing as a result of ill-fitting shoes, poor hygiene, and gait. Continuous pressure results in the formation of an ulcer in the patient, with poor sensation and circulation. They are formed at such points of pressure as the inferior surface of the heel, the ball of the foot under the heads of the metatarsals, and the plantar surface of the great toe. Shoes with pads redistributing the weight away from these areas will assist in correcting the callus. Any abnormality of gait must be corrected. If the callus is very hard and painful, it should be carefully removed by a physician or reduced in size by means of an emery board or pumice stone.

Care of the Feet

Concurrent with the demands of a changing civilization, the functional requirements of the foot have undergone alteration. The uneven, rough ground, trod by primitive man with bare feet, has been changed to a smooth, hard surface. Present-day occupations frequently enforce long periods of standing or of sitting. Covering for the foot is purchased too often with an eye for style rather than for usability. Perhaps a greater advance in this respect has been made by the male than by the female. Men look for comfort more than women do. Protection from heat, cold, and trauma is essential, but at the same time the normal physiologic function of the foot must be satisfied.

A normal amount of exercise is necessary for all parts of the body, and the feet are no exception. Occupation necessitating prolonged standing, with its resultant venous stasis, fatigue, and strain on the ligamentous and muscular supports of the foot, should provide for frequent periods of rest. Similarly, when one must sit for several hours at a time, the foot should be exercised to maintain the normal muscle tonus and circulation.

Stockings have a definite physiologic duty, and not wearing them is harmful. The prerequisites of good hosiery are that they be good absorbents of moisture, nonconductors of heat, and provide adequate protection from heat and cold. Many synthetic products are used in the manufacture of hosiery, but silk and wool remain the only materials which most completely comply with the requirements. Silk absorbs moisture readily, and does not conduct heat. Wool is a better absorbent, and at the same time has a slight elasticity which affords some support for the vascular structure of the legs. It also can be used when more warmth is desired. Combinations of both may be used. Cotton is a poor substitute. Stockings should fit properly, providing enough room, yet not being so large that folds form, creasing the skin and rubbing it to cause blisters and calluses. If they are too short and narrow, the foot will be constricted; stretch stockings may also do this and may be harmful to growing feet. They should be changed frequently. The foot is kept covered for longer periods than any other part of the body, consequently the skin requires special care. Feet should be bathed often, and for this purpose there is no substitute for soap and water. If the feet perspire freely, or the veins remain distended, the bath should be finished with cold water. After bathing, the soap should be washed off thoroughly, the skin dried, and a mild dusting powder applied lightly.

The nails should be kept clean and cut straight across, not curved in the manner of fingernails. Any abrasions, corns, calluses, or blisters should be treated immediately as described.

The rigorous training program in military service and the physical stamina required under battle conditions increase the importance of *foot hygiene*. For this reason, special precautions are taken. Periodic inspection of the feet by a medical officer is necessary to enforce all the hygienic measures mentioned. Trauma is prevented by correctly fitting shoes and socks, and by gradually accommodating the feet to increasing weight bearing until a full pack can be carried for long distances without any discomfort. At no time should a force be applied exceeding the amount which the feet can adequately carry. After long marches, the feet should be washed in cold water, thoroughly dried, and a dusting powder applied. If the feet become tender, they should be bathed in warm salt water, alum water, or a 1 percent solution of formalin. Swollen feet and profuse perspiration will be benefited by soaking them in a 2 percent solution of formalin, elevation, and exposure to air. Shoes should be air-dried, opened to the sun, and stretched, preferably with shoe trees, before being worn again, preferably with a day intervening. Socks should not be worn again until they are washed and dried. Following exposure to cold and moisture, a foot bath with soap and water, cleansing thoroughly, followed by a vigorous massage for at least twenty minutes, and changing to dry socks and shoes is of extreme importance in the prevention of vascular disturbances, such as chilblains, emersion or trench foot, and frostbite.

Fitting of Shoes

Poorly designed shoes, built on the assumption that all feet are alike, together with the public demand that the shoe be fashionable, are responsible for many of the foot ailments. There are certain requirements for a well-fitting shoe.

The *sole* should be of the straight last type; that is, the inner border should be a straight line from heel to toe. The outer flare should have a wide curve to allow room for the lateral toes. The sole should be thick enough to protect the foot from hard and rough surfaces and to support the foot, yet it must be pliable enough to allow for normal flexion of the foot. Leather serves these purposes best.

The *shank* should be wide enough for support, yet it must allow the upper to fit snugly under the longitudinal arch and over the instep when the shoe is laced. A rigid metal shank is not necessary if the sole and shank are strong enough. However, a lightweight metal insert will provide additional support without impeding the normal rolling motion of the average gait. The shank should be slightly higher on the inner side for support of the high medial pillar of the longitudinal arch.

The *toe cap* must provide ample room in the anterior compartment for movement of the toes. It should be rounded and high to avoid pressure on the toes, especially the great toe.

The *heel* should be wide enough for stable support. The average height of the heel for men is about one inch, while it may be two inches or less for women. Although high heels, as in dancing shoes, are harmful if worn continuously, there is no objection to using them intermittently. In this way one may conform to style. A rubber heal is more resilient than leather, and may afford slightly more protection. The *counter* should fit the heel snugly, and there must be no gaping at the top.

For the *upper*, a pliable leather such as calf is preferred. Patent leather is poor because of its lack of porosity. A low shoe will allow more freedom at the ankle, and provides better ventilation. High shoes protect the ankles, and are necessary for rough terrain and when heavy weights are to be carried. The lining of the shoe should be of duck, smooth, and free of wrinkles. The *blucher* style of shoe is indicated, as the seams are on the outside leaving a smooth surface against the foot.

Fitting the shoe must always be done with full weight bearing, because the foot is then expanded to its largest size. Allowance of about one-half inch or a thumb's breadth beyond the great toe is adequate for movement of the toes. The ball of the foot should lie over the widest part of the sole, which is at the metatarsophalangeal joints. There should be ample room across the anterior arch, but it cannot be so wide that the foot can shift in the shoe. If a longitudinal arch support is to be added, extra room is necessary to allow lacing comfortably over the instep.

Fitting of the shoes for heavy labor requires special attention, the same as in the Army. The individual should be carrying a 40-pound pack or its equivalent with all his weight on the foot wearing the shoe. The laces should be tightened. The width of the thumb again represents the correct distance between the end of the great toe and the end of the shoe. The same care is taken to see that the shoe is neither too wide nor too narrow. The shoes must be well softened by manipulation and repeated rubbing with saddle soap before they can be used for either heavy work or long marches. Slippers and sneakers cannot be substituted for shoes. They are to be used only for the purpose that they are intended to serve, lounging and recreation.

Serious medical conditions may first manifest themselves as foot problems, therefore a medical evaluation of the patient is indicated if fairly prompt relief is not secured with first aid measures. Diabetes, gout, arthritis, and peripheral vascular difficulties are among the most frequent of this group of conditions.

Sprains

See Chapter 13, Fractures, Dislocations, and Sprains.

Summary

An attempt has been made to show how the anatomy and physiologic function of the foot can be altered by various factors, such as poor posture, trauma, and ill-fitting shoes. Only those conditions which are commonly met with in civilian and military life are discussed, especially those which can be corrected by simple measures. Too great stress cannot be placed on the necessity for proper exercise, the correct manner of walking, personal hygiene, and the selection and fitting of shoes. The individual with an essentially normal foot, who heeds these preventive measures will seldom have to be reminded that while ailments of the foot may be minor, pain is of major importance.

23 / Medical Emergencies

MAX M. MONTGOMERY AND ROBERT M. POSKE

Medical emergencies during actual warfare or at the scene of a catastrophe are not so numerous as surgical emergencies. However, civil populations subjected to alarms or frequent disruptions of normal routine are bound to present many emergencies of a medical nature. Older people, small children, individuals in poor health, and the handicapped must be given special attention. Large groups of people confined to ill-ventilated rooms lacking adequate temperature and humidity control present numerous problems. The hurrying aspect to any emergency throws an additional load on the cardiovascular systems of older persons. Exposure to weather, the acute infections prevalent at certain times, and many other abnormal conditions precipitate emergencies. There will always be a number of emergencies due to disease present at any given time in certain members of the population.

It is essential that many persons have some training in the recognition and treatment of the more common emergencies. Individuals who urgently need expert medical attention should not be neglected because of erroneous concepts held by first aid workers. Neither should hysterical or neurotic individuals disrupt the work of busy medical personnel. It may be difficult to differentiate such conditions. Needless to say, the patient should receive the benefit of the doubt.

The dictum of *do no harm to the patient* should be uppermost in the minds of those ministering to emergency patients. Often it is difficult to stand by and do nothing. In this chapter an attempt will be made to stress *what not to do* as well as *what to do*. It always should be remembered that an unconscious patient, like a baby, is at the mercy of his environment. Do not injure him by rough handling or forceful manipulation.

The rationale of treatment of emergencies can be appreciated better after the mechanism of their development has been discussed. Such knowledge conditions one's thinking and does away in part with rule-of-thumb therapy.

Calmness in the approach and manner of the responsible person lends assurance to the patient and those near him. One should look for a card, letter, or armband which may give a clue to the cause of the patient's illness. For instance, many diabetics carry a card identifying their disease and giving instructions for their care. This is also true for some epileptic or cardiac patients and for some individuals taking cortisone or other adrenocortical steroids. The purpose of this chapter is to explain the common phenomena seen in people taken suddenly ill and to suggest practical ways of aiding them while awaiting medical help.

Syncope or Fainting

Syncope or fainting is one of the most common medical emergencies. Few clinical conditions present a more dramatic picture. It is an acute, usually transient state in which there is a sudden complete or incomplete loss of consciousness with loss of normal muscular power. Anoxia or lack of a normal oxygen supply to the brain is considered to be the cause. This is frequently brought about by the sight of blood or by some other gruesome sight.

SYMPTOMS AND SIGNS. The onset of the episode varies. The patient may be nauseated, belch, or even vomit. Yawning, giddiness, or a feeling of lightheadedness are often present. The individual feels that he should lie down and often does so, regardless of where he may be. The general appearance preceding the faint is characteristic. The face is deathly white and the exposed portions of the body, especially the forehead, are covered with perspiration. Just before collapse he may experience a sensation of coldness or numbness starting at the lips, fingers, or toes. Things "turn black" before his eyes and he slumps to the ground. He may be vaguely conscious of what goes on about him or lose consciousness completely. At the other extreme is the patient who without any recognized warning collapses suddenly and falls to the ground where he lies motionless or has convulsive movements of the face, extremities, or body. There is probably no other condition which so closely resembles death, and conversely sudden death may simulate collapse or syncope.

During the attack, the pulse may be slow or rapid and thready.

Breathing may be shallow or rapid or cease temporarily. The patient may empty the bladder or rectum. The duration of the attack varies from a few seconds to several minutes. Consciousness returns gradually and the patient usually does not remember the period immediately prior to the attack, hence the comic page query, "Where am I?" Gradually, recovery of muscular power and coordination return, and the patient begins to feel better. However, he may remain pale, perspiring, and weak for a time. Headache and loss of appetite also may persist. Always remember that the patient may injure himself when he falls. Lacerations or fractures may be sustained if the collapse is sudden, or he may fall against a radiator and suffer second or third degree burns.

MECHANISM OF SYNCOPE OR FAINTING. The mechanism of syncope is fundamentally the same in all types, i.e., a cerebral (brain) anemia due to deficient circulation of blood through the brain. Maintenance of an efficient circulation depends upon three factors: 1) the heart, which acts as the motive force circulating the blood; 2) the blood volume; and 3) the vascular system consisting of arteries, capillaries, and veins which act as conduits for the blood. Any one or any combination of these factors may be at fault and so be responsible for syncope. For instance, in syncope of heart disease, the heart fails to function adequately as a pump, either because of marked slowing, standstill, or failure of some other type. Syncope associated with hemorrhage or shock is due primarily to absolute loss of blood volume, while decreased vascular tonus with dilation of the peripheral vascular bed may occur later as a secondary factor. In still other cases, the vascular system may be primarily at fault. The vessels are of varying diameters and their walls are contractile. The smaller vessels or capillaries of the body, when completely expanded or filled, will hold several times the amount of blood contained in the body. The majority of these small capillaries at any one time are contracted, with no blood circulating through them. At intervals, some dilate as others contract, so that at one time only a relatively few contain flowing blood. A widespread loss of this contracted state leads to the collection of a large amount of blood or pooling in some of the dilated vessels and an absence of blood in others. The volume of blood, although normal, has thus become too small to fill this dilated vascular bed. A decreased quantity of blood is returned to the heart, and consequently the cardiac output, or amount of blood pumped by the heart, is decreased. Thus there is insufficient circulation to the brain and fainting or syncope occurs.

A common type of fainting is that having its origin in the higher centers of the brain. This has been spoken of as *psychic shock*. The mere thoughts of a horrible accident or of a gruesome sight may lead to an attack of syncope. Likewise, sensory stimuli such as the sight of blood or the hearing of bad news may initiate fainting. This is due probably to an inhibition of the normal activity of the vasoconstrictor center of the brain by reflex stimuli from the cerebral cortex.

Normally the carotid sinus, a dilation of the common carotid artery located at its bifurcation or division and containing terminations of specialized nerves, and the arch of the aorta are very sensitive to changes in intravascular pressure. An increase in the pressure within these vessels leads to a reflex slowing of the heart and lowering of the blood pressure. A decrease in the pressure leads to a speeding up of the heart and an increase in the blood pressure. Thus, changes of position do not normally cause circulatory disturbances, since these reflexes automatically adjust the blood pressure and blood flow. The failure of this mechanism to function normally or to compensate fully for a loss of circulating blood volume with resulting low pressure leads to insufficient circulation through the brain followed by fainting.

On the other hand, some people have abnormally *sensitive carotid sinus* reflexes, and any pressure on the neck which is transmitted to the sinus, such as a tight collar, pressure with the hand or from a tumor, or turning the head a certain way, is followed by a sudden slowing of the heart with lowering of the blood pressure and fainting. This is called the carotid sinus syndrome. Failure to respond normally to a decrease of pressure in the carotid sinus is especially likely to happen on sudden changes of position and is then spoken of as *postural hypotension* (low blood pressure upon standing).

Inadequate return of blood to the heart due to any circumstance is one of the causes for the decreased output of the heart leading to syncope. Although the pressure within the veins is low, there is a definite force transmitted through the capillary bed which forces the blood on toward the heart. When a man is in the upright position, gravity assists the return of blood through the large veins of the head, neck, and upper chest to the heart. However, the blood from the feet and regions below the level of the heart must rise against the force of gravity. In this it is assisted by the tonus, or state of contraction, of the leg, thigh, and abdominal muscles. The larger veins contain valves, so that the columns of blood are lifted as the leg and thigh muscles contract in walking. If an individual stands still without moving about, there is a tendency for pooling of the blood in the vessels of the lower extremities. The capillaries if not able to obtain fresh blood dilate still further because of a lack of oxygen. Eventually, a considerable quantity of blood is immobilized in the feet and legs. If the weather is warm and the skin and vessels are dilated, the process is further aggravated. When the return flow of blood to the heart is insufficient for the maintenance of an adequate blood flow through the cerebral vessels the individual faints. This type of syncope is seen in individuals who faint while watching a parade on a hot day or while riding in a hot crowded bus. It can be likened to the Roman crucifixion, which is an example of syncope or collapse followed by death. The victim was hung on the wooden cross so that his feet barely touched the ground. A small piece of wood was sometimes placed under the feet to prevent the victim from sliding down. The extremities were either nailed or bound to the cross. If nailed, the bleeding was no appreciable factor in the causation of death for it soon stopped. Some strong men would live for some time while others died within one or two hours. Pooling of blood in the lower extremities was marked because the leg and thigh muscles were relaxed. Thus, the support to the veins was lost and the larger vessels also dilated, thereby producing serious stasis of blood.

The fainting associated with heart disease is due to a decrease in cardiac (heart) output. Acute coronary artery occlusion with *myocardial infarction* may be responsible for sudden decrease in cardiac output and loss of consciousness. Changes in heart rhythm may also be responsible for the alteration of output. These changes include periods of ventricular tachycardia (increase in rate of heart caused by an irritable focus in the ventricles), and periods of asystole (periods in which no heart beats occur). These disturbances diminish the amount of blood leaving the heart and the pressure under which it is circulated, causing a transient loss of consciousness or death. Loss of consciousness due to other heart conditions will be discussed later.

Massive hemorrhage from a peptic ulcer often causes fainting. This is due to acute blood loss with decreased blood volume. The patient may vomit blood or have a number of black tarry bowel movements. Many times the true cause is not at once apparent.

Syncope or Fainting / 361

In general, fainting or syncope is seldom seen in individuals who are seated or reclining. It is apt to occur in people who stand in one place for a long period of time, especially if the environment is warm, for instance, in a crowded bus or shelter. It is more common also in older individuals who have been without adequate food or sleep or in those who are unduly excited or frightened. Pain is a precipitating factor. Suggestion may play a role. One person may faint and then in rapid succession several others. In older people the gradual rising from a chair or bed with a short wait for circulatory adjustment prevents syncope. Even in younger people syncope is common on getting out of bed following a prolonged illness. Certain drugs used for treatment of hypertension produce dilation of smaller vessels. Loss of consciousness may occur in a warm environment or on standing.

TREATMENT. The emergency treatment of this condition is simple and should be applied immediately. Do not attempt to support the patient upright or move him in this position. The body should be placed at once in a horizontal position with the head lowered, or the feet and legs elevated. Turn the head gently to one side and if the patient is vomiting, turn him face down with the head turned to one side and resting on the back of one of his hands. In this position, he has an opportunity to breathe and does not aspirate or inhale the vomitus or "swallow" his tongue. *Do not force fluid of any kind into his mouth.* An unconscious patient often inhales or aspirates these fluids into the trachea and bronchial tree, and this may be followed by pneumonia. Loosen the collar or clothing about the patient's neck. The face may be rubbed with cold water but do not pour large quantities of water over the patient's face or head. The patient should have access to fresh air and excessive crowding about the patient should be prevented. Five percent carbon dioxide in oxygen may be administered if available. Inhalation of spirits of ammonia or other olfactory stimulants may be helpful. The most important thing to remember is that the essential treatment has been initiated when the victim falls to the ground. The lowering of the level of the heart allows venous return, which is followed by resumption of a normal cardiac output and improvement of the cerebral circulation. An unconscious person is helpless. His reflexes are depressed or absent. He cannot swallow and his muscles are flaccid or relaxed. *Handle him gently.*

Often the attack can be prevented by having the patient sit

down and lean forward so that his head approximates his knees. Another position which is helpful, if the patient is able to cooperate, is one in which he kneels on one knee with his head far forward, as in tying a shoelace. This position facilitates venous return to the heart.

Emergencies Due to Heat

Emergencies due to heat are of less importance now because air conditioning equipment cools most modern buildings. However, when this equipment is not functioning the situation may become serious as outside ventilation may be lacking. Power failure may precipitate real trouble. For this reason it is necessary that we understand the basic principles involved in heat loss from the body. As the result of various oxidative processes within the normal body a predictable amount of heat is generated. If this heat is liberated as it is formed, there is no change in the body temperature. If it is liberated more rapidly, the body cools to a point at which the production of heat is accelerated and the excess is available to make up the deficit, thus maintaining the body temperature. Interference with elimination of heat leads to its accumulation and to elevation of the body temperature. The individual is then said to have a fever. It is well known that the speed of chemical reactions is regulated by the temperature of the reacting substances. With an elevation of body temperature metabolic reactions speed up and additional heat is produced. Failure to eliminate sufficient heat leads to a vicious cycle. Not only the normal but additional quantities of heat must be lost.

In the usual environment the heat produced within the body is brought to the surface largely by the blood stream and escapes to the cooler surroundings by conduction and radiation. Air movement or a breeze which strikes the body causes additional heat loss by convection. When the temperature of the surrounding air becomes equal to or rises above that of the body, then all the heat must be lost by vaporization of the moisture or sweat from the skin surfaces. As the air becomes more humid, that is, contains more moisture, the vaporization from the skin surface slows down. A day on which the temperature ranges around 95° to 100° F, with high humidity and little or no breeze, furnishes ideal conditions for the retention of heat. It is on such a day or, more commonly, succession of such days (heat waves) that medical emergencies attributable to heat occur.

Old people and individuals with heart disease have circulatory systems that adjust poorly to such conditions, and they suffer excessively from the heat. Children with unstable vasomotor systems also are quite sensitive to heat. Patients with hyperthyroidism, who are producing excessive quantities of heat because of an increased metabolic rate and who have embarrassed circulations may develop hyperthyroid crises during heat waves. Emergencies due to heat usually are classified under three clinical states.

HEAT EXHAUSTION. This syndrome occurs in individuals working in hot environments and may be associated with heat cramps. This is a form of syncope brought about by the pooling of blood in the vessels of the skin. The heat is transported from the interior of the body to the surface by the blood. The skin vessels become dilated and a large amount of blood is pooled in the skin. This together with the blood pooled in the lower extremities, when in the upright position, may result in an inadequate return to the heart and collapse of the individual. The pulse is weak and breathing is usually shallow. Loss of consciousness is transient. After the patient collapses, the skin changes from red to the very white appearance typical of syncope or fainting. The body surface feels cold and clammy. Pallor of the skin is due to constriction of the skin vessels plus decreased heart output. The rectal temperature if taken will be found to be normal or slightly elevated even though the skin may feel cold. The person looks like an individual who has fainted and responds to the same treatment. However, some of these people do not recover rapidly because vasomotor control of the capillaries is not normal. It often takes a day or so for vascular control to return, and during this period the patient should be protected from heat. This condition is often of such severity that it approaches very closely the shock state. The difference is really quantitative.

Treatment for heat exhaustion consists of lowering the head and moving the patient to a cooler environment. Cool applications to the forehead and skin are of value, as are cool fluids by mouth. Much of the clothing may be removed, since exposure of the skin facilitates the loss of heat. Fanning also results in heat loss by convection. The patient recovers consciousness quickly, although he may not feel well for some time. Salt tablets or intravenous salt solution should be administered. If the condition is very severe, elevation of the feet, legs, and hips above the level of the upper half of the body is advisable. Often the application of light bandages to the extremities, so-called autotransfusion with compression of the more superficial veins, is of great value. The patient should be kept quiet for a few hours or occasionally longer and protected from excessive heat for a few days.

HEAT CRAMPS. Heat cramps are seen in people who work in hot environments and perspire a great deal. It is the loss of salt from the body which causes these very painful cramps of the leg muscles and abdominal muscles. This condition may be associated with heat exhaustion, and patients then complain of weakness, dizziness, and a sense of fatigue. Heat cramps at one time were very common in foundry workers and steelmill workers. However, in recent years the men have been supplied with salt tablets or capsules, or salted drinking water and the condition is not common. The salting of beer, which for many years was a common practice, helped replace the salt loss through excessive perspiration.

The *treatment* of heat cramps is salt, either in tablet form or as salted drinking water. Manual pressure on the cramped muscles gives some immediate relief.

HEATSTROKE (SUNSTROKE). This condition is especially common in alcoholics or elderly individuals exposed to hot environments for prolonged periods. It is associated almost always with a cessation of sweating. This results in a storage of heat so the patient's rectal temperature is high. The skin is dry, red, and hot in contrast to the pale, moist skin seen in heat exhaustion. The pulse is rapid. The patient may be unconscious and remain so for some time. Apparently there is a fatigue of the sweating mechanism. This condition is very serious and in contrast to heat exhaustion, the mortality is high. The history of exposure to excessive heat and headache with loss of consciousness with or without convulsions should suggest the possibility of heatstroke. If the skin is hot, dry, and red and there is a high rectal temperature and no paralysis, treatment should be started immediately. Rectal temperature often registers as high as 110° to 112°F. In confirmation of this, during World War II there were reports from desert training centers of individuals who apparently had a primary disturbance of the sweating mechanism which led to hyperthermia. Recovery was slow, often taking several weeks.

TREATMENT. Medical aid should be obtained as soon as possible. Remove the patient to a cool place. Elevate the head slightly and apply cold applications to the head, neck, and extremities either by cold packs or by a spray, or better still wrap the patient in a constantly moistened cold wet sheet. Gentle rubbing of the skin through the sheet helps maintain the skin circulation. After a few minutes the cold applications can be stopped. If the skin again becomes hot, renew the treatment. Often other modes of treatment, such as ice packs, or placing the patient in a tub of cold water or cracked ice, must be resorted to. The patient should be placed under competent medical supervision as soon as possible. The medical treatment is that of a patient who is in shock and who at the same time has a high fever. He should be supplied with cool solutions of plasma and salt by vein and oxygen by inhalation. Temperature should be obtained frequently and treatment continued until there is a definite reduction of body temperature to 100° F.

Emergencies Ensuing from Heart Disease

There are several types of heart disease but only those likely to cause emergencies will be considered. The treatment is primarily a problem for the physician, and medical aid should be obtained as soon as possible. This is especially true in those cases in which collapse, chest pain, or shortness of breath are the main complaints. Palpitation, rapid heart beat, or irregular heart beat are symptoms which are annoying to the patient but usually are not serious.

ANGINA PECTORIS. This term means "pain in the chest." It is so widely used and understood that its continued use is justifiable even though the term is descriptive of a symptom. This chest pain with the feeling of impending death is not a disease itself but is a manifestation of insufficient blood supply to some portion of the heart muscle. Narrowing of a coronary vessel due to disease may reduce the blood flow. If there is a demand for increased blood flow due to exercise or excitement, this narrowed vessel may be unable to supply the necessary amount. This inadequate blood supply results in an ischemia or local anemia of the heart muscle, and pain is the result. The attacks of pain characteristically occur after exercise or excitement and vary in duration from a few seconds to several minutes. The pain usually is described as "crushing" or "squeezing" in nature, is located in the chest or upper abdomen, and sometimes spreads up into the neck or down the left arm. It may be very severe or just a dull ache. Often the sufferer stops whatever he is doing, stands perfectly still and may press his hand to his chest. His face is ashen gray or pale and may be covered with sweat during the severe attack. He breathes shallowly and is afraid to move lest he increase the severity of the pain. The pain gradually subsides and the patient relaxes. If the attack is severe he may state voluntarily that he was certain he was about to die. Death may occur during the first attack or any subsequent attack, although some individuals suffer from this affliction for years. It is much commoner in men than in women and is infrequently seen in young adults. The occurrence of sudden death is well known in those suffering from this complaint. If the pain persists over a few minutes, myocardial infarction (as described later in this chapter) due to coronary thrombosis must be suspected.

TREATMENT. Prevention of attacks by refusing to hurry or to work or exercise unduly, no matter what the emergency, is the best treatment and sooner or later the patient learns this. Nitroglycerin 0.6 mg in the form of a small tablet is carried by most individuals afflicted by this condition. If the pain is very intense, they may be unable to reach the medication and in such situations, understanding assistance may be of great value. An individual during an attack might only be able to indicate where he carries his medicine. Placing a tablet of nitroglycerin under the tongue of the sufferer may be the most valuable help in the world. Do not attempt or force a patient to hurry or run during a seizure, no matter how urgent the situation. It may be a lifesaving measure to allow him to lie down or sit in the street. One may need to direct traffic around the patient until the attack has ended. After subsidence of the pain, help the patient to a place where he may rest. If the pain does not subside completely or if it is the patient's first experience, see that a physician is called at once.

ACUTE LEFT HEART FAILURE. This condition usually is seen in patients who have had high blood pressure or in older individuals with arteriosclerotic heart disease. The main symptoms are severe dyspnea or shortness of breath, and cough. This may come on after exertion or at the end of the day. Often the shortness of breath wakens the patient from a sound sleep and is accompanied by a paroxysmal cough. If acute pulmonary edema develops, the patient may cough up a large amount of watery, frothy, blood-tinged material. These attacks often are confused with those of bronchial asthma. As a result of failure of the left side of the heart there is a gradual accumulation of blood in the pulmonary circulation. This reduces the available tissue for respiration, and this reduction in vital capacity is one of the main findings. Increased pressure within the small capillaries leads to the exudation of fluid into alveoli, thus producing the pulmonary edema manifested by the profuse frothy sputum.

TREATMENT. The treatment of this condition when well established consists of the administration of morphine. In the milder attacks, the change to the sitting posture with an increase in activity and cough often will lead to an increase in the output of the left ventricle with gradual alleviation of the distress. The administration of oxygen, especially under positive pressure, has been used with success when pulmonary edema develops. In general, help the patient to the position of greatest comfort, usually sitting up and leaning forward. Administer a narcotic, preferably morphine, Demerol, or codeine, or send for someone who can administer the drug. Intravenous aminophyllin is often effective. *Do not attempt to make these patients lie down.* Fresh air and a cool environment are welcomed by the patient. Medical aid should be called as these episodes may prove fatal.

ACUTE MYOCARDIAL INFARCTION. This is death of a mass of heart muscle, due to closure of a coronary artery or one of its branches by *thrombosis* or formation of a blood clot. The pain is similar to that of angina pectoris except that it is more prolonged. Collapse, shock, and sometimes loss of consciousness accompany the severe chest pain or upper abdominal pain which may persist for hours. At the onset, vomiting is often present. The face is pale and perspiration often stands out on the forehead. The pulse may be slow, normal, or rapid in rate. The blood pressure sometimes is elevated, but if the picture is that of shock or collapse, the blood pressure is low. The condition is differentiated from typical angina pectoris by the persistence of the pain. If the patient loses consciousness, one differentiates it from ordinary syncope by its longer duration and the pain in the chest or abdomen complained of after recovery of the sensorium. Acute myocardial infarction is very serious and is followed frequently by sudden death.

TREATMENT. This consists in keeping the patient quiet and warm. Avoid unnecessary moving or examination. A patient with severe chest pain should be given nitroglycerin 0.6 mg on the tongue. If the pain is not relieved, send for a physician immediately. Do not attempt to take the patient to the physician except by ambulance. Oxygen in high concentration should be administered continuously if it is available. If a physician cannot be brought to the patient within a short time, morphine sulfate 15 mg or Demerol (meperidine hydrochloride) 100 mg should be given hypodermically. If a physician is available within a very short time, withhold narcotics until he has seen the patient. There is always the danger of confusing this condition with some surgical emergency such as perforated peptic ulcer.

The administration of a narcotic may lead to confusion in diagnosis. If the condition is typical and medical aid cannot be obtained for some time, morphine or Demerol should be used. External cardiac massage may be spectacularly successful in some patients who have apparently died. Care should be used not to fracture ribs or otherwise injure such patients by the procedure.

STOKES-ADAMS SYNDROME. This is a condition in which the patient loses consciousness for a short time and occurs usually in elderly individuals. It is due to heart block, a condition manifested by very slow pulse rate, less than 40 per minute. As soon as the body adjusts to the slower heart rate, the patient improves. *This patient should be taken to the doctor or to a hospital.* He should be kept flat and oxygen administered if it is available. External cardiac massage may be necessary, but care must be taken not to injure the thoracic cage by overenthusiastic treatment.

RHEUMATIC HEART DISEASE. A patient with rheumatic heart disease may manifest symptoms suddenly due to the onset of an auricular fibrillation. The patient complains of fluttering or irregularity of the heart. The pulse becomes rapid and very irregular. Such irregularity in young persons almost always is due to fibrillation. Another complication of rheumatic heart disease is hemoptysis (coughing of blood). This occurs in patients with rheumatic heart disease of long standing in which the mitral valve opening is contracted to the size of a small buttonhole. The blood accumulates in the lung back of the obstruction.

TREATMENT. The patient with auricular fibrillation should be assured that he is not going to die. He should be allowed to sit up or assume the most comfortable position. *It is safe to move him to a hospital* or to a place where medical treatment can be secured. If the patient is coughing up blood or foamy sputum, morphine should be administered. Having the patient breathe oxygen in high concentration is of value. The patient should be seen by a physician as soon as possible. After the pulmonary edema or hemoptysis subsides, the patient may be moved to a hospital.

PAROXYSMAL TACHYCARDIA. This condition consists of attacks of very rapid heart beats with a feeling of faintness or weakness, and occurs quite frequently in some individuals who are nervous or easily upset. They usually are very apprehensive and alarmed. The heart, between attacks, is apparently normal and transition from normal to rapid beating is sudden. As a rule, a careful history will reveal the fact that the patient has had previous attacks of similar character.

TREATMENT. The attacks can often be stopped by drinking water, pressing with the fingers on one side of the neck, closing the glottis, and straining or pressing on the orbital ridge above the eyeball. Be careful not to injure the eye. The patient should lie down or assume the most comfortable position. He should be assured that the attack is not dangerous and that he will not die. He can be taken to a physician or a hospital for further treatment. Many times sedatives, such as phenobarbital 0.1 g or sodium bromide 1.0 g, will terminate the episode after a time. The oral administration of quinidine and digitalis may be needed, but these drugs should be prescribed by the physician rather than the individual administering first aid. This condition occasionally persists for days and then is dangerous in that the heart may gradually decompensate or fail from fatigue.

In review, attacks of chest pain, attacks of shortness of breath and cough, collapse or syncope, or attacks of rapid and irregular heart beat with a feeling of faintness or weakness are the presenting pictures in the various heart conditions. In general, allow the patient to assume the position which is most comfortable for him. If he is unconscious, one may follow the rule of elevating the head slightly if the face appears red or congested, and lowering the head if the face is pale or white. *All heart patients do not need their heads elevated. In syncope, elevation of the head is dangerous.* Assurance and calm behavior of those administering to the patient are important. Get medical aid to the patient as soon as possible, or see that he is transported to the hospital in an ambulance.

HYPERVENTILATION TETANY. Some individuals who present symptoms of nervousness, tremor, insomnia, and anxiety are subject to episodes which simulate on the one hand heart attacks and on the other hysterical attacks. Following a period of unnoticed, rapid deep breathing, they become panicky, complain of difficulty in getting their breath, tingling and numbness of the hands and feet. If they persist in breathing rapidly, the heart rate increases and they may even lose consciousness. The hands often assume a characteristic position with the fingers extended and with ulnar deviation of the hands at the wrists. This condition is due to alkalosis, resulting from excessive loss of carbon dioxide in the expired air.

TREATMENT. This consists of regulating the patient's rate and depth of respiration by instructing him to hold his breath or to breathe slowly. Rebreathing into a common paper bag held tightly over the nose and mouth is an effective method of terminating an attack.

PULMONARY EMBOLISM. Patients in the postoperative period, on getting up and about, may have a massive pulmonary embolism resulting in loss of consciousness or death. Older bedridden patients, especially those with cardiac disease or those who have thrombophlebitis with edema or swelling of one or both lower extremities, may have pulmonary emboli.

The emboli consist of blood clots which break loose from thrombi which form in the veins of the pelvis or lower extremities. They are carried to the lungs and lodge in the pulmonary vessels. If the embolus is large and occludes one of the pulmonary arteries, sudden death may result; or cyanosis and severe chest pain may result in death after several hours; or the patient may recover. A smaller embolus often causes chest pain similar to that of pleurisy, with cough and bloody sputum. The differentiation from pneumonia may be difficult.

There is no simple first aid treatment. Attempts at cardiac resuscitation and artificial respiration should be carried out in patients who collapse. In less severe cases the patient should be moved to a hospital as soon as possible.

ENDOTOXIC SHOCK. Older men occasionally have a chill and fever about one and one half to two hours following catheterization or a surgical procedure of the genitourinary tract. This represents a bacteremia and is usually transient. In some instances, however, it is followed by shock. Such patients should be kept warm and, if possible, intravenous fluids should be started. Removal to a hospital as soon as possible is essential.

Convulsions

Convulsions are paroxysms of involuntary muscular contractions. They may be localized to one part of the body or be generalized, and involve both sides of the body, face, arms, trunk, and legs. In the typical convulsion, the patient is unconscious. If the onset is sudden, he may fall and injure himself. If the muscles of the face and jaws are involved, the mouth foams, and if the tongue or cheek is bitten, the foam becomes bloody. The breathing is loud and labored due to the clenched jaws. Contraction of the neck muscles interferes with venous return and the face becomes congested and cyanotic or bluish in color. The movements of the muscles are jerking in character, purposeless, and the amplitude of movement is dependent on the rigidity of the muscles. Convulsions are seldom fatal in themselves. However, the patient may fall or be fatally injured during such an attack. Death may also be due to underlying conditions such as cerebral hemorrhage or eclampsia.

EPILEPSY. This disease is probably the most common condition in which convulsive seizures are seen. These attacks may be preceded by a sensory aura, a peculiar smell, sound or visual sensation, which warns the patient of an impending attack. In such cases he may be able to lie down in anticipation of the onset. Patients who have no forewarning may fall or throw themselves on the floor or ground with a hoarse cry. The muscles usually are tense for 5 to 30 seconds during which time breathing stops. Then the legs, arms, head, and body jerk spasmodically. The face usually is pale just prior to the attack but blue or cyanotic at the height of the seizure. The tongue often is bitten, and frothing at the mouth is common. The patient may involuntarily empty the bladder and rectum. Usually the seizure subsides in a few minutes, although there is a type, *status epilepticus*, in which the patient passes from one seizure to another until anesthetized or until given deep sedation. The patient usually sleeps for a variable time after the attack, although following mild seizures, some patients awaken immediately. It may be difficult to judge the nature of attacks of this type but if the tongue is injured or the patient involuntarily empties the bladder or rectum, it is usually epilepsy.

Treatment of epilepsy consists essentially in protecting the patient. A gag between the teeth to protect the tongue may be used. This should be of wood, such as a pencil covered with a handkerchief. Insert it with care. Do not break the patient's teeth. Place a pillow or coat under the head to protect the face or head from injury. Do not attempt to hold the patient still but move surrounding objects so he will not injure his extremeties. *Do not attempt to pour liquids into his mouth.* If the seizure lasts for some time or the patient passes from one convulsion to another, *summon medical aid.* As previously mentioned, anesthesia or heavy sedation occasionally is needed to control the convulsions.

CONVULSIONS IN CHILDREN. General convulsions in infants and young children have various causes. In infants convulsions usually are due to birth injuries, or tetany. In older infants and young children they may mark the onset of acute infectious disease, gastrointestinal upsets, or possibly epilepsy. They often represent the child's reactions to a sharp elevation in temperature.

The *treatment* consists of keeping the child quiet until medical aid arrives. This is best accomplished by immersion in a tepid tub of water. Be sure the water is not too hot as many fatal burns have resulted from such treatment. Test the water with the elbow or upper arm, not with your hand. Do not pour water into the tub without first removing the infant. In older children, if the skin is hot, as in the onset of an acute infection, lukewarm or tepid sponging of the body may reduce the temperature and stop or prevent recurrent convulsions. If the child is not a known epileptic, every effort must be made to obtain medical aid.

ECLAMPSIA. This condition manifests itself in the later months of pregnancy, during labor or soon after delivery of the child, by convulsive seizures. This is a very serious condition and is an acute emergency.

TREATMENT. Call a physician immediately. Keep the patient absolutely quiet and make no attempt at examination between seizures. Darken the surroundings if possible. During the convulsion protect the patient by placing a gag between the teeth. Move surrounding objects and place some protective material such as a blanket or coat beneath the head and body.

HYSTERIA. Hysterical attacks usually occur in young women. Unconsciousness is not present but the patient may be in a trancelike state. This can be distinguished from coma by the fact that the body is held rigid. The eyes are closed tightly and there is a definite resistance when an attempt is made to raise the upper lid. Convulsive seizures also may be seen. These are atypical and not characteristic of true convulsions. The voice may be lost. The patient may complain of blindness or of being able to see only two small fields directly in front of the eyes, so-called tube vision. There may be a lump in the throat which the patient is unable to swallow. Anesthesia or loss of sensation of the hands and forearms, feet and legs, so-called glove and stocking anesthesia, is common. Laughing and crying fits do not present much difficulty in diagnosis. However, the diagnosis of hysteria is dangerous and unjustifiable unless all other conditions have been excluded and should be made only by an experienced physician.

TREATMENT. If the patient is known to have attacks, the best emergency treatment is a word to the patient as to their known nature and then strict neglect. If no attention or alarm is manifested, the attack tends to subside.

LOCAL CONVULSIONS. Local convulsions or convulsive movements involving a group of muscles or muscles of one extremity usually are due to habit spasm, tic, hysteria, malingering, or a brain lesion due to depressed bone or a tumor.

TREATMENT. There is no practical first aid treatment for such local convulsions. They are not serious. Sedation with 30 mg phenobarbital may control them to some extent. Send the patient to a physician.

Coma

Coma is a state of unconsciousness. The diagnosis of the cause of coma often is difficult even when one has diagnostic facilities available. However, a few conditions cause the majority of cases and these will be taken up briefly with emphasis on the characteristics which enable one to recognize them. An unconscious patient must be looked over carefully for signs of injury. He may have a *skull fracture*. An alcoholic odor to the breath may or may not mean that the patient is intoxicated. One should look closely at the face to see if one side is flattened or pulled over. The size of the two pupils should be compared. One should examine both arms and legs and compare the rigidity or tenseness of the muscles of the two sides.

SKULL FRACTURE OR CONCUSSION. These conditions usually follow an injury and often are associated. There may be a cut on the head or a bump at the site of injury. Inequality of the pupils indicates brain damage. Bleeding or discharge of a clear fluid from the ears almost certainly means skull fracture. The pulse rate and blood pressure depend on the amount of brain damage and whether or not the patient is in shock. Paralysis or weakness of the muscles of one side of the face or of one or more extremities indicates severe brain damage. This condition is dealt with in detail elsewhere.

UREMIC COMA. This is seen in advanced kidney disease. The onset of uremic coma is gradual and such a patient usually is found at home in this state. He does not develop it on the street. Neighbors and friends usually will tell you that he recently has been unable to see well, has had headaches, or been mentally confused or drowsy. The breathing is of the acidotic type, that is, forced, deep, and rapid. The pulse is full and hard. There is an extremely unpleasant odor to the breath, the so-called uremic odor. There may be small white crystals of uremic frost on the patient's nose or forehead. The tongue is dry and the skin is not only dry but often cold. The blood pressure usually is high.

TREATMENT. There is no adequate first aid treatment. Keep

the patient warm and move him to a hospital. Renal dialysis may be necessary.

DIABETIC COMA. This is due to an acidosis arising from uncontrolled diabetes mellitus. The patient often has a card or notice on his person stating that he is a diabetic or he may have a friend or relative who volunteers this information. At the onset, the patient can be aroused but usually is confused and unable to cooperate. The characteristic breathing of acidosis is present. This is deep, forced, pauseless, rapid respiration in which the abdominal and accessory muscles may share. There is no evidence of obstruction of the air passages. The patient may or may not have fever. The red, warm, dry skin often suggests a febrile reaction. The odor of the breath is that of acetone. This has been described as a sweetish or fruity odor. The breath in uremia has an entirely different odor. In diabetic coma, the amount of sugar in the blood is increased markedly.

TREATMENT. These patients should be moved to a hospital immediately. They require careful expert attention including urine tests, blood tests, and insulin therapy. There is no adequate first aid treatment. If insulin is available a physician may be contacted by telephone concerning its use.

HYPOGLYCEMIC COMA. This is due to an overdose of insulin, to a failure to obtain food after taking insulin, or more rarely to pancreatic tumors. The term hypoglycemia means a decreased amount of sugar in the blood. An emergency might arise in time of war or catastrophe which would prevent the diabetic patient from obtaining his food after taking his insulin. If a patient is found comatose and has a diabetic card in his pocket or is a known diabetic, hypoglycemic coma must be considered. The respirations of coma due to acidosis have been described, those due to hypoglycemia in contrast are slow and shallow. The patient is pale. The tongue is moist; the skin often cool but not infrequently moist and bathed in sweat.

TREATMENT. This is one condition under which the rule of withholding liquids from stuporous patients may be broken. If the patient has sugar in his pocket, he still may be sufficiently cooperative to swallow this or some other food. If not, no time should be lost in securing a physician who should at once inject glucose (a form of sugar) intravenously. Time is valuable, prompt action may be lifesaving. Such patients should not be allowed to exert themselves since any exertion aggravates the hypoglycemia and deepens the coma. The subcutaneous injection of adrenalin (1 ml of 1 to 10,000 solution) may terminate the reaction or coma. These cases should be moved to a hospital or be seen by a physician immediately.

CEREBROVASCULAR ACCIDENT. This is often called apoplexy or a stroke of paralysis. Cerebral hemorrhage generally occurs in elderly patients who have had high blood pressure for some time. Arteriosclerosis with a low blood pressure often leads to a cerebral thrombosis in which the onset is gradual. In the common stroke due to *cerebral hemorrhage,* the onset is sudden. The patient falls off a chair or falls to the ground. For a time he may maintain consciousness but there usually is a paralysis of the face, of an upper extremity, lower extremity, or both. Consciousness may be lost within a short time. The breathing is slow and deep, the face is congested, and the pulse is strong and slow. One side of the body is limp, and the arm or leg falls flaccidly when dropped. The face may be flattened or pulled over to one side. One pupil may be larger than the other, or the eyes or head may turn to one side. In typical *cerebal thrombosis* the onset is slow with a feeling of numbness in one extremity, mental confusion, and inability to concentrate. Later the patient lapses into unconsciousness with or without paralysis. This is due to a clot in a vessel. The symptoms of cerebral hemorrhage and cerebral thrombosis are very similar.

Treatment of this condition is one of inaction. Elevate the head slightly; place cold cloths or an ice bag to the head; do not move the patient any more than is absolutely necessary until medical aid arrives; do not attempt to give the patient anything by mouth and do not give stimulants by hypodermic injection. If the hemorrhage is massive the patient may die within a short time.

CORONARY THROMBOSIS. This has been discussed under heart disease. If a large segment of the coronary artery is involved, an infarction of the myocardium will develop. If there is massive infarction of the myocardium with profound collapse and shock, the patient may lose consciousness and be seen in coma. If there is a history of severe chest pain prior to the loss of consciousness, coronary thrombosis may be suspected. The blood pressure usually is very low and the patient may have a rapid pulse. Breathing may be intermittent or shallow and rapid. The treatment has been discussed.

ALCOHOLIC INTOXICATION. Excessive indulgence in alcohol is one of the commoner causes of coma. One should look over the patient very carefully for injury before deciding that his condition is solely due to alcohol. The odor of alcohol is not proof that the patient is intoxicated. The patient may be semiconscious. Early, the face is flushed, the pulse is slow and bounding, and the breathing is even and fairly deep. More recently, determination of the alcoholic content of the blood has been used as a diagnostic procedure. If feasible, such a patient should be taken to a hospital for medical attention.

TREATMENT. Washing the stomach removes unabsorbed alcohol and may be valuable in establishing the diagnosis. Intravenous glucose and oxygen often revive patients more rapidly than other measures. Stimulants administered subcutaneously, such as caffeine sodium benzoate, often will bring the patient around in a short time. If the pulse becomes weak or the patient collapses, oxygen and artificial respiration should be used. Summon medical aid since the alcoholism may be incidental to some other condition.

Drug Addiction

In recent years a number of drugs have been popular with a segment of our population. These include LSD, marihuana, amphetamines, as well as barbiturates. Even more dangerous and addicting drugs have been reported as being used by so many in certain localities as to constitute "epidemics." Natural opiates, synthetic opiate-like drugs, and mixtures of drugs known by various slang names are used. Since these narcotics are obtained through illegitimate channels accurate information concerning their preparation is lacking. The practice of "cutting" or diluting results in products of varying and unknown potency so that fatalities from overdosage occur even among experienced users. Treatment for overdosage is mandatory and such a comatosed individual must be given expert medical attention as soon as possible. Artificial respiration should be carried out while the patient is being taken to the hospital. Pulmonary edema frequently occurs. Tracheal intubation or tracheostomy is often necessary. Intravenous Nalline treatment must be started as soon as possible (see section on Opium Poisoning).

Barbiturates of many kinds, known as goof balls, downs, fool pills, blue heaven, tooies, yellow-jackets, reds, red birds, devils, and so on are frequently used by the same individuals taking amphetamines. Barbiturates are used to induce sleep and amphetamines to wake up. Overdosage occurs when the patient is under the effects of the drug and does not realize how much he takes (see section on Barbiturate Poisoning).

LSD. (d-lysergic acid diethylamide) or "acid" frequently causes bizarre behavior, preoccupation with various trivia, or hallucinations often dealing with colors. Psychotic episodes are not uncommon. These individuals should be taken to a hospital and sometimes must be restrained for their own protection. Sedation may be necessary. Psychotic behavior may last for protracted periods.

MARIHUANA. Marihuana, known as grass, hemp, hash, pot, weed is used by some "in" members of the young generation. Occasionally an acute psychosis manifested by hallucinations and a paranoid state lasting hours to several days occurs. These individuals so affected should be restrained if necessary until given care at a hospital.

AMPHETAMINES. Amphetamines (Benzedrine, Dexedrine, methadrine, or Desoryn) and several amphetamine-like drugs (Diethyltryptamine, Dimethyltryptamine) are known as "ups" by addicted users. Other slang terms for these preparations include Bennies, splash, peaches, dexies, co-pilots, oranges, footballs, meth, speed, crystal, DET, and so on. These stimulants taken by mouth or intravenously in excessive quantities cause headache, marked agitation, tremulousness, incoherent speech, and often auditory and visual hallucinations. Rapid heart rate, often with irregularities of rhythm, dilated pupils, tremor of the body, and diarrhea also occur. The individual should be taken to a hospital or physician as soon as possible. A sedative such as one of the barbiturates may be given if necessary and external stimulation should be avoided.

Chemical and Drug Poisoning

Poisoning by ingestion of various substances, either by accident or with suicidal intent, is frequent. Poison Control Centers have been established in most large communities. Call the nearest one for first aid advice, and take the patient there or to the nearest hospital as soon as possible. Accidental poisoning invariably is due to carelessness. Children are attracted by colored capsules, tablets, or liquids, and will swallow them if they are left within reach. One should always read the label on any bottle before taking or administering its contents. *Do not use the contents of an unlabeled bottle.* If there is any question about the dosage of medicine, inquire before using it. Poisonous drugs should be kept separate from other drugs or medications. This applies to lay people as well as to druggists, doctors, dentists, or first aid workers. Do not put any caustic or poisonous substance in a used bottle without destroying the old label and applying a new one. The practice of putting such substances as muriatic acid or turpentine in an old whiskey bottle has been responsible for many severe burns and poisonings. Individuals under the influence of sedatives such as the barbiturates may without realizing it take an additional excessive dose. They may then be under suspicion as potential suicide victims.

The more common drugs taken with suicidal intent or by accident are phenol or carbolic acid, tincture of iodine, lysol or some other cresol antiseptic, barbiturates, and mercuric chloride. The barbiturates include barbital, Veronal, Luminal, phenobarbital, Sodium Amytal, Sodium Ortal, Allonal, and Seconal. Corrosive acids, caustic alkalies, phosphorus, arsenic, chloroform, methyl alcohol, strychnine, belladonna, atropine, morphine, and codeine are some of the other drugs and chemicals which may cause poisoning. *Vomitus or stomach contents should be saved for later examination when poisoning is suspected.* A large number of proprietary preparations used in the home and in industry as cleaners, solvents, or other reagents are poisonous when ingested. A list of the ingredients may appear on the label of the preparation or one may be able to obtain such information by telephone from a Poison Control Center. Advice as to first aid may also be printed on the label.

The symptoms and signs of chemical and drug poisoning depend upon the substance taken. Strong corrosive acids (hydrochloric, sulfuric, and nitric acids) or caustic alkalies (lye and caustic potash) cause very painful discolored burns of the lips, tongue, and mouth as well as abdominal pain and severe systemic symptoms, if swallowed. Barbiturates or alkaloids, on the other hand, cause no local action but have profound systemic action after absorption causing drowsiness and coma.

UNKNOWN POISON. If the ingested poison is unknown, the object of the treatment is to dilute the substance and remove it from the stomach. Large quantities of fluid, such as water, milk, or tea are given, and these are removed by use of the stomach tube or by induced vomiting. If a stomach tube is not available, stimulating the back of the throat may induce vomiting. If this fails, give an emetic such as a tablespoon of mustard in a cup of warm water. Apomorphine 6 mg by hypodermic injection or one tablespoon of syrup of ipecac in a cup of warm water are often used. It is next advisable to give the whites of several raw eggs or milk or both. The so-called *universal antidote* consisting of two parts of activated charcoal, one part of tannic acid, and one part of magnesium oxide is widely advocated. The charcoal will absorb phenol and strychnine. The tannic acid precipitates alkaloids, certain glucosides, and many metals. The magnesium oxide neutralizes acids. After each dose of one or two teaspoons in water, vomiting should be induced. There are proprietary preparations very similar to this universal antidote.

If symptoms of shock develop, keep the patient warm and use artificial respiration if necessary. Continue for several hours, even though the patient may be apparently dead. The use of a respirator is especially valuable. Oxygen or 5 percent carbon dioxide in oxygen should be administered even though a respirator is being used. Needless to say, it is imperative that an open airway be maintained.

PHENOL OR CARBOLIC ACID. Cresol, lysol, creosote, and guaiacol poisoning are treated the same as phenol poisoning. If seen early and a stomach tube is available, olive oil should be given by mouth. The stomach should then be washed out several times with more olive oil. Because of the local effect of the phenols, a tube should not be passed if the quantity taken was large or if the patient is seen late and is having severe epigastric pain. Sodium sulfate or magnesium sulfate (Epsom salts) in concentrated solution, 1 or 2 tablespoons in a cup of water, may be given by mouth. Vomiting should be induced. Then a demulcent drink such as milk, egg white in water, barley water, or flour in water should be administered. Alcohol may be used to remove phenol from local burns. However, it should not be administered internally for treatment of phenol poisoning. If the patient is in a state of collapse, follow the treatment for shock outlined above.

IODINE. The mouth and lips are usually burned and stained in iodine poisoning. Vomiting and pain are the usual symptoms. Later there may be thirst and a suppression of urine. A solution of starch in water should be taken by mouth. Induce vomiting or wash out the stomach. Repeat this process several times. Morphine may be needed to relieve pain.

BARBITURATES. These include barbital or Veronal, Luminal or phenobarbital, Sodium Amytal, Sodium Ortal, Allonal, Seconal, Nembutal, and others. The symptoms of poisoning are headache, mental confusion, staggering gait, incoordination, drowsiness, and finally coma. Occasionally nausea, vomiting, excitement, and hallucinations are seen. If a very large dose is taken, deep coma with cyanosis and circulatory collapse appear quickly. The deep reflexes and pupillary reflexes remain for a relatively short time. Pneumonia, due to shallow breathing and aspiration of secretions, is the common cause of death. Respiratory paralysis due to medullary depression is seen in severe poisoning.

The treatment in the early stages consists of prompt evacuation and washing of the stomach. Vomiting may be induced, but a stomach tube is usually needed since the patient is drowsy or comatose. An ounce of two of Epsom salts in four ounces of water should be left in the stomach to act as a purge. Respiratory depression may be treated by inhalation of 5 percent carbon dioxide in oxygen. Artificial respiration may be necessary. The patient in coma should be moved to a hospital as soon as possible. Intravenous fluids, diuretics, and other specialized treatment such as dialysis may be essential.

NONBARBITURATE HYPNOTICS. Glutethimide (Doriden) and Methyprylon (Noludar) in overdosage cause lethargy, low blood pressure, and respiratory depression. Convulsions and coma occur later. Alternating periods of coma and relative alertness are evidence of Doriden overdosage. Treatment is similar to that of barbiturate poisoning.

BICHLORIDE OF MERCURY. The symptoms appearing within a short time consist of vomiting, abdominal pain, diarrhea (often bloody), and collapse. Somewhat later, the mouth and throat show swelling, bleeding, and ulceration. Death is usually due to kidney damage. Occasionally, complete suppression of urine for several days is followed by recovery.

Haste is all important in the treatment of this condition. Give the whites of 2 eggs and a pint of milk. Induce vomiting or empty the stomach with a tube. Leave an ounce of Epsom salts in solution in the stomach. If eggs or milk are not available, give soap and water. Finally, ground or chopped meat may be given in water. Later induce vomiting. Treatment of the later stages is a medical problem. Intravenous salt solution, sodium thiosulfate solution, colonic irrigations, and many other forms of therapy are used. *The patient should be taken to a hospital or a physician immediately, since early treatment with BAL (British anti-lewisite) is imperative.*

ARSENIC. Paris green and Rough on Rats are the common sources of arsenic in poisoning. The chief symptoms are intense pain in the upper abdomen, vomiting, diarrhea, and collapse. Treatment consists of rapid removal of the substance from the stomach by vomiting or by stomach tube. Egg whites and milk should be given. Magnesium oxide (2 teaspoons) and tincture of iron (1 tablespoon) to a cup of water should be given. This converts the arsenic trioxide into an insoluable arsenate. After the above treatment (which requires very little time) the patient should be hospitalized at once for BAL treatment.

ORGANIC PHOSPHATE TYPE OF INSECTICIDES. These include HEPT (hexaethyltetraphosphate), Malathion, OMPA (octamethylpyrophosphoramide), Parathion, and TEPP (Tetraethylpyrophosphate). These are too dangerous for use about the home but are employed in farming. They interfere with normal nerve impulse conduction. Nausea, vomiting, abdominal cramps, diarrhea, sweating, constriction of pupils, productive cough, difficulty in breathing, anxiety, restlessness, mental confusion, difficulty in speaking, twitching of the muscles of the face and neck, and generalized muscular weakness follow exposure to excessive amounts of these sprays or dusts. In severe poisoning, convulsions and coma occur and death may result from respiratory or circulatory failure.

TREATMENT. Intramuscular injection of 2 mg of atropine sulfate hourly until the full effects of atropine are obtained may be lifesaving. Maintenance of an airway is important, and use of oxygen inhalation and artificial respiration may be necessary. If the substance is taken by mouth, the stomach should be emptied and activated charcoal or universal antidote should be administered.

CORROSIVE ACIDS. The most common acids in this group include hydrochloric, sulfuric, and nitric. These cause painful discolored burns of the tongue and mouth, or marked swelling and edema of the tissues. Abdominal pain and collapse follow if they are swallowed in any quantity. Give no emetics and do not risk using a stomach tube.

Alkalies are given in an attempt to neutralize the acids; milk of magnesia, milk with borax, chalk or calcium carbonate, or lime water are used. Soda bicarbonate and soapsuds may be given. Later, milk, olive oil, and frequent feedings of bland foods are given to neutralize the gastric acidity. The patient should be kept warm. Morphine is usually needed for pain. Stimulants may be necessary. If there is intense edema of the mucous membranes of the pharynx, get the patient to the nearest hospital so intubation or tracheotomy may be performed if necessary.

CAUSTIC ALKALIES. Lye or caustic potash are occasionally swallowed accidentally. The mouth and pharynx are damaged by the corrosive action of these substances. Bloody vomitus is present if much is swallowed. Avoid using the stomach tube. These substances must be neutralized with a large amount of weak acid, such as diluted vinegar, lemon juice, or grapefruit juice. Milk or egg white should also be given. Morphine is usually needed for pain. Stimulants such as caffeine or strychnine may be necessary. Keep the patient warm and in the recumbent position. Get him to a hospital as soon as possible.

PHOSPHORUS. Phosphorus is found in many rat pastes and also in matches. The best treatment is to wash the stomach with a pint of 0.5 percent solution of copper sulfate. This should be repeated several times. An ounce of Epsom salts should be administered. Later a demulcent such as egg whites in water or milk is given. It may be necessary to administer morphine to relieve pain.

OPIUM AND OPIATE-LIKE DRUGS. Morphine, codeine, Pantopan, laudanum, paregoria, heroin, Dilandid, Metapon, Demerol are some of the opium derivatives or opium-like synthetic drugs. Cocaine can also be included in this group. Accidental poisoning due to taking these drugs by mouth will be considered here. The use of these drugs by addicts and those members of our society "experimenting" with drugs often taken intravenously make up the largest number poisoned by overdosage. The triad of coma, pinpoint pupils, and depressed slow breathing are characteristic of poisoning. If the patient is seen early before coma is deep, mustard in water may be tried as an emetic. Usually it is unsuccessful. A stomach tube should be used to empty the stomach as soon as possible. Wash with a 1 to 1,000 solution of potassium permanganate. Some advocate leaving a small amount of this solution in the stomach. Give strong coffee and keep the patient awake if possible. Strychnine and caffeine given as stimulants may be necessary. Cold applications often stimulate respiration. All such patients should be removed to a hospital which has a respirator available, since artificial respiration may have to be continued for a number of hours. Inhalations of 5 percent carbon dioxide in oxygen are helpful. Do not give these patients whiskey or brandy. A narcotic antagonist, nalorphine, which is given parenterally, is often very effective. However, this is also a respiratory depressant so it may still be necessary to use artificial respiration after its administration. An acute narcotic withdrawal syndrome sometimes follows use of nalorphine. Mixtures of heroin and cocaine do not result in pinpoint pupils and the cause of coma may not be obvious until needle "tracks" along the veins are noticed. Opiate-induced pulmonary edema with cyanosis occasionally occurs. These patients should be taken to a hospital as soon as possible.

SALICYLATES. Salicylate or aspirin poisoning occurs most often in children from ingestion of "candy" aspirin tablets, or an Oil of Winter green preparation. Onset of symptoms is usually delayed 12 to 24 hours. Irritability, restlessness, coma, or sometimes convulsions occur in small children. Older children and adults have ringing in the ears or dizziness, often followed by delirium. Rapid deep breathing is the most characteristic sign. Hemorrhage into the gastrointestinal tract or into the skin may occur. The patient should be hospitalized as soon as possible. If it is known or suspected that the patient has taken a large amount of salicylate, the stomach should be emptied by use of the somach tube or by making the child vomit. The stomach should then be washed out with tap water. This may prevent absorption of the drug and the development of severe poisoning.

IRON. Preparations of iron have been reported as causes of poisoning in children. Nausea, pallor, and restlessness are often followed by vomiting, bloody diarrhea, and shock, with associated drowsiness and coma. The stomach should be lavaged thoroughly with soda bicarbonate solution as soon as possible. It is essential that the victim be transported to a hospital or to a physician immediately.

TRANQUILIZING DRUGS. These drugs are not as dangerous as most other depressants. The most common effect of overdosage is deep sleep or coma. The initial depression of excessive amounts of the phenothiazine derivatives (Promazine and chlorpromazine) has sometimes been followed by restlessness and convulsions. In addition, respiratory depression and a marked fall in blood pressure sometimes occur.

TREATMENT. The stomach should be emptied if the patient is seen immediately after taking the drug. Otherwise, and if deep sleep is the only finding, parenteral fluid administration may be the only treatment needed. Amphetamine and epinephrine should not be given. Barbiturates should not be used except by a physician as they may potentiate the depressive effect of these drugs.

STRYCHNINE OR NUX VOMICA. The symptoms of poisoning are those of central nervous system stimulation. The face and neck muscles feel stiff, respond violently to stimulation, and within a short time there are muscle twitchings involving the entire body. A mild sensory stimulus such as a noise or movement of an extremity may precipitate a convulsion. This seizure is due to tetanic contraction of all the muscles, and the action of the stronger ones predominates. The typical position is that of hyperextension, known as opisthotonus. The body is arched so that only the crown of the head and the heels touch the floor or bed. The legs are extended, the feet turned in, the arms flexed on the chest or extended, the fists clenched, and the jaw and face muscles strongly contracted producing a grimace known as risus sardonicus. Such seizures usually last about a minute during which the patient stops breathing, becomes cyanotic or blue, and may lose consciousness. Further seizures follow immediately or somewhat later. Consciousness is maintained between the attacks. The victim is apprehensive and suffers severe pain during the muscular contractions. Death may occur during the first convulsion and if untreated, the patient usually survives only two to five seizures.

TREATMENT. In case it is known or strongly suspected that strychnine has been taken and no convulsion has appeared, give strong tea or a solution of one teaspoonful of tannic acid in one-half glass of water. Induce vomiting and make every effort to get a physician. If convulsions are present, slow intravenous injection of 10 percent Sodium Amytal (0.4 to 1.0 g) or phenobarbital sodium (0.3 to 0.7 g) is the treatment of choice. The dose should be given slowly and just sufficiently to keep the patient asleep. A stomach tube should not be used unless the patient is anesthetized. Artificial respiration and oxygen inhalation should be used if necessary. The intravenous injection of glucose tends to combat the severe anoxia and prevents irreversible changes in the brain cells.

ATROPINE OR BELLADONNA. This drug is used extensively and minor forms of poisoning are not uncommon. In the more severe types the thirst, dry mouth, and dry throat become so severe that talking or swallowing is impossible. The skin is red, dry, hot, and a rash is often present over the face and neck. The pupils are widely dilated and do not react to light. The pulse is weak and rapid. The respirations are increased. The breath sounds are dry and harsh. There is restlessness, insomnia, disorientation, excitement, hallucinations, delirium, and mania. These individuals are often thought to have an acute psychosis. Circulatory collapse and death follow the rapidly rising temperature which may reach 108° F.

TREATMENT. If the drug is taken by mouth give tannic acid solution, strong tea, or the universal antidote (described earlier), and induce vomiting or wash the stomach. Get the patient to a hospital or physician so that pilocarpine can be given and intravenous Sodium Amytal can be used to control extreme excitement and restlessness. Artificial respiration or inhalation of 5 percent carbon dioxide and oxygen may be needed. Ice bags and alcohol sponges, also cold intravenous solutions, should be used to control the high temperatures. It is usually necessary to empty the bladder by catheterization.

CHLORAL HYDRATE. When combined with alcohol this is known as knock-out-drops or a Mickey Finn. An overdose renders the victim helpless. The early symptoms are burning in the throat, nausea, upper abdominal pain, and vomiting. Later there is deep stupor with cyanosis, slow breathing, low blood pressure, and low body temperature.

TREATMENT. The stomach should be emptied by an emetic or the stomach tube. Keep the patient warm and give artificial respiration if needed. If the patient is conscious after the stomach is emptied give strong black coffee. If in a coma, give 0.5 g of caffeine-sodium benzoate subcutaneously. The intravenous injection of 10 mg or 20 mg of picrotoxin may be lifesaving. Intravenous glucose solution should be given to protect the liver from injury.

TRINITROTOLUENE (TNT). Poisoning with this substance is usually seen in munition workers or members of the armed forces. The poison is removed from the skin by washing with a solution of sodium hyposulfite. Move the patient into the open. Keep him at absolute rest. Administer large amounts of water with alkaline salts, such as sodium citrate and sodium bicarbonate.

CARBON MONOXIDE POISONING. Sufficient carbon monoxide may be inhaled to cause unconsciousness and death in a few minutes. It is odorless and is found in automobile exhaust gas, illuminating gas, sewer gas, and smoke from fires or furnaces. In wartime, especially during bombing, it is important that one be on the alert for the detection of carbon monoxide arising from broken gas pipes. The carbon monoxide unites with the hemoglobin of the red blood cells 250 times as readily as does oxygen and prevents the formation of oxyhemoglobin. As a result the transport capacity of blood for oxygen is reduced. Exposure to this gas, even in low concentration over a prolonged period of time leads to an anoxemia (lack of oxygen) which may cause death. The brain is most susceptible to anoxemia.

SYMPTOMS. There may be headache or dizziness but usually there are no symptoms until the individual collapses, or he finds he is unable to walk. He soon lapses into a stupor and dies. The skin has a peculiar cherry red color in distinction to the color seen in asphyxiation from other causes.

TREATMENT. Get the victim into the fresh air immediately. If the weather is cold, use a gas-free room elsewhere in the building or adjacent building. If breathing has stopped or is irregular, start artificial respiration (see Chap. 14), and continue until breathing is regular or a respirator arrives. Artificial respiration should be continued although the case may appear hopeless. Call a physician as soon as possible. Inhalation of 5 percent carbon dioxide in oxygen is the accepted method of treatment. The carbon dioxide stimulates respiration and facilitates the oxygen exchange in anoxic states.

In large industrial plants where carbon monoxide poisoning is often encountered, trained personnel including physicians are usually immediately available. Utility workers and lifeguards at beaches are unusually well trained in the art of administering artificial respiration over long periods of time.

GASOLINE, BENZENE, NAPHTHA POISONING. This usually results from inhalation of fumes or accidental swallowing of the chemical. The symptoms resemble those of acute alcoholism. The victim may become maniacal and later lose consciousness. Transfer him at once to the open air, remove gasoline or benzene soaked clothing, apply external heat, and give treatment for carbon monoxide poisoning.

CARBON TETRACHLORIDE. Inhalation or ingestion causes dizziness, headache, mental confusion, and coma. Death may result from respiratory or circulatory failure or from kidney or liver failure.

TREATMENT. If the substance was inhaled, move the victim into the open air, administer oxygen, and give artificial respiration. If ingested, the stomach should be emptied by lavage or emetics. Alcohol should not be given. The patient should be moved to a hospital as soon as possible.

Food Poisoning

Food may cause poisoning when contaminated by a toxic substance derived from a container, or when contaminated by bacteria, such as the staphylococcus or a member of the salmonella group. The staphylococcus may multiply in the food, producing an enterotoxin responsible for the symptoms of poisoning while members of the salmonella group multiply in the bowel and produce dysentery.

Substances in which toxic products occur naturally are not

foods. Poisonous mushrooms or toadstools normally contain a poisonous alkaloid, muscarine. Certain fish also produce a product which is poisonous to man. When taken as food these articles cause illness.

STAPHYLOCOCCUS FOOD POISONING. The symptoms are due to enterotoxin produced by the organisms growing in food. Meats, cream, milk, cheese, bakery goods, and other foods kept at room temperature or in large containers in a refrigerator have been the cause of outbreaks of poisoning.

Nausea, vomiting, abdominal pain, and diarrhea appear within two to six hours after the ingestion of the food. Often headache, muscular pain, and collapse occur.

TREATMENT. Vomiting and diarrhea are usually very severe and it is unnecessary to pump the stomach or give a cathartic. Intravenous fluids are often necessary to combat the severe shock resulting from excessive fluid loss. There is no specific treatment.

SALMONELLA FOOD POISONING. This is an infectious process and usually occurs in epidemics. It is due to ingestion of heavily contaminated foods. The symptoms may appear within a few hours or be delayed for several days. The attack is often ushered in by a chill followed by fever. Vomiting, diarrhea, and abdominal pain incapacitate the victim. If the diarrhea is severe, muscular pains and collapse may follow due to loss of large amounts of fluid or blood. The symptoms may be mild or severe with extreme prostration. The diagnosis can be established by culturing the causative organism from the blood and stools or later by blood serum reactions. In these outbreaks, a search should be made for a carrier among the food handlers.

TREATMENT. The patient should be kept at rest and given fluids as soon as nausea and vomiting subside. If diarrhea has been severe, two teaspoonfuls of paregoric or morphine sulfate 15 mg subcutaneously will usually check the loss of fluid. Heat to the abdomen, bed rest, and restriction of food are advised. A patient in collapse should be kept warm; in such cases medical aid should be obtained at once since these patients need intravenous saline solution and plasma to combat the loss of fluid. The patient should be left recumbent if he feels faint. Antibiotics may be needed but should be prescribed only by a physician.

BOTULISM. This poisoning results from the ingestion of canned foods contaminated by botulinus spores. The canning sterilization does not destroy the spores included with the vegetables or meat. These change to the vegetative form which produce a true toxin. Home canned vegetables are especially likely to be contaminated unless they are sterilized in a pressure cooker. Canned foods which are softened, show bubbles, or have a rancid odor should not be used. Uncooked foods or fresh foods do not contain this toxin.

Symptoms appear in from 4 to 48 hours. These are mainly referable to the motor nervous system. Weakness, dizziness, double vision, paralysis of the eye muscles, incoordination, difficulty in swallowing and in breathing appear. There are no sensory disturbances. Constipation and retention of food in the stomach is common. Death in from one to eight days results due to cardiac and respiratory failure. The severity of symptoms varies greatly, but at least half the victims die.

TREATMENT. If suspected food is inadvertently taken, the stomach should be emptied and Epsom salts should be given. If or when symptoms occur, the patient should be moved to a hospital where antitoxin can be given and artificial respiration can be continued as long as signs of life remain.

FISH POISONING. This is of two types. Physiologic products of the glands of some fish are toxic to man. Certain species resembling the sturgeon used in parts of Russia and the "tetrodons" used in China and Japan are toxic, and their ingestion may cause death. Bacterial infection of canned fish may be responsible for poisoning. The fish may be contaminated before packing or after the can is opened.

MUSSEL POISONING. This is due to the ingestion by the mussel of certain small unicellular organisms which during the summer months are very numerous in the ocean. These organisms contain a strong alkaloid, harmless to the mussel but very toxic to man. Ingestion of such mussels is followed immediately by toxic symptoms such as a prickly sensation and numbness of the lips, fingertips, and tongue. Muscular incoordination (ataxia) develops, and within 2 to 24 hours is followed by paralysis and respiratory failure. Most of those affected die. There are no antidotes. Apomorphine should be given immediately to induce vomiting. Artificial respiration and the respirator should be used to combat respiratory paralysis. This type of poisoning has been reported from the Pacific coast, Nova Scotia, and the European coast.

MUSHROOM (TOADSTOOL) POISONING. The symptoms of severe abdominal pain, nausea, retching, vomiting, and diarrhea appear from a few minutes to 18 hours after partaking of poisonous mushrooms or toadstools. Confusion, convulsions, or coma may eventually appear.

TREATMENT. Empty the stomach and give a cathartic immediately. The victim should be moved to a hospital.

GRAIN AND VEGETABLE POISONING. Ergotism is the most common entity in this group. It is caused by the prolonged use of grain contaminated by ergot fungus. It has occurred in epidemics in Europe. Acute ergotism is manifested by slight fever, weakness, headache, and tingling sensations in various parts of the body. Diarrhea with nervous symptoms such as spasm of the muscles and occasionally convulsions occur. Mental depression is common.

In the chronic form of poisoning, there is gangrene involving the fingers, toes, nose, or ears, and occasionally convulsions.

Treatment consists of elimination of the offending food. Nausea and vomiting may be relieved by 1.0 mg atropine sulfate, and the nervous symptoms by 10 ml or a 10 percent solution of calcium gluconate given intravenously.

POTATO POISONING. This is rare though a number of outbreaks after the use of sprouted potatoes have been reported. The toxic substance is salamin, produced by bacterial action. Chills, fever, headache, vomiting, diarrhea, colic, and prostration are the symptoms. Some patients become jaundiced. All recover.

Treatment consists of emptying the stomach and bowel.

LATHYRISM OR LUPINOSIS. This has been reported in North Africa and India where chickpea meal is used in the preparation of food. The condition is a spastic paraplegia or paralysis of the lower extremities.

AKEE POISONING. This illness of Jamaica, also known as the vomiting sickness, is caused by eating immature or spoiled akees. The symptoms are vomiting, convulsions, and coma. The mortality is high. Alcohol followed by an emetic has reduced the death rate.

Contagious Diseases

The problem of contagion is one which increases in importance as people are together under abnormal environmental conditions. In air raid shelters or temporary quarters of any type, the exposure incident to contagious or infectious disease is increased. While efficient isolation of suspected individuals is impossible under such conditions, much can be accomplished if a close watch is maintained. Care in maintaining a clean, safe supply of drinking water and emergency rations will help in keeping down the incidence of gastrointestinal disorders and infections due to the various dysentery organisms. Immunization against typhoid, paratyphoid, diphtheria, and smallpox should be given to those portions of the population exposed to disruption of their normal mode of living.

Any child or individual with a high fever, rash, or other skin lesion should be isolated or kept from the rest of the group. A physician should be called to see the patient; persons exposed should be isolated when the proper diagnosis has been made. Individuals with acute upper respiratory infections should stay as far away from others as possible. They should cough or sneeze into a handkerchief. Infants and young children who have not had whooping cough should be immunized. Those who come in contact with patients having rashes, skin lesions, sore throats, or fever should wash their hands carefully after waiting on them. Attendants should not allow such a patient to breathe or cough in their faces.

Chills

The chilly sensation arising from a cold skin is usually due to a deficient circulation through the skin vessels which stimulates the "cold" end organs. This is followed by an increased muscle tonus with increased heat production. A true chill often is indicative of the onset of an acute infectious disease or of a foreign protein reaction as in a transfusion of incompatible blood. It is accompanied by clonic muscular contractions. The skin feels cold, the teeth chatter, and the patient shakes or shivers. The cold skin is due to vasoconstriction which results in a decrease in blood flow to the skin. Transfer of heat to the body surface is in this way decreased. The extra heat produced by shivering or shaking is stored and the body temperature rises. Eventually the skin vessels dilate, the skin warms up, and the chill stops. Perspiration follows and evaporation facilitates the loss of the stored heat. Thus at the start of the chill the skin is pale and at its termination, it is flushed, warm, and red.

The *treatment* of a chill consists of the application of heat, warm blankets, hot water bottles or pads, and administration of warm drinks. Application of heat is especially indicated in posttransfusion chills or in serum reactions. In general, any patient who feels chilly or has a definite chill should be warmed up, since the increase in blood flow through the skin, incidental to the storage of heat or decreased loss of heat, stops or diminishes this chilly sensation. Warm blankets, newspapers, or coats should be placed under the individual as well as over him. A patient can lose a tremendous amount of heat through conduction if he is lying on a cement floor or the cold ground. Do not burn the patient. Always test a hot water container on the forearm, especially if it is metal. All hot water bottles or flatirons should be wrapped with cloth or paper so that they do not come in immediate contact with the patient's body.

The treatment described above is largely symptomatic. Since chills are usually caused by infections of a serious nature, the patient should seek medical care, and examination should be performed to find the cause so that specific therapy may be instituted.

Exposure to Cold

The effects of cold on the individual are of great interest at the present time. With subzero temperatures within a few miles of the earth's surface, even at the equator, the problem becomes a universal one.

The symptoms of exposure to cold are well known. There occurs first a sensation of chilling with the reaction of "goose pimples." If heat production is increased sufficiently or if heat loss is reduced by protection of clothing or shelter from wind, the reaction stops. Otherwise the chilling is accentuated and there is a progressive fall in the temperature of the extremities. They become stiff and numb. Mental changes similar to those seen in anoxic states follow shortly. Errors in judgment and inability to make decisions are among the early defects. The heat loss from the trunk leads to further constriction of the vessels of the extremities and to freezing of the hands, feet, ears, or nose in spite of apparently adequate protection. If the trunk is warmly clothed so heat loss is at a minimum, the blood flow through the extremities is maintained, and frostbite even at low temperatures may be minimized. Adequate clothing, especially of the trunk, is very important in withstanding the cold. The clothing must not be tight. Lanolin rubbed into the skin twice daily is said to be helpful.

TREATMENT. The exposed individual should be moved into a protected room and the wet and frozen clothing removed. Artificial respiration should be used if necessary. Warm stimulating drinks add heat internally. Inhalation of 5 percent carbon dioxide in oxygen may alleviate the mental confusion. Do not subject frostbitten tissues to friction. Local effects of cold are considered in Chapter 10.

Starvation

An individual deprived of food derives energy first from his carbohydrate stores (glycogen). Then fat is utilized, and eventually the body proteins are metabolized. If plenty of water is available, life is maintained for a number of weeks. The rate of destruction of body tissue is dependent on the activity of the individual.

During the first few days of starvation the subcutaneous fat and other fat deposits in the body suffer. There is also a loss of extracellular water. The rate of muscle destruction is dependent on the availability of carbohydrate and fat. When the stores of carbohydrate fail, the body utilizes acetone bodies for sources of quick fuel. When these are no longer available, the muscles and other proteins are the sole source of energy.

The symptoms of inanition are weakness, loss of weight, lethargy, and inability to tolerate exertion. The symptoms of specific vitamin deficiencies do not occur in starvation when no food is available. After the first few days hunger is not noted. The pulse and respirations grow gradually weaker, complete exhaustion supervenes, and the victim frequently dies of pneumonia.

Vitamin deficiency states occur when certain foods are available in limited quantities but constitute an incomplete diet. As vitamin stores are exhausted, the individual develops single or combined deficiency states.

TREATMENT. The patient should be kept at absolute bed rest. Intravenous dextrose solutions furnish immediately available energy. Their use should be continued until the victim is able to swallow without danger of aspirating food into the lungs. Nutritious liquids are first given by mouth in fairly small quantity; later, readily digestible food is given. The administration of vitamins especially B and C should be started at once. They can be given by hypodermic injection until the victim is able to take them by mouth. Protein can be given intravenously in the form of a protein hydrolysate.

Dehydration

Water holds the body salts, proteins, and other solutes at a level exerting a constant osmotic pressure. Theoretically, if water should be added to the body fluids there would be a dilution and a lowering of the osmotic pressure. If water should be abstracted the osmotic pressure would rise. All of the physiologic reactions, and indeed the preservation of life, are dependent on the maintenance of a constant osmotic pressure. Practically, secondary adjustments within the organism prevent any significant variations in the body fluids due to the addition or abstraction of water.

Water is required for the elimination of heat. It is vaporized from the skin and lung surfaces. If the individual is engaged in hard work he develops extra heat which has to be eliminated. If he is surrounded by hot air he will have to vaporize more water, since heat loss by radiation is reduced. Water requirements are then increased by work and exposure to hot conditions. Water is also used to carry out through the kidneys and bowels the end products of protein metabolism and salts of various types.

Thirst is a symptom of water deficiency, but it is not a guide to the quantity required. The dry parched tongue, the dry scaling skin which wrinkles easily, and the sunken soft eyeballs indicate that the extracellular supplies of water have been requisitioned and are now reduced. In severe dehydration states the individual's tongue is so dry that he is unable to chew food. Swallowing becomes impossible. The urinary output is decreased to such an extent that urination is painful due to deposition of salts in the bladder. At this time if the blood volume were measured it would be found reduced.

TREATMENT. It is obvious that individuals engaged in work will require more water in hot than in temperate climates. Thirst is not a reliable guide to the amount of water required. Chewing of gum or the holding of pebbles in the mouth promote the flow of saliva and frequently reduce thirst. Water incorporated with food which contains salts of various types is absorbed more readily than the same quantity of water taken alone. Further, the salts tend to expand the blood volume and hydrate the tissues.

The more active treatment of dehydration consists of the intravenous injection of physiologic salt solution with or without glucose. When the dehydration is severe it is often best relieved by the addition of base, in the form of sodium lactate, to the fluids. The increase in urinary output and the changes in the appearance of the tongue are satisfactory indices of the adequacy of the treatment. The appearance of edema denotes the use of excessive quantities of salt solution.

ALLERGY AND ANAPHYLAXIS. Allergy manifests itself in many ways. The common diseases such as hay fever, asthma, and hives are, in reality, types of allergy which in general represent sensitization of the patient to some substance. This offending agent may be plant pollen, food, and in fact most any conceivable substance. Penicillin, one of the more commonly used antibiotics, is an agent which may give rise to allergic and even anaphylactic reactions; if the latter type of reaction is not treated immediately by such urgent measures as administration of epinephrine, institution of artificial respiration, or cardiac resuscitation, a fatality may result. An adequate airway should be maintained. Intravenous hydrocortisol is also of value. (See also anaphylaxis due to injection of serum (see below). Hay fever and asthma will not be discussed, since they are chronic disease.

HIVES. As stated above, hives are produced because of sensitization. When they occur in supposedly healthy people, they are usually secondary to food. Seafood is a very common etiologic factor. The hives occur a few hours to a few days after exposure to the offending substance. They develop as indurated areas which itch but rarely produce pain. Occasionally they develop about the face and produce moderate swelling of the lips, eyelids, and so on, although these swellings usually are known as angioneuroedema, a definite manifestation of allergy. Sensitization of this mild type usually clears itself spontaneously and no radical therapy is indicated. Application of calamine lotion containing 1 percent phenol or 1 percent menthol is quite effective in relieving the itching. Epinephrine (Adrenalin) and antihistamine compounds may be helpful.

SERUM REACTION. Serum reaction manifests itself in one of two ways. The most common manifestation and by far the less serious is the development of hives two to six days after the administration of serum, such as that given for lockjaw or diphtheria. In addition to the hives, such manifestations as nausea, vomiting, mild fever, and restlessness likewise appear. The intramuscular injection of 5 or 6 minims of epinephrine (Adrenalin) usually causes rapid subsidence of the symptoms.

The severe reactions (anaphylaxis) following injection of serum are very rare, but are extremely serious. They usually come on within a few seconds or minutes after the injection and require immediate therapy to prevent lethal outcome. The patient usually complains first of pain in the chest and difficulty in breathing. The pulse may be rapid and irregular. The patient becomes weak, pale, and may actually collapse to the floor. The blood pressure may drop and in fact be unobtainable. The best treatment for patients with such reaction is the administration of epinephrine. Such patients may receive 8 to 15 minims of epinephrine diluted in 10 cc of distilled water intravenously. It has been administered into the heart with markedly beneficial and dramatic effects. This dose may be repeated in an hour or two if the blood pressure fails to rise.

Although such reactions are rare, they are sufficiently serious to make it necessary to determine whether or not a patient who is to receive serum might be sensitive to it. In sensitive patients the administration of a fraction of a drop into the skin will produce a tiny wheal, indicating sensitivity.

POISON IVY AND POISON OAK. One of the most important phases of these conditions is the *prevention of the skin reaction* after exposure or contact with either of two plants. Frequently, people discover the presence of poison ivy or poison oak during their trip into the woods, but only after they have come in contact with it. Proper treatment, if resorted to within a few hours, will prevent development of the disease. One of the simplest and most effective procedures in preventing the skin lesions after exposure is washing the contaminated areas with soap and water. After thoroughly washing these areas with soap and water, gently washing it with some solvent such as benzene will add to the effectiveness of the prevention.

The skin lesion develops 12 to 48 hours after contact with the plant, and manifests itself first as reddened areas which itch considerably. Very soon small blisters or vesicles appear. These vesicles may rupture or be ruptured by scratching and are apt to become infected. In severe cases, actual ulceration may be present. The condition is spread by the patient who scratches an affected area and transfers some of the poisonous material to other areas. Considerable edema of the subcutaneous tissue may develop under the affected areas. In serious cases the condition may last for weeks in spite of seemingly adequate treatment.

Although the prophylactic treatment is very effective, the treatment of the actual lesion, once it develops, is not so effective. However, certain remedial agents are of distinct benefit and should be used. In the early stages of the disease the application of calamine lotion containing 1 percent phenol or menthol will be quite effective in relieving the itching which at times is extremely aggravating. In the exudative or ulcerative stages the application of 10 percent aluminum acetate is advisable.

SEA OR AIR SICKNESS. The mechanism of production and the manifestations of these two types of sickness are relatively the same, although the former occurs at sea whereas the latter occurs in the air. In either case it is the reeling and tossing of the boat or plane and the deleterious action on the semicircular canals of the ear which give rise to the symptoms. Unquestionably, fear of development of the condition, and neurotic tendencies increase the severity of the symptoms and are actually responsible for the development of some. However, in most people seasickness or airsickness is a true condition not to be spoken of as resulting from neurotic characteristics.

The patient is apt to feel a heavy uncomfortable sensation in the upper abdomen followed soon by *intense* nausea. Salivation is apt to develop. Vomiting usually occurs and at times is so severe that the patient can retain no food. Vertigo is fairly common. The skin is pale and cold and frequently covered with a "cold sweat." There is mental and physical lethargy. In serious cases there may be actually a drop in the blood pressure with tachycardia (elevation of the pulse rate).

Dramamine is usually effective in preventing sea or air sickness, and often effective in relieving it, if given after the sickness develops. Fresh cold air is usually helpful. Occasionally an abdominal support applied rather snugly will help relieve symptoms. Alcohol may relieve the symptoms for a short time but usually aggravates them later on and for a much longer period than the relief obtained. Alcohol is, therefore, contraindicated. Sedatives such as phenobarbital (30 mg) are usually helpful; this dose may be repeated two or three times per day.

ALTITUDE SICKNESS. The manifestations of altitude sickness slightly resemble those produced by air or sea sickness but are produced by a different mechanism. As one ascends in the air the percentage of oxygen becomes less, and the oxygen needs of the body are not met completely. Symptoms usually develop in the average individual if he goes higher than an altitude of 13,000 or 14,000 feet. Early symptoms are weakness, headache, vertigo, nausea, occasionally vomiting, prostration, and mental confusion. The patient usually has difficulty in getting his breath, which is explained not on the basis of obstruction to the respiratory system, but on the rarefied atmosphere which deprives the body of sufficient oxygen. He may actually be cyanotic.

The most effective method of treatment is to have the patient return to a low altitude. The administration of oxygen will likewise be effective in correcting the symptoms. The patient should be put to rest, preferably in the recumbent position, and should confine his activities to a minimum.

CAISSON DISEASE. This is a condition encountered in caisson workers or divers when they have been subjected to decompression too rapidly. The cause of the symptoms is liberation of bubbles of nitrogen into the tissues. During compression, the blood going through the lungs becomes saturated with nitrogen; this results in absorption of nitrogen by the tissues. When the pressure is released, or when the individual returns to normal atmospheric pressure, the tissues give up the nitrogen to the blood stream. If this nitrogen accumulates in the formation of bubbles, symptoms develop. The nitrogen is found first in the venous blood and fatty tissues, but bubbles may actually develop in bones. Within one half to 3 hours after leaving the caisson, symptoms will develop unless decompression has been effected slowly. Common symptoms are severe pains in the extremities frequently associated with nausea, vomiting, and abdominal pain. Weakness of the lower extremities is a common complaint and has given rise to the lay term "the bends." This weakness may progress to actual paralysis followed by coma and death.

The most effective treatment is to submit the patient to pressure as is routinely done in a pressure chamber when the worker returns from the caisson. When he is subjected to increased pressure which is released slowly over a period of hours the symptoms usually disappear. Symptomatic treatment including hot fomentations, morphine, and so on, may be indicated.

24 / The Prostrate Patient

WARREN H. COLE

The term "prostrate" is applied to a group of patients with varying degrees of delirium, mental confusion, or collapse. The patient may or may not be able to respond intelligently to questions. If he is markedly confused mentally, the condition is spoken of as *delirium*. If he is incapable of any sensory perception or motor function, the term *unconscious* or *comatose* is applied to his mental state. The terms unconscious and comatose are synonymous as far as the patient's mental incapacity is concerned, but the term *coma* is usually applied when the patient is unconscious because of physiochemical reasons, such as diabetic coma and coma from uremia (kidney disease). All patients in shock will be prostrate, but not unconscious, until late severe stages.

The prostrate patient will afford the first aid worker an extreme amount of difficulty in the application of intelligent care, largely because the diagnosis frequently will be so difficult. There are so many conditions which will produce this type of physical and mental disability that even trained physicians have difficulty at times in arriving at the correct diagnosis and intelligent therapy. Naturally, one of the difficulties in reaching a diagnosis will lie in the fact that frequently the patient is incapable of furnishing any history. If the patient is conscious, he will very often be able to supply the diagnosis through the history. It is naturally important that the diagnosis be made as soon as possible, because on many occasions life will depend upon correct immediate action.

Many of the conditions producing prostration are so complicated, as is also their first aid therapy, that the discussion and treatment presented in this chapter are largely directed toward physicians or those having medical training. *The aid of a physician must be sought at once.*

Causes of Prostration

Fortunately some of the most common conditions causing prostration are the least serious; the first one mentioned below is an example.

FAINTING. Fainting is perhaps the most common cause of severe prostration or unconsciousness. It is discussed in detail in Chapter 23.

SHOCK. The development of shock secondary to severe injury with or without hemorrhage is, of course, common in these days of advanced mechanization (see Chap. 8).

ACUTE ALCOHOLISM. When too much liquor is consumed, mental confusion will be encountered, and if the quantity is sufficient, total unconsciousness will develop. Unfortunately it is quite common, but infrequently fatal in the acute bout. Chronic alcoholism often leads to premature death due to cirrhosis of the liver, esophageal hemorrhage, and so on.

HEART DISEASE. During the past two or three decades, it has been apparent that heart disease is becoming more frequent and is attacking younger people than were afflicted by it a few decades ago. One of the important causes of acute prostration due to heart disease is obstruction of the coronary artery due to thrombosis or arteriosclerotic plaques (angina pectoris), as is discussed in Chapters 14 and 23.

DIABETIC COMA. Attacks of unconsciousness resulting from uncontrolled diabetes are not as common as before the introduction of insulin. However, they still occur, partly because patients frequently are unaware of the presence of the disease or fail to adhere to their diet as prescribed by the physician. Diabetic coma results from too much sugar in the circulating blood, but it must be remembered that the opposite condition (that is, too little sugar in the blood) resulting from too much insulin or from certain tumors of the pancreas may likewise produce prostration.

ASPHYXIA. This condition may be produced by numerous causes, perhaps the most common of which are carbon monoxide poisoning, fires, and near drowning. Usually the asphyxia resulting from carbon monoxide is produced by exposure to exhaust fumes in small garages where automobile motors are running. Unfortunately, suicide is frequently attempted by carbon monoxide asphyxiation, achieved by turning on a jet in a gas stove or exposing oneself to fumes of a motor. Fires may cause fatal asphyxia because all oxygen is consumed and replaced by noxious fumes. Electric shock may cause serious depression of respiration. In many instances these victims may be revived by artificial respiration (see Chap. 14).

INJURY OR DISEASE OF THE BRAIN. Another common cause of severe prostration or unconsciousness is a lesion of the brain. Of this group, injury is one of the most important, insofar as a fracture of the skull with associated laceration and hemorrhage into the brain is so frequently sustained in automobile accidents. Another common cause of acute prostration is apoplexy (commonly known as a stroke), which is produced by a rupture or thrombosis of a blood vessel in the brain, usually occurring in elderly people; it is discussed in Chapter 17. Occasionally, rupture of blood vessels is associated with tumors of the brain, producing unconsciousness or serious mental disturbances.

POISONING. Prostration due to poisoning is usually the result of suicidal intent. Mercury (bichloride), sedatives (barbital compounds), and morphine are the drugs commonly used. Details of this complication may be found in Chapter 23.

UREMIA. Delirium and coma may be caused by advanced kidney disease. It comes on gradually, and rarely will patients afflicted with it be found prostrate on the street. Prodromal symptoms such as headaches, drowsiness, and mental confusion are usually present (see Chap. 23).

MISCELLANEOUS CAUSES. There are numerous miscellaneous conditions which may cause acute prostration. In hot weather, heat exhaustion may be a likely cause. There are numerous types of insanity which may produce mental confusion and prostration. Epilepsy which may produce total unconsciousness associated with convulsions is not infrequent. Hysteria, which is a functional mental disease presumably not caused by an organic lesion, may be encountered. Prostration may accompany serious acute infections, such as meningitis and pneumonia. But the first aid worker will rarely encounter prostration of this type (i.e., due to infection), since the patient will have had symptoms for a variable length of time before prostration occurs and will not venture out. However, collapse might occur (though knowing of his condition) if he overtaxed his weakened physique.

Procedures in Examination of the Prostrate Patient

OBSERVATION AND INSPECTION. Careful observation of the surroundings in respect to the patient will lead to the correct diagnosis in a great many instances. Perhaps the first observation to be made is to determine whether or not the patient is in need of immediate aid, such as control of hemorrhage and relief of respiratory obstruction. Discovery of a dead person in the ruins of a wrecked car is obvious proof of an automobile accident, but this circumstantial evidence, conclusive as it may seem, does not disprove the possibility of the person's death *before* the accident. For example, he may have been shot by gangsters or may have had a heart attack. If the patient is still alive it is obviously important from the standpoint of therapy that the proper diagnosis be made; if dead, this responsibility does not concern the first aid worker, since the diagnosis will be made by the coroner. However this factor is mentioned to illustrate the many complications which must be studied in accident cases.

Observation of the surroundings may reveal evidences of a struggle or weapons. The victim's clothing may be torn, indicating that the cause of his prostration was due to violence and not a medical disease. Obviously, the presence of wounds would be proof of violence. Regardless of whether or not there is evidence of injury, the first aid worker should smell the patient's breath. If there is alcohol on the patient's breath, acute alcoholism may or may not be a prominent factor in the patient's prostration. If the patient has an acetone breath (fruity odor), he may be suffering from a condition such as diabetic coma. Burns on the lips might indicate that he had taken poison.

HISTORY AND DETERMINATION OF MENTAL STATUS. The first aid worker may be able to make a diagnosis if history is obtainable from the patient or bystanders. However, the patient may be totally unconscious; if so, no history will be obtainable from him. If he is merely confused or delirious, history may be obtainable, but it may be inaccurate. It is important, therefore, that the degree of mental confusion be analyzed as accurately as possible in order that proper evaluation of the patient's replies to questions be made. The type of mental confusion and delirium may be very important in arriving at a diagnosis. For example, the euphoria and typical speech difficulties encountered in an intoxicated person are fairly easy to recognize. The speech center of patients who have had an apoplectic stroke is frequently damaged by the hemorrhage in the brain. They may appear conscious but are unable to talk; on other occasions they are observed to make strenuous effort to talk but succeed only in mumbling certain words or parts of words. Patients with uremic (diseased kidney) coma frequently talk a great deal, pronouncing words fairly accurately, but speak in a completely irrational manner.

DETERMINATION OF CIRCULATORY STATUS. The state of the patient's circulation should be determined immediately so that shock, if present, may be treated promptly. The first aid worker should feel the patient's pulse, count the rate, and feel the skin for increased perspiration and decrease in temperature. He should likewise take the patient's blood pressure, if a blood pressure machine is available. These examinations will rapidly detect the manifestations of shock which have been described elsewhere. An irregularity in the heart rate would suggest that the collapse was due to an acute cardiac accident, such as coronary occlusion. If cyanosis (bluish discoloration of skin) is present, there will be indication of either respiratory obstruction or failure of the circulatory apparatus. This failure in the circulatory mechanism may be due to a primary heart disease, to respiratory obstruction, or to acute trauma of sufficient degree to interfere with the heart and its circulatory function.

DETAILED EXAMINATION. After a preliminary examination is made, and the urgent first aid needs, such as control of hemorrhage and establishment of a satisfactory airway, are taken care of, the first aid worker should proceed with a detailed examination as described in Chapter 2. This examination will be directed particularly toward discovery of fractures (by detection of deformity or abnormal mobility), hemorrhage from the ears, contusions about the body, and other manifestations. Since it is much more difficult to arrive at a correct diagnosis in the absence of a history, it is obviously essential that the examination be as thorough as possible, thereby taking advantage of every possible bit of information discernible.

Treatment of the Prostrate Patient

The first aid worker must first look for the urgent possible causes such as obstruction of air passages, or hemorrhage, and treat them if found. If a radial pulse is absent, cardiac arrest must be suspected; lack of a radial, temporal or brachial pulse may support this possibility, and cardiac resuscitation will be indicated (see Chap. 14). If none of these is present, the patient should be sent immediately to the hospital, where careful examination and effective therapy may be carried out. Regardless of whether any of the three conditions just mentioned as requiring immediate treatment on the spot is present, an ambulance must be called as soon as possible. If bystanders are present, one of them should be asked to call one. If no bystanders are present, the first aid worker should attend first to such duties as control of hemorrhage, elimination of obstruction to the airway, or institution of artificial respiration or cardiac resuscitation before taking the time to call an ambulance. Poisoning is one of the many conditions which require immediate action (e.g., evacuation of the stomach).

As stated above, one of the most urgent considerations is to control hemorrhage, which is done according to instructions given in Chapter 9. Practically as important will be relief of any respiratory obstruction. There may not be any foreign bodies obstructing the pharynx, yet it may be obvious that the patient has an obstruction to breathing. As described in Chapter 14, this obstruction may be due to the fact that the tongue has fallen back against the posterior part of the pharynx. This happens in unconscious patients and may be so acute as to produce death by suffocation. Another condition which may result in serious obstruction due to the tongue falling back against the pharynx is a fracture of the jaw, which allows shortening of the structures in the floor of the mouth in a backward direction. If the patient is unconscious and having a respiratory stridor, he should be changed from the supine position to a prone or semiprone position. This in itself may be sufficient to restore an adequate airway. If not, the first aid worker should elevate the jaw anteriorly by pressing the ramus of the mandible forward. This is usually effective in establishing an adequate airway. Secretions should be removed from the mouth. It may be necessary to insert some sort of makeshift mouthgag, such as a stick of wood wrapped with a handkerchief, to obtain access to the mouth and perhaps sponge out an excess of saliva, vomitus, and so on (see also Chaps. 14 and 19). False teeth, loose dental plates, and so on should be removed in the unconscious person lest he aspirate them back into the larynx. If respirations still appear to be obstructed, the mouth may be pried open with the stick protected with gauze and the tongue grasped by the fingers covered with gauze to aid in traction. Pulling the tongue forward in this manner will almost certainly remove any obstruction in the posterior pharynx except that produced by foreign bodies. The patient must be watched closely for vomiting if he is unconscious, since vomitus is so apt to be aspirated. Placing the patient in a semiprone position will aid considerably in prevention of aspiration of vomitus, but the first aid worker should be prepared to sponge the mouth out repeatedly and remove food particles which might be aspirated back into the trachea.

If there is no evidence of shock, the patient will usually be more comfortable if his head is elevated slightly. If he is in shock the head must be kept down level with the body, and in fact preferably, the head and chest should be lower than the lower extremities.

Manipulate the patient as little as possible lest injury sustained by him be exaggerated. It is usually desirable, however, to move the patient to a comfortable position, and to correct obviously awkward positions of extremities and other parts created by the accident.

Keep the air circulating about the patient, particularly if he is having trouble breathing or is warm. It may be necessary to fan him, or open windows and doors in case the accident has occurred inside a building. If he is obviously seriously injured and exposed to cold atmosphere, he should be kept warm by applying blankets over and under him. Hot water bottles are dangerous because unconscious or semiconscious people will not detect the heat of a hot water bottle which may be too hot. Chemical heating pads which will generate heat with the addition of a few milliliters of water may be very useful, and are safe if directions are followed regarding the amount of water to be added.

While awaiting the ambulance or physician, the first aid worker may proceed with the splinting of fractures regardless of whether or not the patient is conscious. Before the patient is transported, the fractures should be immobilized as described in Chapter 13.

25 / First Aid in Industry

BURTON C. KILBOURNE AND EUDELL G. PAUL

Industry has recognized the value of efficient first aid for many years. Prompt first aid to the sick or injured may permit the employee to continue safely at work, or, with a more serious emergency, provides assistance until medical or surgical treatment is available. In spite of constant safety education and a lowering of accident rates, 2,200,000 workers of the United States in 1968 incurred injuries at work: 14,300 fatalities resulted (National Safety Council Accident Facts, 1969). More appalling were the 3,100,000 injuries and 41,700 deaths of workers occurring away from work. These figures denote very definitely the need for continued provision for first aid in industry and in the community.

The highest incidence of injuries is found in the construction, transportation, and mining industries. Trade, manufacturing, and utilities show a lower frequency rate. Studies of the source of injuries (Table 1) are of great importance to the safety worker in preventive programs and to the first aid worker in anticipating the need for first aid in a specific industry.

There are few injuries in industry not duplicated in nonindustrial experience. First aid, therefore, as applied in industry differs only in that it is more highly organized. Where a large number of workers are concentrated in a relatively small plant area, well-equipped first aid stations staffed by nurses and doctors are provided. This staff will train first aid teams in various work areas and disperse emergency stretchers and supplies throughout the plant. The training stresses the importance of prompt, proper care for all injuries and when and how to move the seriously injured. Workers become more safety conscious when participating in such periodic training.

TABLE 1. *Source and Cost of Compensable Work Injuries.*

Source of Injury	All Cases % of Cases	All Cases Ave. Cost*	Fatal % of Cases	Fatal Ave. Cost*	Permanent % of Cases	Permanent Ave. Cost*	Temporary % of Cases	Temporary Ave. Cost*
TOTAL	100.0	$ 783	100.0	$18,575	100.0	$1,925	100.0	$265
Handling objects, manual	22.6	725	13.9	20,900	9.6	1,940	28.5	265
Falls	20.4	1,075	17.4	18,700	18.5	3,000	21.2	310
Struck by falling, moving objects	13.6	550	9.3	16,800	19.3	1,260	11.1	230
Machinery	10.2	810	3.1	25,000	19.2	1,650	6.3	175
Vehicles	7.1	1,150	20.7	19,300	7.1	2,650	6.9	300
Motor	*5.0*	*1,280*	*18.0*	*19,300*	*4.3*	*2,800*	*5.2*	*300*
Other	*2.1*	*900*	*2.7*	*19,500*	*2.8*	*2,300*	*1.7*	*310*
Stepping on, striking against objects	6.9	350	2.3	22,800	5.6	840	7.6	115
Hand tools	6.1	540	1.5	21,000	8.1	1,225	5.3	185
Elec., heat, explosives	2.5	840	7.7	17,300	2.2	1,800	2.6	185
Elevators, hoists, conveyors	2.2	1,150	3.6	19,000	3.8	2,400	1.5	325
Other	8.4	800	20.5	15,500	6.6	2,100	9.0	285

* Compensation only.
Source: Reports from state labor departments.
(From Accident Facts. National Safety Council, 1969)

In the transportation industry, the first aid service must plan for the emergencies of traveling employees and passengers. The possibility of delay in reaching the nearest medical and hospital facility makes necessary the provision for appropriate first aid equipment and personnel training.

In the mining industry, first aid and mine rescue work are taught hand in hand. It is occasionally necessary for a medical attendant to be transported to the scene of an accident while the release of an injured miner is progressing. The majority of casualties, however, are given first aid by their group and brought out to the first aid station or hospital.

First Aid Stations

In any large industrial plant there will be one or more main dispensaries completely equipped and staffed by physicians and nurses. Also there will be outlying first aid stations; in small industries these will be the only medical centers in the plant. Of these facilities, the first aid stations concern us most in this discussion. Each of these should consist of one room for dressings and a small consulting room. There should be two rest rooms for injured or ill employees who must lie down and await either ambulance or medical care by a physician; adjoining each of these rooms there must be a toilet. The doors must be so arranged and of such size that a stretcher can be taken in and out without difficulty. Figures 1 and 2 show the arrangement of a first aid room. Because these rooms are apt to be small, it is essential that the rest rooms have outside windows, lest injured or sick employees lying in them develop a feeling of claustrophobia. In hot humid climates air conditioning is a necessity. Obviously these stations will be located where they are accessible to the greatest number of employees for a minimum loss of time and outdoor exposure. The furniture in the room should be comfortable, neat, and preferably of all metal construction. There should be no unnecessary pieces of furniture. A simple bed, a straight chair in each of the rest rooms, a small table, a small desk, two chairs in the consulting room, one specialist type of chair with head rest which can be lowered into a reclining position (in the dressing room), a metal stool for the first aid worker, a screen, instrument cabinet, and two small dressing tables would constitute the bare minimum of furniture.

X-RAY FACILITIES. Frequently the question is asked just how large must a factory or industrial plant be before x-ray facilities are justified in the first aid setup. The answer must depend on several different factors. The first relates to the medical policy of the company, i.e., whether or not routine chest x-rays for preemployment are required, and whether these pictures are repeated at periodic examinations. Ordinarily one x-ray machine will be ample unless the main dispensary and first aid station are located far apart. If the plant is small and there is no x-ray equipment in the main dispensary, then the number of employees which will justify investment in the x-ray machine will vary between 500 and 1,000. In a plant which is a little more prone to accidents and where routine chest pictures are taken, 500 employees will warrant the installation of an x-ray. On the other hand, if it is a plant where accidents are not common and not so many chest pictures are taken, 1,000 employees should be the dividing point. It is assumed here, of course, that the first aid installation is visited daily or at least frequently by regular medical attendants.

EQUIPMENT FOR DRESSING STATIONS. Each first aid station should have several trays in readiness for the care of a lacerated or open wound. Each tray should be about 12 × 18 inches; it, as well as

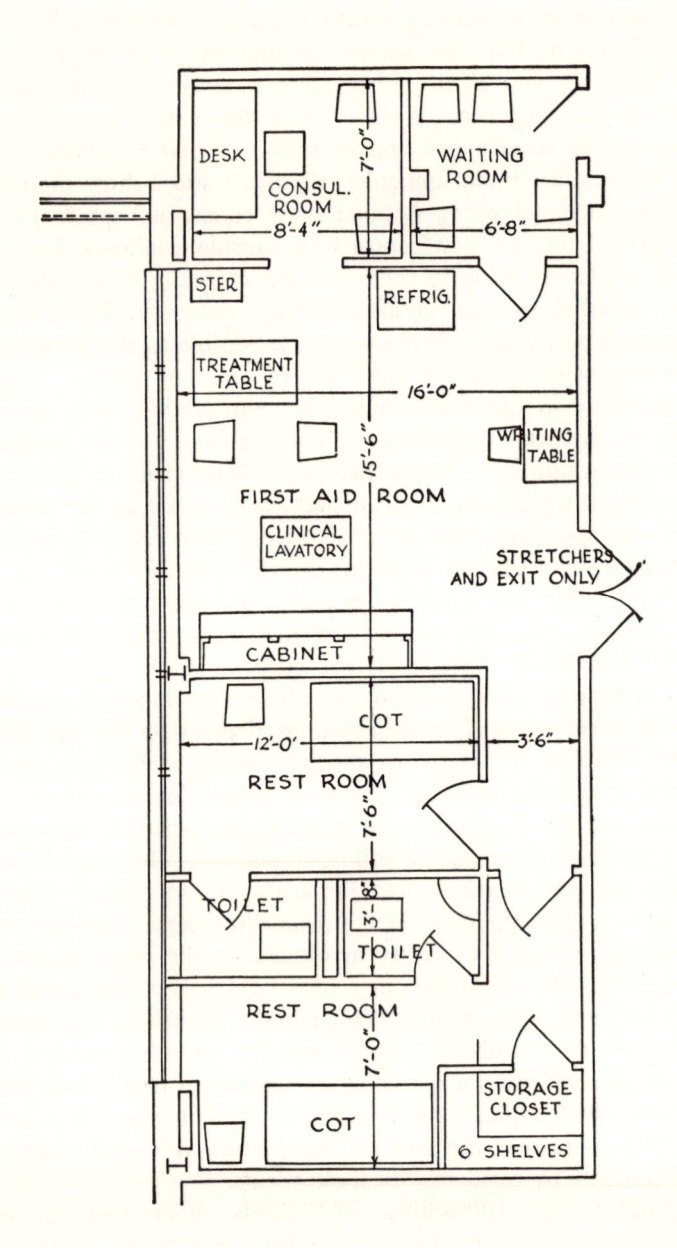

Fig. 1. Essential rooms for a satisfactory first aid installation. Rooms are minimal in size but adequate if volume of work is not too great.

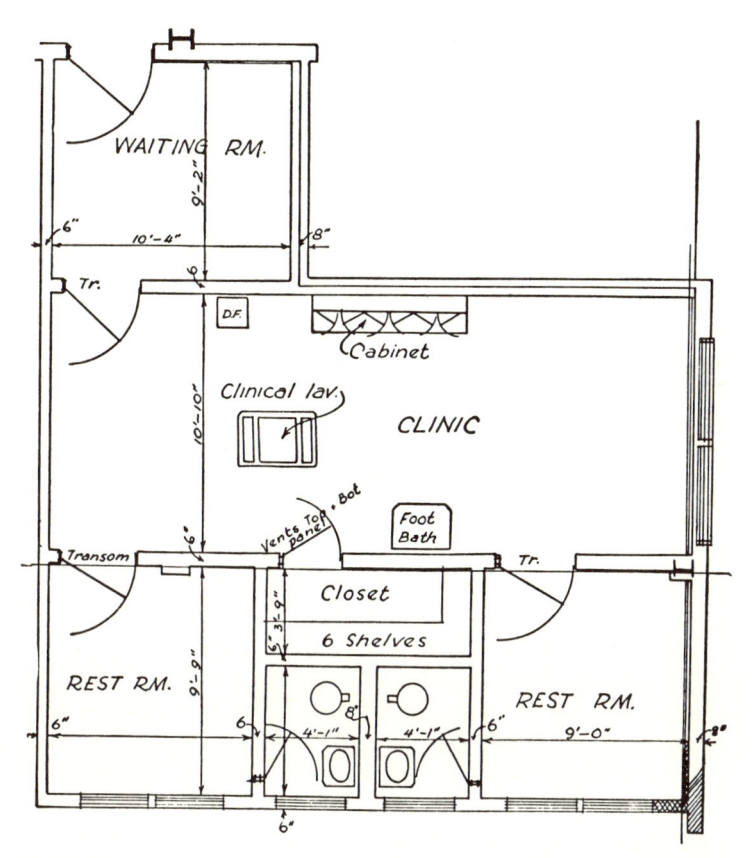

Fig. 2. Alternate plan for a first aid installation. In this sketch the consulting room has been sacrificed as such to permit a larger clinic for the first aid room. One of the rest rooms can be used as a consulting room when necessary. In both sketches, nurses use one of the rest rooms as their change room and for relaxation.

its contents, should be sterile and enclosed in a sterile pillow slip or towel. Each time it is sterilized the date should be put on the cover and it should be resterilized at regular intervals of about one month. The following items are suggested for the contents of the tray: cap, mask, gown, rubber gloves, several sterile towels, sutures, small and large sponges, applicators, local anesthesia solution, syringe and needles, scissors, knives, small straight and curved hemostats, needle holders, tissue forceps, small self-retaining retractors, and any special instruments or other equipment desired by the attending physician. Since it takes considerable time to set up and sterilize such trays, even the smallest first aid station should have at least two available at all times. More may be required if accidents are common. In addition to these trays of sterilized materials, which are kept ready for use at any time, the dressing tables in the first aid room should contain several jars adequately covered in which will be kept cotton pledgets, small and large gauze squares, and applicators. Besides these jars there must be a sterile forceps for taking contents out of the jars; this forceps must be kept in one of the sterilizing, noncorrosive solutions such as are now available commercially. Bandage scissors, pointed scissors, splinter forceps, and tissue forceps of several kinds should be kept sterilized in an instrument tray and resterilized after each use. Several sizes of adhesive compresses or similar ready-dressings should be within easy reach, as well as a roller containing several rolls of adhesive tape of different widths. On a lower shelf of this dressing table there should be a supply of bandages of various sizes and widths, as well as some elastic bandages and a few rolls of plaster bandage varying in width. Also in this shelf can be kept a few board, aluminum, or plastic splints to be fashioned and used as necessary. While it is true that every first aid station must have a few drugs on hand, these should be kept to an absolute minimum, and the list should, of course, be prescribed by the attending physician and given out only in accordance with his written instructions. Although aspirin and a few syrettes of morphine are probably the two absolutely indispensable drugs for a first aid station, a selection of antibiotics, injectable and oral for treatment of infections is desired. Muscle relaxant medications for back or muscle spasms are also useful. Tetanus toxoid for a booster dose on wound inception is essential, and presumes that a program of immunization is conscientiously followed. As indicated in Chapter 2, the safest cleansing agent for any wound is soap and water; however, in some work the skin of the patient will be covered with so much grease that a grease solvent, such as benzene, will have to be used to cleanse the skin around the wound.

RECORDS. Because of the unique position in industry of the first aid worker, as well as the medical department, with responsibility both to the injured employee and to management, complete and accurate records of all injuries are essential. Even a minor scratch may, under certain unfavorable circumstances, result in major temporary or permanent disability. A brief but accurate account of the manner in which the wound was received with a note as to its location (extremity, right or left, and digit involved), appearance of the wound (fresh or several days old), and the treatment rendered should be recorded in every case. Whatever system is used, it should be well indexed and accessible to the first aid worker or nurse for notations each time the patient is seen.

First Aid Treatment of Industrial Injuries

GENERAL PRINCIPLES. In most industrial plants the majority of injuries occur within a few minutes travel distance of the first aid station or medical dispensary. Depending upon the seriousness and location of the injury, many employees will be able to walk to the first aid station. The more seriously injured must be brought in by stretcher.

For those injuries of a minor nature the first aid treatment rendered will also be the definitive treatment. In all cases this treatment must serve the best interest of the injured employee. If the condition can be handled adequately in the first aid station and the employee safely allowed to return to work, this course should be followed.

If there are uncertainties as to the extent or nature of the injury even though apparently minor, the nurse or first aid attendant should not assume responsibility, but after rendering such temporary care as indicated, should call a physician or see that the patient is transported to the hospital. A similar procedure in serious cases is obviously indicated. The ability to evaluate each situation correctly and a realization of the limitations of the first aid function are the most important qualities of the industrial nurse or first aid worker.

Earlier surveys have shown hand and finger injuries to occur more frequently. These are still quite common but have been surpassed by trunk injuries in this report (Table 2). This is apparently

TABLE 2. *Location of Injury.*

Head, face and neck	7	Trunk	27
Eyes	4	Leg	11
Arms	8	Feet	9
Hands	9	Toes	3
Fingers	16	General	6

(Accident Facts 1969)

due to the reporting of many more back strains which, in earlier years, did not cause loss of time from work. Referring to Table 3, we note a relatively low incidence of infections. This reflects the emphasis in industry generally on good first aid.

TABLE 3. *Nature of Work Injuries, 1961, Illinois.*

Cuts and Lacerations	24.7
Fractures	20.7
Sprains and Strains	14.1
Bruises and Contusions	7.7
Burns	4.5
Hernia	3.2
Amputations	1.7
Inflammations	1.0
Infections	1.1
Punctures	2.0
Others	8.9
Occupational Diseases	0.8
Heart Diseases	0.2
Not Reported	11.4

CLOSED WOUNDS. Contusions to the extremities are most common, and if more than very minor, the part must be x-rayed to rule out fractures. The treatment described in Chapter 6 is carried out (i.e., cleansing the area, application of cold, and application of a pressure dressing) as indicated. The indication for this therapy depends on the degree of swelling and discoloration; cold and pressure are particularly indicated if a hematoma is present, as would be suggested by a fluctuant swelling. Contusions to the head, accompanied by more than very transient headache, or by even a short period of unconsciousness, must be considered potentially serious, and the patient is to be seen by a physician (see Chapter 17). In instances of contusion to the chest, aggravation of pain on breathing, coughing of blood, shortness of breath, pain intensified by compressing the ribs, and crackling of air under the skin upon palpation with the fingers are symptoms and signs of more serious injuries (see Chapter 15).

Frequently contusions to the abdomen do not at first produce symptoms of sufficient discomfort to suggest that underlying organs may have been injured. Should there be any question as to whether the trauma has caused an internal injury, a physician must be called or the patient hospitalized. While making the initial survey and examination, the pulse and blood pressure should be recorded and all such information forwarded to the hospital for comparison with subsequent readings and observations (see Chap. 16).

Contusions to the back and flank may produce kidney, as well as musculoskeletal injury. A urine specimen which is tinged with blood indicates injury to the kidney or some other organ in the genitourinary tract, such as the bladder or urethra. Hospitalization is mandatory for such injuries.

In all contused wounds, the first aid attendant should be more concerned with the possibilities of more serious underlying injury than with the relatively unimportant treatment of the obvious surface injury. When doubt exists, he must err on the side of safety for the injured employee.

OPEN WOUNDS. Abrasions should be cleansed and protected by a suitable dressing. Such minor injuries are ideally treated by use of a single layer of fine mesh gauze directly over the area, with or without a thin application of a bland ointment, an overlying gauze compress held in place by suitable outer bandage and left undisturbed until the skin has healed. For abrasions to the fingers and hands, frequent dressings will be necessary because of soiling. Should there appear to be any delay in healing, or if the abrasion is deep, a splint to restrict motion is indicated.

Serious hemorrhage is not frequent in industrial injuries. However, a sufficient number of employees must have first aid training to provide effective aid if it does occur. Such measures are described in Chapter 9. The first aid attendant can bring to the scene supplementary materials such as the large wound dressing, a good blood pressure cuff, or pneumatic tourniquet. Many dispensaries have Dextran or Ringer's Lactate on hand, and these should be started as an intravenous infusion if the patient shows any evidence of shock. It is best to have the physician present to supervise this and the transportation of these patients; however, if this is not practical, prompt removal to the closest hospital is essential after control of the bleeding.

The first aid treatment of an open wound consists primarily of application of a pressure dressing to stop hemorrhage (if present) and adequate coverage or protection by a bandage (see Chap. 6 for details). For definitive care open wounds must be cleansed and irrigated, their depth and extent determined, devitalized tissue and foreign material removed, underlying structures repaired, and the skin closed within an interval of time considered to be safe from the standpoint of infection if prompt, clean healing and maximum function is to be obtained. In the well-organized industrial medical department this is nearly always feasible. The first aid attendant should recognize the minor incised wounds or lacerations which will require only cleansing, dressing, and splint, and he may become expert in the use of adhesive bridging to overcome slight degrees of gaping of wound edges. In occasional instances metal skin clips are appropriate as a first aid procedure to close a small laceration. Usually, however, such gaping wounds should be handled by the doctor;

sutures are tolerated better than clips about the extremities. Unless the plant dispensary has a well-equipped operating room with adequate nurses and assistants for the surgeons, the care of injuries involving more than a few skin sutures should be given in a hospital. The physician or hospital should be notified, and the patient sent ahead without delay. The lapse of time from the first aid station to the hospital operating room is cumulative, and may easily exceed the four-hour "safe period" for preferred treatment if there is delay at any point. Definitive treatment given after a greater interval is more frequently complicated by wound infections. Because of this danger, the primary operation often must be limited to wound cleansing and debridement, and the repair of underlying structures deferred until a later time. Very often this loss of opportunity for primary repair in compound injuries means the acceptance of an inferior result.

Examples of serious, deep wounds common in industry are as follows.

Deep tearing *lacerations and avulsions* may be caused by forcible contact with blunt objects, with the extremity or object in motion. There may be extensive skin, muscle, or ligament injury, but major blood vessels, tendons, and nerves are frequently spared due to inherent toughness and mobility. Large flaps of skin may be stripped up, ranging in extent from a small portion to a major injury, such as the glove type avulsions in which the skin of the hand is pulled off much in the manner that a glove is removed. First aid consists of sterile pressure dressings and splint. Definitive treatment calls for careful cleansing, excision of contaminated and mangled tissue, and closure by opposing the edges or immediate skin grafting. In some instances, the skin which has been peeled off can, after proper preparation, be used as a graft.

Crushing injuries are caused by a great variety of machines and other mechanisms in which the extremity or body is caught between or thrown against heavy objects. In such instances open fractures are frequent. The surface lacerations are of a bursting type and may be less extensive than the disruption of the underlying tissues. These injuries frequently produce such damage to the walls of the blood vessels that thrombosis occurs, and gangrene may ensue. In wringer type injuries this may occur even though no fractures are evident, and the skin may be intact. In all this group, voluminous, evenly applied pressure dressings as a first aid measure may help to prevent the extreme congestion with venous blood which may be more damaging than actual hemorrhage. Needless to say, the same type of dressing is indicated following the definitive repair. Postoperative management often includes the use of anticoagulant drugs, such as heparin (to further guard against the tendency to thrombosis) and a lidocaine block of the sympathetic nerve supply to the part to improve the blood flow.

Traumatic amputations, particularly of the fingers, though not nearly as common since the advent of safety guards on machines, are still frequent. A pressure dressing is sufficient as a first aid procedure, and prompt definitive treatment makes possible the saving of maximum length either by immediate flap closure or by primary skin grafting. The latter is particularly useful in closing the stump of an amputation through the distal phalanx in order to save length and preserve the fingernail. Occasionally an arm or leg may be crushed off or cut off by machinery. Tourniquet and pressure dressing are the first aid measures indicated for control of hemorrhage. Morphine should be given for pain, and plasma for shock; hospital treatment is urgent.

Emery wheel grinds are a combination of laceration or avulsion and burn. This injury is known to first aid attendants in industry for its slowness in healing and the tendency to deeper involvement than was at first evident. Bleeding is minimal because the friction burn has, in effect, cauterized the tissues. Minor wounds of this type may be treated by cleansing, petrolatum dressing, and splint. More extensive treatment should include cleansing, thorough exploration, the immediate excision of all exposed tissue to a depth of one eighth of an inch, followed by primary suture. Such wounds must never be sutured unless the burned tissue has been cut away. The prominence of the knuckles of the back of the hand make this a common site of the injury, and frequently tendons and joints may thus be injured. These involvements make doubly important the prompt removal of the patient to the hospital for early adequate treatment in order to avoid infection and permanent impairment of use of the fingers.

Sharp edges of sheet metal or metal turnings, in addition to cutting tools, are responsible for most *deep incised wounds and severed tendons and nerves.* The skin wound is often small and bleeding minimal; yet the first aid worker must exercise constant care in examining not only the immediate wound, but also the function and sensation of the extremity beyond the point of injury. If there is any question of ability to flex or extend the extremity or digits distal to the laceration, the tendon is probably cut. Similarly, if sensation is impaired, nerve injury should be suspected. Because of the very meager blood supply to tendons, infection is very prone to develop unless the primary repair can be accomplished within four hours of the time of injury. If there is delay in suspecting the tendon injury or in getting hospital care, the patient must wait six to eight weeks or longer before the tendon can be repaired. If infection occurs, the chances for a functional result from either primary or secondary repair are very poor. Although the presence of infection in nerve repair is slightly less damaging to the result, there is no doubt that the earlier such injuries are cared for the better. The greatest service in first aid in these cases is the prompt recognition and arrangement for adequate care. Sterile dressings and splints are used as indicated.

Foreign bodies are very apt to be found in wounds sustained in industry. These may be slivers of wood or steel, glass, graphite, carbon, cloth, and various types of metals. If steel or glass, the foreign body proper is not as important as the effect it has had in damaging the underlying structures. They do not often produce infection and are innocuous unless they lodge adjacent to or in a nerve, tendon, muscle, or blood vessel of the extremity, or penetrate an organ of the abdomen or chest. X-rays should be taken for diagnosis, but the decision for or against removal rests with the physician and is determined after weighing the risk of infection or future trouble against the trauma of removal. Generally, superficial steel chips can be removed easily if seen early. If nerves have been damaged or blood vessels injured, the immediate repair is indicated and the foreign body removed if encountered. Irritation of tendons may not be diagnosed until active use is begun, and secondary removal may then be done. Steel chips deeply imbedded in muscle are best left alone. Wood slivers and cloth should be removed because of the danger of infection. Carbon particles should be scraped out to avoid tattooing in superficial skin wounds. Graphite from pencil points causes chemical destruction of tissue; therefore, early excision and irrigation are indicated. Another foreign substance with very detrimental effect is the grease injected forcibly through a puncture by the tip of a grease gun. Here immediate evacuation by the physician of as much of the material as possible using numerous incisions is indicated, followed by treatment of any subsequent infection or necrosis. The depth of penetration and the experience of the attendant are the criteria for deciding whether foreign bodies can be handled in the first aid station.

BURNS. Burns of all types are encountered among industrial accidents and range from the minor superficial to complete cremation.

Obviously, the latter are not seen in the first aid dispensaries. Of the minor varieties, first aid treatment similar to that mentioned under abrasions can be applied. Cleanliness and protection by rest are the principles involved here. As the seriousness increases, first aid treatment, as described in Chapter 10, should be applied. It should be remembered that the depth of involvement is frequently difficult to assess correctly from appearance alone. Hot metal burns are usually third degree. Burns from ignition of clothing saturated with gasoline are deep second and third degree. Hot water burns are variable. Acid and strong alkali burns are very deceptive at first and often develop into third degree burns due to continuing action of the chemical long after exposure. Patients presenting small areas of deep second or third degree involvement of the upper extremity and trunk can be treated adequately in the first aid dispensary under a physician's supervision, but if the same involvement were present on the foot or leg, this person should be hospitalized or kept in bed. Small superficial burns treated by early, gentle cleansing, bland ointment, pressure dressing, splint, rest, and infrequent changes of dressing usually heal readily. For extensive burns of any area equivalent to that of an upper extremity, immediate hospitalization for treatment of anticipated shock is indicated. Skin grafts are indicated when third degree burns are more than an inch in diameter (see Chap. 10).

FRACTURES, DISLOCATIONS, AND SPRAINS. The frequency of fractures varies somewhat among various industries, but generally, fractures of the fingers and toes are most common, with fractures in the hand, wrist, and foot next in frequency. Ankle, heel, and leg fractures appear with slightly greater frequency than fractures of the forearm, elbow, and arm. Rib fractures are not uncommon. Spine and pelvic fractures occurring as a result of collapse of rock or walls are frequently seen in the mining industries. The first aid treatment of these varieties is covered specifically in Chapter 13. A proper backboard is especially indicated for transportation. A supply of useful splints of aluminum, wood, or plastic should be kept in every first aid station for the common upper-extremity types. Inflatable air splints are useful in forearm fractures. Pillows are very effective for the fractures about the ankle. This pressure, evenly applied, helps minimize the swelling and is comfortable. Inflatable or half-ring splints should be available for fractures of the leg and femur. The first aid worker or nurse should proceed to the scene of the accident with suitable splints for major lower extremity fractures and apply these before allowing the patient to be put on a stretcher. Most patients with upper extremity fractures may be allowed to self-support the injured arm in a manner which is comfortable and be brought to the first aid station for additional splinting. Morphine should be given as directed by the physician for relief of pain, and arrangements for hospital care effected if necessary. We have previously stressed the importance of early definitive treatment of open fractures. While many of the closed fractures do not require urgency, some, because of associated dislocation with injury or compression to the major blood vessels, may require immediate treatment if the limb is to be saved. In minor closed fractures, thorough soap and water cleansing prior to the application of a splint is indicated; this serves to prevent infection of blisters which tend to appear with subsequent swelling. Pressure dressings and elevation of the part help to minimize the swelling.

Sprains of the wrist and ankle are most frequently encountered and can be diagnosed only after adequate examination by the physician. X-rays are essential. Treatment may be given on a presumptive basis in mild conditions, but subsequent examination by the physician is necessary (see Chap. 13). Sprains of the back are of importance because of their frequency and ensuing disability. The first aid worker may easily underestimate the seriousness of this condition and should be cautious in allowing patients to return to work without first seeing the physician. Rest, in a reclining position, and heat are helpful. Many mild back sprains are aggravated by ill-advised attempts to return to stooping and lifting.

HERNIA. Table 3 reveals that 3.2 percent of work injuries are hernias. It is important that the first aid worker obtain an accurate history of possible injury and symptoms. The common accidents reported by the worker are unusual lifting, straining, or slipping which forces the injured into a stretched or awkward position. The first aid attendant should note and record such complaints as groin pain, low back pain, periumbilical pain, scrotal or testicular pain, nausea, and the sudden appearance of inguinal swelling. Often the swelling does not occur immediately. It is in these cases that the initial notation of presenting symptoms is of greatest importance. In most states compensability of the hernia is based on an injury or unusual strain at work, no previously know hernia, and a report to a superior or the medical department within a limited time following the accident.

The pain incidental to a newly protruded hernia can be relieved by placing the patient in a reclining position which will result usually in spontaneous return of the contents into the abandoned cavity. When this fails to produce relief, or the hernia cannot be reduced, incarceration or strangulation should be suspected and a physician called immediately.

EYE INJURIES. Foreign bodies in the eye are of daily occurrence in industrial first aid stations. The first aid attendant will find that a good light and magnifying lenses are necessary in the treatment of these patients. By shifting the light beam to strike the corneal surface from different directions, very few foreign bodies or abrasions of the corneal surface will be missed. The method of inspecting for foreign bodies is depicted in Chapter 18, Figure 2. The eye is then irrigated with sterile physiologic saline solution which will frequently flush out the particle. Moistened cotton-tipped applicators are used gently to wipe out the particle. If, as is frequent in industry, the particle is embedded in the cornea or sclera, a physician should be called. The reddening of the sclera should be recognized as evidence of eye infection and proper medical referral advised. Occasionally, in spite of the use of safety glasses (much more common when glasses are not worn) flying chips of steel lacerate or penetrate the cornea or sclera. Such wounds must receive expert care from an eye specialist as soon as possible if the vision is to be saved. First aid consists in covering the eye with a sterile gauze patch. The treatment of burns of the eye is described in Chapter 18.

Miscellaneous Types of Emergencies

Electric shock and asphyxiation by gases are serious emergencies, and must be treated quickly by artificial respiration and closed chest cardiac massage as outlined in detail in Chapter 14, if respirators are not available. Portable resuscitators are useful when of accepted type and their operation is understood. A small emergency oxygen tank for use with a mask is extremely valuable in conjunction with artificial respiration, or after such patients resume respiratory activity. Other medical emergencies such as acute coronary occlusion (see Chap. 23) can be materially benefitted by oxygen as a first aid measure. Heat exhaustion and heat cramps (see Chap. 23) should be well understood by the first aid worker in industry, and protection of the workers by salt administration carried out systematically.

Finally, the first aid worker in industry serves an important function when he can apply such treatments as he may be called upon to perform with efficiency, good judgment, understanding, and a desire to help in every situation to the best of his ability.

26 / Military and Civil Defense Aspects of Mass Casualty Management

JOHN J. KOVARIC

There can be dramatic differences between the types of casualties produced in warfare and those that may occur during a natural disaster or in a nuclear holocaust. However, there are important lessons that can be translated from man's experience during war to prepare his community for almost any tragedy. Triage is normally associated with battle casualties, but the art of sorting and treatment by priority is such an integral part of every emergency clinic that the association of everyday accident victims with "combat" is frequently overlooked.

Accidents of all types in the United States now claim over 50 million victims a year. Of these over 112,000 die, and 10 million are disabled, if only temporarily, and need some type of bed care, while over two million need hospitalization. These patients constantly occupy one out of every eight hospital beds available, taxing the medical capabilities of most communities. The development of over one million convalescent/nursing home beds has been a necessity to back up the 800,000 hospital beds. This continuous heavy drain on our manpower and economy is more serious as an everyday problem than it is in the theatre of war. The treatment of specific wounds has been well covered in the preceding chapters, and although there are some specific differences in the management of combat trauma in contrast to civilian trauma, the missions of both military and civilian mass casualty care are similar: to conserve the fighting strength, and to provide the greatest good for the greatest number.

Military Medical Preparation and Support

During the peak manpower strength in Vietnam, about 15,000 medical personnel were included in the 550,000 troops. Twelve thousand of these comprised the U.S. Army's 44th Medical Brigade, and Surgeon's Office (Division personnel). The remaining 3,000 was comprised of U.S. Navy and U.S. Air Force medical personnel.

About one in every 40 troops in Vietnam was involved in patient care. U.S. Army medical personnel maintained 22 hospitals with 6,300 beds,* a number of dispensaries, dental clinics, laboratories, and depots. The professional help necessary included 800 physicians, 800 nurses, and 150 pilots. During one year of maximum involvement, these personnel and installations were responsible for the care of 123,000 admissions, plus an outpatient load of six times that amount (Table 1).

TABLE 1. *Total Admissions to U.S. Army Hospitals in 1968.*

Battle casualties (IRHA) *	41,163
Disease and non-battle injuries	81,636
Total hospital admissions	122,799
Total wounded but not admitted	34,000+ †

* IRHA—injured as a result of hostile action.
† Includes only U.S. Army personnel.

In the initial stages of planning to care for large numbers of patients, it is only natural to focus attention on trauma—and in warfare, on combat casualties. However as the figures will demonstrate, battle casualties constitute only one third of all hospital admissions. Another one third are due to accidents, and the remaining one third to disease. Among the outpatients are those who were wounded, but not seriously enough to warrant hospitalization.

Following a natural disaster, such as a flood, hurricane, or tornado, the medical treatment necessary is not limited to those patients who need major surgery. It must include all those who can be treated and released, and all other patients unfortunate enough to be ill at the time plus those who have had unrelated accidents or surgical problems.

In any mass casualty situation, the medical profession must consider the return to duty, or return to work, rate. Since not all patients need be admitted to a hospital, they can be returned to work

* This includes 1,200 convalescent beds.

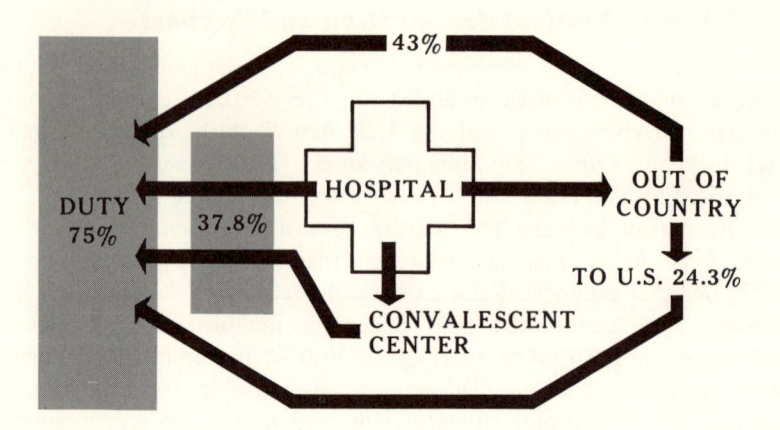

Fig. 1. The disposition of wounded patients admitted to the hospital.

in a short time. In Vietnam, those who are returned to duty from hospitals are normally returned within 30 days. In spite of the seriousness of many wounds, less than 3 percent of the combat casualties died after admission to a hospital; and three out of every four patients were eventually returned to duty, either in Vietnam or in the United States (Fig. 1). Table 2 shows data obtained from the U.S. Army

TABLE 2. *U.S. Army Personnel Casualty Figures, January 1965-April 1969.*

Total wounded	138,454
Admitted to hospital	70,694
To duty in Vietnam	26,745
To duty after evacuation	26,664
Total patients to duty	53,389 = 75.5%

Surgeon General's Office, which pertain only to U.S. Army Troops. It is important to point out that during this same four-year period, over 203,000 patients were admitted to hospitals because of disease and nonbattle injuries; and an additional 200,000 with minimal-care needs were either put on quarters or kept in dispensary-sized treatment facilities.

A major difference between the use of facilities in handling military mass casualties and those in a civilian disaster is the enormous military hospital bed reserve. The hospital capacity in Vietnam is fortunately backed up by many of the 37,000 bed spaces throughout the military hospitals in the continental United States. In addition, this separation of care for the acutely ill on the one hand, and chronically ill on the other enables the Medical Department to concentrate specialty manpower and supplies where they will be needed most. The most recent and largest civilian effort analogous to this type of evacuation was undertaken by the Air National Guard following Hurricane Camille in Mississippi. Three hundred already hospitalized bed patients were flown to interior hospitals to allow local facilities to concentrate on the expected storm casualties.

If the number of civilian personnel involved in patient care were proportional to that in the military, it would total a staggering 10 million. (There are currently about 2.5 million people involved in hospital patient care.) This is arrived at by applying a 1 to 40 ratio for military personnel in the combat zone, plus all those military personnel functioning in similar capacities in the States. Although this proportion tends to be ideal for disaster-type situations, it is too high for the reality of everyday trauma. Still another major difference between combat wounds and everyday civilian trauma is the severity of the injuries. This may be best demonstrated by the difference in mortality rates. In Vietnam, the ratio of Wounded in Action to Killed in Action is about 6 to 1. The ratio of civilian accidents requiring hospitalization to resulting deaths per year is about 20 to 1; and if the higher figure of 10 million temporary disabilities is used, the ratio increases to 100 to 1.

It must be emphasized that these civilian casualties are based on a business-as-usual workload and their care requires peak performance from the medical communities. The provision of additional manpower, supplies, and facilities should be a matter of constant concern and planning. Without adequate preparation, the burden of an additional 100 or 1,000, or even thousands of casualties in one area could be chaotic and would result in a "medical-care disaster."

Preparation in a Military Hospital

One of the busier Evacuation Hospitals in Vietnam had a 400-bed capacity and an average daily census of 220 patients. During 1968, almost 14,000 patients were admitted. The monthly admission rates varied from 1,000 to 1,400 patients. These were divided into medical, surgical, and psychiatric admissions. Throughout the year, medical patients constituted about one third of the admissions, and surgical patients about two thirds. The latter could be divided equally into battle casualties and other surgical patients (such as accidents). There was no neurosurgery performed. In addition to the admissions, over 6,000 outpatients were seen per month. The psychiatric unit admitted 70 patients per month.

The total hospital staff varied from 300 to 340. Depending upon circumstances, the total included 25 to 35 physicians, most of whom were specialists, 55 nurses, 12 administrators, and over 210 enlisted men who worked on the wards, in the labs, in supply, on vehicles, and as clerks.

Hospital Staff—400 Bed Evacuation Hospital

General surgeons	8
Thoracic surgeons	2
Orthopedists	4
Urologists	1
Opthalmologists	1
Internists	4
Anesthesiologists	2
General medical officers	3
Physchiatrists	4
Dentists	2
Nurses and anesthetists	55
Administrative staff	12
Enlisted men	210

In the light of experience at this hospital several problems warrant reemphasis.

TRIAGE. Although the emergency room may be manned around the clock, it is imperative that qualified surgeons are always on call to triage casualties whenever they arrive. Resuscitation, diagnosis, evaluation, and the time of treatment are all critical steps that should be undertaken by the best qualified. Surgical teams are called and additional operating rooms opened as the need arises, and surgical specialists requested as needed.

PATIENT FLOW. When the number of casualties appear to be on a large scale, the entire hospital staff must be notified and act according to PREARRANGED plans. There is a place and need for everyone assigned to the hospital. For example, the psychiatrists can handle the wards and evacuation of patients who could be moved; the internists can use outpatient clinics to handle minor injuries; the general medical officers and dentists can be put on surgical teams, or substituted as anesthetists (if experienced); and the entire staff should be put on 12-hour shifts if the situation appears to be prolonged.

BLOOD. The average amount of blood given a casualty who receives blood is six units. For planning purposes however, the blood procured is about two units per casualty admitted to the hospital. Even though the master plan calls for blood to be shipped from the United States, it is still desirable that a hospital have access to a "walking blood bank." This is invaluable when fresh blood is needed to correct a hemorrhagic diathesis.

X-RAY. This hospital takes between 6,000 and 10,000 exposures per month. When this critical area is at its busiest, it must have enough personnel, equipment, and physical space to perform its mission as smoothly as it does when it operates under normal circumstances.

MEDICAL SUPPLIES. In any disaster, transportation and personnel may not be available to obtain essential items. To prevent a supply crisis, adequate planning involves the advance procurement of all stocks necessary to maintain a hospital at its peak load for 30 days. This stock should be in addition to the normal requirements of the installation. Perishable drugs can be rotated from the Emergency Stockpile and replaced as necessary.

The manner in which plans for troop medical support are evolved is not unlike the manner in which local community needs are met by a medical society and/or by following the recommendations of the American Medical Association. The plans do not develop by accident and a great deal of experience and organization is necessary for both civilian and military hospitals. The logistic advantages of a military organization under the circumstances are obvious and need not be ennumerated. Among the more important factors in determining the size and location of an Army hospital in a combat zone are:

1. The number of troops (population) being supported.
2. The type and amount of disease encountered in the area.
3. The number and type of accidents that might be expected.
4. The number and type of combat casualties that could occur.
5. The number of specific surgical and medical specialists necessary to treat all the previously mentioned patients.

6. The amount of other critical manpower essential to the unit—nurses, corpsmen, administrative assistance.
7. The supplies and equipment essential to the task: blood, fluids, dressings, medicines, anesthesia and x-ray machines, tables, generators, vehicles, and so on.
8. Medical evacuation and communications are also an integral part of treatment. Perhaps the major reason that evacuation is so expedient is that the U.S. Army Medical Department, singularly among all the medical services throughout the world, owns and operates its own ambulances, buses, helicopters, and radio net.
9. And, a factor that is not referred to frequently enough: the constant TRAINING of all these personnel to function appropriately when the occasion arises.

Civilian Medical Preparation and Support

In an effort to reinforce the drugs and medical supplies essential to hospital care in civilian disasters or in event of attack, the components of 2,500 hospitals, each with 200 beds, have been assembled and placed around the Nation. It is hoped that more medical personnel in local communities will become aware of the potential need for this equipment and organize a plan of action to utilize it should the occasion arise. These Packaged Disaster Hospitals constitute an inventory of almost $100 million and are monitored by the Division of Emergency Health Services (DEHS) of U.S. Public Health Service, Department of Health, Education, and Welfare (DHEW). Each unit contains equipment and drugs to care for 200 patients for 30 days.

In addition to these, a stock of pharmaceuticals is available to any hospital that will participate in another of DEHS's program. A Hospital Reserve Disaster Inventory, depending upon its size, contains the drugs essential to treat 50, 100, or 200 patients for one month during a catastrophe. This $4 million investment can provide medications for 10,000 patients. The only requirement on the part of the requesting hospital is merely to use and replace various drugs before they expire.

In order that certain localities have mobility and effectiveness in small local disasters, the Division of Emergency Health Services designed a Natural Disaster Hospital. Twenty-five of these, each valued at $4,800,000 have been distributed to areas where tornadoes and floods are likely to occur. The 50 beds and 48 litters in these units make them valuable, short-term assets.

The Office of Civil Defense, Department of Defense, has stocked and marked public fallout shelters to protect much of the population against radiation in case of a nuclear holocaust. There are currently enough medical kits, sanitation kits, and food and water in these locations to provide the bare essentials for life for 64 million people for two weeks; or 100 million people for one week. The medical contents of these survival kits were specifically designed not to reinforce treatment facilities, but to provide the public with some basic requirements for day-to-day living. Local civil defense directors are responsible for administering these shelters and for care of the supplies.

For the past seven years, the Office of Civil Defense has funded a training program for Medical Self-Help, which has been operated by the Public Health Service's DEHS. During this time over 10 million people have been given a 16-hour course in first aid. This ambitious undertaking has as its goal the training of one out of every five Americans. In reaching this goal, it should be mandatory that certain personnel, such as ambulance and medical attendants, firemen and policemen, have this training—just as it is for their counterparts in the military.

Medical Disaster Planning

No single plan of action could possibly cover all situations or communities. It is therefore the responsibility of local leaders to provide the best possible insurance for the survival of themselves and their neighbors. The following checklist is intended as a guide to provide the reader with additional background for consideration when preparing to meet the needs for medical assistance during a natural disaster or nuclear holocaust. To complete this list, names, locations, phone numbers, and coordination should be checked and verified.

Emergency Medical Care Resources Checklist

Medical personnel:
    Doctors———Nurses———Dentists———Veterinarians———
Medical transportation:
    Ambulances———Rescue trucks———
Treatment areas:
    Hospital———Convalescent/Nursing home———
Medical clinics:———

Surgical and medical supplies:
    Pharmacies———Drug wholesaler———Drug manufacturer———
Blood banks———
Clinical laboratories———
Fire department———
Police department———
Medical society———
Dental society———
Nursing society———
Red Cross———
Large industries (personnel and vehicles)———
Public Health Office———
Local civil defense director———
Power and Light Company———
Public transportation———
Department of highways———
Telephone Company———
All communication nets———

Summary

No single master plan can possibly cover all eventualities for mass casualty care, either civilian or military. However, when consideration is given both circumstances there are basic rational steps that can be taken, which can be modified to fit most occasions. The optional use of personnel—both medical and paramedical—for patient care is usually preplanned. Other factors, however, may not be given serious enough consideration because they seem insurmountable. These may include the stockpiling of thousands of dollars worth of drugs and medical supplies, the rapid evacuation of large numbers of patients, and the establishment of an all-inclusive communications network over which the responsible agencies can be contacted. During a disaster of large magnitude, the effectiveness of previous follow-through on each of these problems could be as important as patient-care itself.

Index

Abcess, 92, 96
  bullet, 81
  tooth, 102
Abdomen, 252
  injury, in fracture, 165
    symptoms and signs, 258
    tenderness, 258
    vomiting, 258
  pain, 261
  wound
    nonpenetrating, 257
    penetrating, 256
Abdominal injury, first aid, 259
Abrasion, 69
  infection, 94
  treatment, 76
Accident, cerebrovascular, 375
Acid
  carbolic poisoning, 379
  in eye, 294
  phenolic, poisoning, 379
  poisoning, 381
Addiction, drug, 376
Airway, 205
  equipment for mouth-to-mouth resuscitation, 223
  obstruction, in resuscitation, 219
Airsickness, 296
Akee poisoning, 389
Alcohol, in snake bite, 86
Alkali, in eye, 294
Allergy, 393
  to bee sting, 88
Allonal poisoning, 379
Altitude sickness, 396
Ambu bag, in assisting ventilation, 239
Ambulance service
  equipment, 141, 142
  organization, 139
Amphetamines, 377

Amputation
  of hand, 323
  traumatic, 415
Anaphylaxis, 88, 393
Angina pectoris, 365
Ankle
  bandage, 56, 57
  fracture, 194
  splinting, 188
Anoxic shock, 105
Antibiotics, in treatment of wounds, 77
Antihistamine, in bee sting, 88
Antivenin
  bee, 88
  in treatment of snakebite, 87
Apophysis, calcaneal, 347
Apoplexy, 375
Appendicitis, acute, 261
Arachnoid bite, 87
Arch, of foot, pain, 333
Arm, 26
  splinting, 173
Arrest. *See also* Cardiac arrest.
  cardiac, 203, 247
  cardiopulmonary, 201
  with chest injury, 249
  pulmonary, 202
Arsenic poisoning, 380
Artery
  bleeding, 115
  brachial, pressure point, 118, 119
  common carotid, pressure point, 117, 119
  femoral, 118, 119
  injury in fracture, 165
Asphyxiation, 419
Aspirin
  poisoning, 383
  in sunburn, 132
Asystole, 204

429

430 / Index

Athlete's foot, 348
Atropine poisoning, 384
Axilla, bandage, 58, 59

Bag, Ambu, in assisting ventilation, 239
BAL, as antidote, 380
Bandage
  in abdominal injury, 259
  ankle, 56, 57
  axilla, 58, 59
  Barton, 61
  Esmarch, 120
  eye, 63, 65
  figure-of-eight, 53
  finger, 53, 54
  forearm, 56
  groin, 64
  hand, 60
  head, 63, 64
  hip, 64
  jaw, 61, 62
  neck, 58, 59, 60
  open wound, 52
  scalp, 61, 63
  spica, of hip, 64
  spiral reverse, 53
  with stocking, 66, 67
  tight, 53
  thorax, 60
  thumb, 55
  triangular, 50, 51
  wrist, 55, 60
Bandaging, 50
  technique, 51
  tight, 53
Barton bandage, 61
Bee sting, 88
Benzene
  as cleanser, 81
  poisoning, 386
Bichloride of mercury poisoning, 380
Bite
  bat, 84
  black widow spider, 87
  brown spider, 88
  cat, 85
  chigger, 88
  dog, 84
  fox, 84
  of hand, 325
  human, 89, 99
  insect, 87
  snake, 85

  spider, 87
Black eye, 288
Black widow spider bite, 87
Bladder injury, 315, 316
Blank cartridge wound, 82
Blast, nuclear, 149
Bleeding. *See also* Hemorrhage.
  arterial, 115
  capillary, 116
  venous, 116
Blepharospasm, 290
Blister, foot, 350
Blood
  circulation, 35, 36, 37, 38
  clotting, 34
  coughing. *See* Hemoptysis.
  description, 33, 34
  in military hospital, 425
  vessels, 35
    injury, 115
Board, spine, 183
Bone
  broken, 161
  swallowed, 263
Botulism, 387
Brachial artery, pressure point, 118, 119
Brain
  contusion, 71
  injury, 277
Breathing, absence, 7
  in heart-lung resuscitation, 296
British anti-lewisite, as antidote, 380
Brown spider bite, 88
Bullet, removal, 81
Bunion, 349
Burn, 123
  chemical, 131, 134
    of eye, 293
  classification, 126
  early care, 131
  eye, 292, 307
    acid, 294
    infrared, 293
    radiation, 293
    ultraviolet, 293
  in electric injuries, 135
  first degree, 127
  hand, 325
  head, 307
  hydrochloric acid, 134
  hydrofluoric acid, 134
  industrial, 417
  lime, 134
  minor, initial management, 132

Index / 431

Burn (*cont.*).
 mustard gas, 134
 neck, 307
 nitric acid, 134
 phenol, 134
 phosphorus, 134
 potassium hydroxide, 134
 prevention, 124
 second degree, 127
 sodium hydroxide, 134
 sulfuric acid, 134
 tear gas, 134
 third degree, 127
 transportation of patient, 129
 trichloroacetic acid, 134
Bursitis, heel, 344
Butterfly dressing, 80

Caisson disease, 397
Calcium, in eye, 295
Calcium gluconate, in diagnosing black widow bite, 87
Callus, 351
Carbon monoxide poisoning, 385
 with burn, 125
Carbon tetrachloride poisoning, 386
Carbuncle, 98
Cardiac arrest
 massage, closed, 248, 249
 shock, 105
 standstill, 204
 tamponade, 245
Cardiopulmonary arrest, 201
Cardiovascular collapse, 204
Carpal bones, 27
Cavity, in tooth, 102
Cellulitis, 92, 96
Cerebrospinal fluid, leakage, 270
Cerebrovascular accident, 375
Chest
 defect in wall, 240
 firm blow in cardiac arrest, 215
 injury, 235
  with cardiac arrest, 249
  pain, 236
 sucking wound, 241
Chill, 390
Chloral hydrate poisoning, 385
Chlorpromazine poisoning, 383
Circulation, artificial, 208
Civil Defense, 420
 Packaged Disaster Hospital, 17
Clavicle, 26
Cleanser, makeshift, 81

Closed-chest cardiac compression, 208
Cold, 391
 in extremity, in tight bandaging, 53
 injury, 137
Colic
 gallbladder, 262
 renal, 263, 319
Collapse, cardiovascular, 204
Collar, in splinting cervical spine, 182
Colles' fracture, 27
Coma, 373
 diabetic, 374
 hypoglycemic, 374
 uremic, 373
Common carotid artery, pressure point, 117, 119

Diaphragm, 32
Digestive system, 43
Dilandid poisoning, 382
Dilated pupils, in shock, 107
Diphtheria, 390
Disaster planning, 17
 medical, 427
Disease, contagious, 389
Dislocation, 161, 186
 ankle, 192, 193
 elbow, 187
 finger, 189
 foot, 193
 hip, 188, 190
 industrial, 417
 intervertebral disc, 282
 knee, 191
 mandible, 302
 shoulder, 187
 thumb, 189
 toes, 193
 wrist, 189
Distension, gastric, in mouth-to-mouth resuscitation, 217
Drainage, in deep wounds, 80
Dressing, to control hemorrhage, 74
 pressure, to control hemorrhage, 116

Earache, 101
Eclampsia, 372
Edema, in contused wounds, 68
Elbow, splinting, 173
Emergency
 abdominal, 252
 cardiorespiratory, 196

Emery wheel injury, 415
Emphysema, subcutaneous, 244
Epidermophytosis, 348
Epilepsy, 371
Epinephrine in bee sting, 88
Ergotism, 389
Eryspelas, 97
Evisceration, 259, 260
Exhaustion, heat, 363
Exposure, 391
Eye
 abrasion, 290
 alkali in, 294
 blunt injury, 288, 304
 burn, 133, 292, 293. *See also* Burn, eye.
 concussion, 288
 contusion, 288
 dendritic ulcer, 292
 first aid, 297
 hemorrhage, 304
  subcutaneous, 288
 injury, 286
  blunt, 288, 304
  electric, 293
  industrial, 419
  penetrating, 289
 laceration, 289, 306
 lewisite, 295
 lye, 294
 mace, 295
 mustard gas, 134
 pain, 296
 pupils, 8
 silver in, 295
 tear gas, 295
Eyelid, laceration, 289

Face, 30
 blunt injury, 303
 laceration, 306
Failure, acute left heart, 366
Fainting, 357, 399
 treatment, 361
Femoral artery, pressure point, 118, 119
Femur, 28
Fever, 9
Fibrillation, ventricular, 204
Fibrosis, perineural, 339
Fibula, 29
 splinting, 177
Finger(s), 27. *See also* Bandage; Dislocation.

Fire, rescue, 125
First aid
 kit, 15
 station, industrial, 406
Fish poisoning, 388
Flail chest, 388
Flatfoot, 333
Food poisoning. *See* Poisoning.
Foot
 athlete's, 348
 care, 352
 injury, 329
 march, 341
 splinting, 180
 strain
  acute, 334
  chronic, 334
Forearm, splinting, 176
Forehead, 30
Foreign body, 81
 in ear, 83
 in esophagus, 389
 in eye, 82, 290, 309
 in genitourinary tract, 320
 in larynx, 308
 in mouth, 308
 in nose, 83
 swallowed, 263
Fracture, 161
 with abdominal organ injury, 165
 with arterial injury, 165
 avulsion, 162
 cervical vertebra, 282
 closed, 72, 161
 Colles', 27
 comminuted, 161
 compound, 72, 161
 compression, 162
 with contusion, 71
 depressed, 163
 diagnosis, 164
 femur, 166, 176
 first aid, 167
 greenstick, 162
 and hemorrhage, 167
 impacted, 161
 industrial, 417
 jaw, 303, 304
 mandible, 303
 march, 341
 maxilla, 304
 metatarsal bone, 341
 with nerve injury, 165
 nose, 304

Fracture (cont.).
 oblique, 161
 open, 72, 161, 185
 pathologic, 163
 rib, 238
 segmental, 161
 and shock, 167
 simple, 161
 skull, 270, 271, 373
 spiral, 161
 splinting, 167, 172-184. See also Splinting.
 sprain, 162
 temporal bone, and paralysis, 48
 transverse, 161
 vertebra, 279
Freezing, 137
Frostbite, 137
 of hand, 326
Furuncle, 98

Gangrene, from tourniquet, 111
Genitourinary tract, 310

Hand, 27
 crushing injury, 322
 laceration, 322
 puncture wound, 307
 splinting, 176
 tourniquet, 326
 wringer washing machine injury, 322
Head, 30
 injury, 299
  infection in, 302
  shock in, 301
 puncture wound, 307
Heart
 contused wounds, 70
 description, 35
 disease, 365
  rheumatic, 368
 failure, 366
 injury, 245
Heat
 cramp, 364
 exhaustion, 136, 363
Heatstroke, 136, 364
Heel, painful, 343
Hematoma, 69
Hemoptysis, 8
Hemorrhage, 6, 7
 arterial, 65, 111, 115

Hemorrhage (cont.).
 brain, 270
 cerebral, 375
 control, 1, 116, 117
 in deep wounds, 78
 femoral artery, 65
 in fracture, 167
 groin, 64
 head, 301
 neck, 301
 in open wound, 71
 scalp, 266
 and shock, 103, 108
  treatment, 109
 venous, 111, 116
Hemorrhoid
 prolapsed, 101, 264
 thrombosed, 264
  infected, 100
Hemothorax, 24, 243
HEPT poisoning, 381
Hernia, 418
 strangulated, 263
Heroin poisoning, 382
 in shock, 107
Hexaclorophene, in soap, 77
Hexaethyltetraphosphate poisoning, 381
Hiccough, 247
Hip, 27. See also Bandage; Dislocation.
 joint, 27
 splinting, 176
History, in treatment of shock, 109
Hives, 394
Hornet sting, 88
Human bite. See Bite, human, of hand.
Humerus, 26
Hydrochloric acid, 134
Hydrofluoric acid, 134
Hypotension, postural, in fainting, 359
Hypovolemic shock, 105
Hypoxia, in shock, 104
Hysteria, 372

Ilium, 27
Incised wound, 70
Infarction, myocardial, 367
Infection
 abrasion, 94
 avulsion, 95
 with colon baccilli, 73
 in deep wounds, 80
 fingernail, 98

Infection (cont.).
  with gas baccilli, 73
  hand, 323, 325
  in head injury, 302
  human bite, 99
  laceration, 95
  lymph node, 97
  middle ear, 101
  in neck injury, 302
  of open wound, 73
  puncture, 95
  scalp, 268
  sebaceous cyst, 96
  staphylococcal, 73
  streptococcal, 73
  surgical, 91
  tetanus, 73
  treatment, 92
  with Welch bacillus, 74
  wound, 73, 80, 94, 95
Inflammation, in infection, 91
Injury
  abdominal, 258
  by biologic agent, 159
  bladder. See Bladder injury.
  chemical, 156, 157
  electric, 113, 114
  eye. See Eye, injury.
  face. See Face.
  foot, 329
  head, 299, 302
  kidney, 313, 314
  mouth, 302
  neck, 299, 302, 305
  nerve, in fracture, 165
  nervous system, 266
  penis, 318
  prostate, 316
  scalp, 266, 267
    shaving, 267
  scrotum, 319
  skull, 266, 269
  spinal cord, 167, 279, 284
  spine, 266
  thermal, 123
  ureter, 315
Innominate bone, 27
Insecticide poisoning, 381
Intervertebral disc, dislocation, 282
Intestinal obstruction, 262
Intoxication, alcoholic, 375
Iron poisoning, 379
Ischium, 27

Kneecap, 29
Knock-out drops, 385

Laceration, 70, 306
  brain, 270
  eye, 289
  infection, 95
  mouth, 306
  neck, 307
Lathyrism, 389
Leg, 27. See also Splinting.
Leukocytosis, 33
Lewisite, 158. See also Eye.
Lighter fluid, as cleanser, 81
Lime, 134
Liver, rupture, 70
Lockjaw. See Tetanus.
LSD, 377
Lung
  collapse, 241
  defect, 242
Lupinosis, 389
Lymphadenitis, 97
Lymphangitis, 97

Mace, in eye, 295
March foot, 341
Marihuana, 377
Mass casualty management, military aspects, 420
Medical service, emergency, 139
Metacarpal bone, 27
Metatarsalgia, 337
Mickey Finn, 385
Military hospital
  blood, 425
  patient flow, 424
  preparation, 423
  supplies, 425
  triage, 424
  x-ray service, 425
Mouth-to-mouth resuscitation. See Resuscitation.
Muscular system, 24
Mustard, distilled, injury, 157
Mustard gas, 134
  in eye, 295
Myocardial infarction, 367

Nausea, in abdominal injury, 258

Neck, 31
  injury, 299
    blunt, 305
    shock in, 301
Needle, broken, 81
Nerve(s)
  peripheral, 285
  severed, 415
  spinal, distribution, 281
Nervous system, 48. *See also* Injury.
Neurogenic shock. *See* Shock.
Nitrogen mustard, 158
Node, lymph, infection, 97
Nodular poisoning, 380
Nose. *See* Foreign body; Fracture.
Nosebleed, 304
Nuclear weapons, effects, 149
Numbness, in tight bandaging, 53
Nux vomica poisoning, 383

Obstruction
  intestinal, 262
  respiratory, 299
Octamethylpyrophosphoramide poisoning. *See* Poisoning, OMPA.
Oil of Wintergreen poisoning, 383
Open wounds, 69
Oxygen, in treatment of shock, 112

Packaged Disaster Hospital, 17
Pain
  abdominal, 261
  chest, 236
  eye, 296
  heel, 343
  in renal colic, 319
  in tight bandaging, 53
Paralysis, 7
  and fracture of temporal bone, 48
Paraphimosis, 320
Paratyphoid, 390
Paronychia, 98
Patella, 29
Pelvis, splinting, 181
Penetrating wound, 70. *See also* Wounds.
Periastitis, 347
Pericardial tamponade, in shock, 108
Pericardium, description, 35
Peritonitis, 256
  and shock, 258

Phalanges, 27
Phenol, 134
Phosgene, 158
Phosphorus, 134. *See also* Poisoning.
Plantar digital neuroma, 340
Pneumothorax, 241
  tension, 242
Poison ivy, 395
Poison oak, 395
Poisoning
  acid, 381
  akee, 389
  allonal, 379
  arsenic, 380
  aspirin, 383
  atropine, 384
  barbiturate, 379
  belladonna, 384
  benzene, 386
  bichloride of mercury, 380
  carbolic acid, 379
  carbon monoxide, 385
    with burn, 125
  carbon tetrachloride, 386
  caustic potash, 381
  chemical, 377
  chloral hydrate, 385
  chlorpromazine, 383
  cocaine, 382
  codeine, 382
  creosote, 379
  cresol, 379
  Demerol, 382
  Dilandid, 382
  Doriden, 380
  drug, 377. *See also* specific drug.
  fish, 388
  food, 386
  gasoline, 386
  Glutethimide, 380
  guaiacol, 379
  HEPT, 381
  heroin, 382
  hexaethyltetraphosphate, 381
  hydrochloric acid, 381
  iodine, 379
  iron, 383
  laudanum, 382
  luminal, 379
  lye, 381
  lysol, 379
  Malathion, 381
  mercury, 380

Poisoning (*cont.*).
  Metapon, 382
  Methyprylon, 380
  morphine, 382
    in shock, 107
  mushroom, 388
  mussel, 388
  naphtha, 386
  Nembutal, 379
  nitric acid, 381
  Noludar, 380
  nux vomica, 383
  Oil of Wintergreen, 383
  OMPA (octamethylpyrophosphoramide), 381
  opium, 382
  Pantopan, 382
  Parathion, 381
  paregoria, 382
  Paris green, 380
  phenobarbital, 379
  phenolic acid, 379
  phosphorus, 382
  potato, 389
  promazine, 383
  Rough-on-Rats, 380
  salicylate, 383
  salmonella, 387
  Seconal, 379
  sodium amytal, 379
  sodium ortal, 379
  staphylococcal, 387
  strychnine, 383
  sulfuric acid, 381
  TEPP (tetraethylpyrophosphate), 381
  TNT (trinitrotoluene), 385
  toadstool, 388
  tranquilizing drug, 383
  unknown, 378
  Veronal, 379
Police, 6
Position, in diagnosis of shock, 107
  in treatment of shock, 112
Position of function, in care of hand, 324
Potash, caustic, poisoning, 381
Potassium hydroxide burn, 134
Pressure, central venous
  finger, to control hemorrhage, 117
  in shock, 108
Pressure point(s), arterial, 111, 117, 118, 119
Prostate, injury, 316

Prostration, 398–414
  treatment, 402
Pulmonary arrest, 202
Pulse, 8
  rate, low, 368
  in shock, 107
Puncture wound, 70
  head, 307
  infection, 95
  neck, 307
Pupils, 8
Pus, 92
  in ear, 101

Rabies, 84
Radiation
  effect in nuclear blast, 152
  illness, 155
Radioactivity, 20
  screening, 21
Radius, 26
Rattlesnake bite, 85
Rescue, fire, 125
  from electrical injury, 113
Respiration
  artificial, 207
    in electric injury, 114
  irregular, 7
Respiratory obstruction, 299
Respiratory rate, increased, 7
Respiratory system, 41, 42
Resuscitation
  cardiac, 208, 215
  cardiopulmonary, in children and infants, 214
    complications, 212
  in drowning, 236
  emergency, 231
  equipment, 223
  heart-lung, 205, 208
  mouth-to-mouth, 207, 248, 249
    gastric distension, 217
    vomiting, 217
Resuscitator
  automatic, 228
  mechanical, 230
Retention, urinary, 320
Rib, fracture, 238
Rule of nines, 128

Sacroiliac joint, 267
Safety pin, swallowed, 264
Scapula, 26
Scorpion sting, 88

Scrotum injury, 319
Seasickness, 396
Septic shock, 105
Serum reaction, 394
Shaving. *See* Injury, scalp.
Shock, 103, 104, 399
  anoxic, 105
  in crush injury, 89
  cardiac, 105
  diagnosis, 106, 107
  dilated pupils, 107
  electric, 419
  endotoxic, 370
  in fracture, 167
  in head injury, 301
  and heroin poisoning, 107
  hypovolemic, 105
    replacement therapy, 111
  and hypoxia, 104
  in neck injury, 301
  neurogenic, 104
  oxygen, in treatment, 112
  pathology, 105
  and pericardial tamponade, 108
  in peritonitis, 258
  position in treatment, 112
  psychic, in fainting, 359
  and pulse, 107
  secondary, in electric injury, 114
  septic, 105
  in serum reaction, 394
  unconsciousness, 107
Shotgun wound, 82
Shoe fit, 353
Shoulder, 26. *See* Dislocation; Splinting.
Skeletal system, 24, 25
Skin, color and condition, 7
Skull
  compound, 271
  depressed, 271
Sling, 51
Smallpox, 390
Snakebite, 85
  treatment with antivenin, 87
Snake, poisonous, 85. *See also* specific snakes.
Sodium hydroxide. *See* Burn.
Spasm
  abdominal, in black widow bite, 87
  muscle, in abdominal injury, 258
Spider
  black widow, 87
  brown recluse, 88

Spinal cord
  injury, 279, 283
  in fracture, 167
  treatment, 284
Spine, 31
  board, 183
  injury, 266
  splinting, 181
Spiral reverse bandage, 53
Spleen, rupture, 70
Splint
  for dislocation, 187
  improvised, 175
  inflatable, 170, 171
  traction, 170
Splinter, 81
Splinting
  coaptation, 169
  in deep wounds, 80
  emergency, 174
  of fractures, 167, 172–184
    elbow, 173
    femur, 176
    hip, 176
    humerus, 173
    knee, 176
    leg, 177
    neck, 181
    pelvis, 181
    shoulder, 173
    spine, 181, 182
    tibia, 177
    wrist, 176
Sprain, 161, 193
  industrial, 417
Spur, heel, 346
Stocking, as bandage, 66, 67
Standstill, cardiac, 204
Staphylococcus aureus, 96
Starvation, 392
Station, first aid, 15
Sting
  bee, 88
  scorpion, 88
Stokes-Adams syndrome, 368
Strain, foot, 334
Strangulation, of hernia, 263
Streptococcus, 96
Stroke, 375
Sunburn, 132
Sunstroke, 364
Supplies, for military hospital, 425
Suppuration, 92
  ear, 101
Syncope, 357. *See also* Fainting.

Tachycardia, paroxysmal, 368
Tamponade, cardiac, 245
Tarsal bone, 29
Tear gas, 134
Teeth, blunt injury, 302
Temporal bone fracture, and paralysis, 48
Tenderness, abdominal, in injury, 258
Tendon, Achilles
 inflammation, 344
 rupture, 345
 severed, 415
Tenosynovitis, 344
Testicles, torsion, 320
Tetanus, 73
 prophylaxis, 93
 in shotgun wound, 82
Tetany, hyperventilation, 369
Tetraethylpyrophosphate poisoning. See Poisoning, TEPP.
Therapy, replacement, in hypovolemic shock, 111
Thermal effects, in nuclear blast, 150
Thorax, 32
Thrombophlebitis, acute, 100
Thrombosis, cerebral, 375
Tibia, 29
 splinting, 177
Tingling, in tight bandaging, 53
Toe(s), Morton's, 339
Toenail, ingrown, 350
Toothache, 101
Tourniquet, 111, 120
 in deep wounds, 79
 errors in application, 122
 and gangrene, 2, 111
 in hand injury, 326
 in snake bite, 86
Tracheostomy, 222, 223
Tracheotome, 221
Tracheotomy, 2
Tranquilizing drug poisoning, 383
Triage, 17
 in military hospital, 424
Triangular bandage, 50, 51
Trichloroacetic acid, 134
Trinitrotoluene poisoning. See Poisoning, TNT.
Typhoid, 390

Ulcer
 dendritic, of eye, 292

Ulcer (cont.).
 peptic, perforated, 262
 varicose, 100
Ulceration, infected, 99
Ulna, 26
Unconsciousness, 7. See also Shock.
Ureter, injury, 315
Urethra, injury, 316
Urinary retention, acute, 320
Urinary system, 47

Vein, bleeding, 116. See also Hemorrhage.
Ventilator, automatic, 228
Vertebra fracture, 279
Vision, sudden loss, 297
Vomiting, 8
 in abdominal injury, 258
 in mouth-to-mouth resuscitation, 217

Whooping cough, 390
Wound(s)
 abdominal, 257
 antibiotics in treatment, 77
 blank cartridge, 82
 bullet, 81
 closed, industrial, 412
 contused, 68, 76
 deep, 78
 drainage, 80
 hand, 307
 head, 307
 heart, 245
 incised, 70
 lacerated, 70
 open, 69, 71, 76
  bandage, 52
  industrial, 413
 penetrating, 70
 puncture, 70
  hand, 307
  head, 307
 infection, 95
 neck, 307
 shotgun, 82
 throracoabdominal, 257
Wringer washing machine, injury to hand, 322
Wrist, 27
 bandage, 55, 60
 dislocation, 189
 splinting, 176
Wristdrop, 283

RD
131
C62
1972

**NO LONGER THE PROPERTY
OF THE
UNIVERSITY OF R. I. LIBRARY**